A POPULAR GUIDE TO MEDICAL LANGUAGE

A POPULAR GUIDE TO MEDICAL LANGUAGE

Edward R. Brace

VNR VAN NOSTRAND REINHOLD COMPANY
──────────────────── *New York*

Copyright © 1983 by Van Nostrand Reinhold Company Inc.

Library of Congress Catalog Card Number 82-6877

ISBN 0-442-21353-0

All rights reserved. No part of this work covered by the copyright hereon may be reproduced or used in any form or by any means—graphic, electronic, or mechanical, including photocopying, recording, taping, or information storage and retrieval systems—without written permission of the publisher.

Printed in the United States of America
Designed by Tere Loprete

Published by Van Nostrand Reinhold Company Inc.
135 West 50th Street
New York, New York 10020

Van Nostrand Reinhold Company Limited
Molly Millars Lane
Wokingham, Berkshire RG11 2PY, England

Van Nostrand Reinhold
480 Latrobe Street
Melbourne, Victoria 3000, Australia

Macmillan of Canada
Division of Gage Publishing Limited
164 Commander Boulevard
Agincourt, Ontario M1S 3C7, Canada

16 15 14 13 12 11 10 9 8 7 6 5 4 3

Library of Congress Cataloging in Publication Data

Brace, Edward R.
    A popular guide to medical language.

    1. Medicine—Dictionaries. I. Title
R121.B69   610'.3'21   82-6877
ISBN 0-442-21353-0

INTRODUCTION

Most patients want to know a lot more than their physicians have time to tell them. In the rush of the average office visit, they may also be reluctant to ask detailed questions about a specific medical problem, or why certain diagnostic tests and procedures are necessary, exactly how they are performed, and what they can tell the doctor.

Physicians often toss off medical terms quickly or, even worse, give cursory and opaque "popular" explanations. The patient then leaves the doctor's office with a vague feeling of ignorance and confusion about the terms used and the precise nature of the disease or disorder.

Medical jargon is the specialized vocabulary used by physicians, nurses, and others in the field of health care; by its very nature, it is largely unintelligible to those not directly involved in the medical sciences. The purpose of this book is to explore, in a clear and methodical manner, the special language of the medical profession.

Presented here in one continuous alphabetical listing are the most important technical terms of interest to the layman. Also explained are diagnostic tests, the nature of major diseases and how they are treated, the more commonly used abbreviations, and what physicians mean by such terms as *CAT scan, intravenous pyelogram, syndrome, diabetic retinopathy, patent ductus arteriosus, slipped disk, spina bifida, fetal monitoring,* and *myocardial infarction.*

Because entries are alphabetized and extensive use is made of cross-references, no general index is necessary. In addition, some popular or common names of various subjects (such as *lockjaw*) are listed to direct the reader to the appropriate entry under the subject's medical or technical name (such as *tetanus*). Most words printed in *italics* within an entry are separate entries, as are all *italicized* words found at the end of an entry. No technical terms essential for understanding are used within a particular entry unless they too are given an individual entry, although

Introduction

only the most relevant terms for increased understanding are italicized—in any entry. The reader is invited to look up these terms to obtain additional knowledge.

The information contained in most entries goes far beyond that provided in even the largest medical dictionaries. After a brief definition or description of the entry, background information is offered that helps answer those questions a patient might ask a physician—if time and courage permitted.

Modern medicine and the men and women who practice it are somewhat mysterious to most people; the white coat and stethoscope are not unlike a priest's robes and chalice. Medical jargon is particularly mysterious. We fear or are intimidated by what we do not understand. This is a book of understanding; a book that will, it is hoped, unravel the riddle of medical jargon and explain exactly what doctors do and how they do it.

Impossible though it may seem, doctors are people—people with special skills, just like automotive mechanics or carpenters. All doctors were once little boys or girls; they had measles and chickenpox, fights after school, read comic books under the covers, were afraid of the dark, wrote on walls, tracked mud into the kitchen, "borrowed" items that were not theirs, got dirty, had bloody noses, were spanked, cried, laughed, fell hopelessly in love at the age of eight, collected rocks, rocked dolls, made mudpies, lied to their parents, waited nervously for the arrival of Santa Claus, believed in the tooth fairy, fell out of trees, dreamed special dreams, and (in most cases) finally grew up. Just like the rest of us.

Why is it that we tend to think of doctors in images normally reserved for godlike or superhuman beings? Basically, it is a lack of communication, knowledge, and understanding. We should learn to ask more questions and gain a basic knowledge about how our body works and the types of problems that can occur when the body temporarily malfunctions. Or, in the case of a potentially fatal illness such as cancer, we should be prepared to know what treatment options are available. The human body is complex, and we are conditioned to place a physician in charge when something goes wrong. Doctors are not solely to blame for our thinking of them as the high priests of health, although some may encourage this attitude. The uninformed patient is also at fault.

A physician's education and training involves many years of preparation: four years of college, three or four years of medical school, and at least one additional year after the M.D. degree working under close supervision as an intern in a hospital. Then, after passing a state examination to practice medicine, he or she is given a license and can begin

Introduction

seeing patients as a general practitioner, join other doctors in a group practice or clinic, remain at a hospital, or continue medical education and become a specialist.

We were all once children, but some doctors continue to treat their patients as if they were still children. They sometimes withhold information they think is too complicated for their patients to understand, or they may oversimplify to the point of absurdity. ("Don't worry about that, Mrs. Jones. Just take these [unidentified] pills and everything will be fine.") Unless a patient knows what to expect from his or her physician under various circumstances, it is very difficult to know how to ask intelligent questions. *A Popular Guide to Medical Language* is designed in part to ease this difficulty.

A few doctors seem to resent patients who know how to ask intelligent questions about their medical problems. This is most unfortunate. The feeling seems to be that "knowledgeable" patients are hypochondriacs: people who are obsessed with illness or who imagine that they are ill. The fact is that patients who take the time to understand how the body works and the general nature of their specific disease can be of great help to their doctors. Good doctors understand this and encourage their patients to learn more about the vast realm of modern medicine and diagnostic procedures. Good doctors have a healthy sense of humor, understand their role in treating their patients not just as "cases" but as *individuals* with specific needs, and are always willing to answer questions.

We go to a doctor for a service. We want his or her skill in identifying a specific problem. What do we have? How can it be treated? What is the outlook for a speedy recovery? The patient has the right to know what the doctor discovers about any health problem. We pay for that service, either directly or through a health insurance plan. There should be no mystery about what doctors do for their patients. When we pay a mechanic for hours of work on our car, we have the obvious right to know exactly what problems were discovered and how they were fixed. The same general principle applies to doctors. We pay them for a service. If they do not tell us all we want to know, we have the right—and duty—to ask.

Doctors are not gods. They are real people with real problems. They, too, bleed when they are cut. They laugh when they are happy. They also tend to rush you out of the office before you have had a chance to ask the questions that have been on your mind. Don't let them get away with it. You are paying for their time and knowledge.

Any car owner knows that there are good and bad automotive mechanics; occasionally, one finds a superior mechanic. The same is true

Introduction

in the medical profession. Any mediocre mechanic can repair a car if the problem is known. The identification (diagnosis) of a patient's problem is perhaps the most important service a doctor can provide. If the diagnosis is incorrect, the treatment will probably also be incorrect. Should that happen, the patient's condition may worsen. Once an accurate diagnosis is made, the rest is relatively straightforward—providing the identified disease or disorder can be treated. Medicine is an art as well as a science. Professional judgment is essential.

A Popular Guide to Medical Language is not meant to replace the essential counsel and advice of medical professionals, but to enhance the doctor-patient relationship by encouraging patients to become better informed about a wide variety of medical terms. This book attempts to remove the mystery and confusion that surrounds more than a thousand words and phrases commonly used in modern medical practice. By so doing, perhaps it can improve the communication and understanding between medical practitioners and the people who provide their livelihood. A knowledgeable patient is a better patient.

A

abdomen The part of the body below the thorax (chest) and above the pelvis. The abdominal cavity contains the lower part of the esophagus, stomach, intestines, liver, gallbladder, pancreas, spleen, kidneys, and urinary bladder; in females it also contains the uterus and ovaries.
SEE ALSO *abdominal pain, peritoneum*

abdominal pain Any pain felt within or around the *abdomen*. The nature of the pain may be sharp, stabbing, dull, gnawing, aching, intermittent, or persistent. Valuable diagnostic clues to the possible source of the problem are often revealed by the type of pain.

Among the most common causes of abdominal pain are indigestion (dyspepsia), heartburn (pyrosis), menstrual cramps (dysmenorrhea), and distension or powerful contractions of abdominal organs such as the stomach or intestines. The exact area of the pain may be difficult to specify, although it is commonly more severe around the middle of the abdomen.

Sudden attacks of sharp abdominal pain, especially if the pain persists and is accompanied by nausea and vomiting, may indicate a potentially more serious condition that requires prompt medical attention. The possibilities include *appendicitis*, gallstones, kidney stones, *peritonitis*, partial or complete obstruction of the intestinal tract, *peptic ulcer*, or severe inflammation of the intestines.

The sensation of abdominal pain is not always associated with a problem within the abdomen itself. At times the *pain* may be "referred" from another part of the body that has closely interconnected nerve pathways. Referred pain in the abdomen may be caused by a problem within the chest, such as a mild heart attack, pleurisy, or pneumonia. Only a physician can make an accurate diagnosis.
SEE ALSO *cholecystitis, cholelith-*

abortion

iasis, colic, diverticulitis, gastritis, intussusception, pylorospasm, salpingitis

abortion The termination of pregnancy by the expulsion or deliberate removal of a fetus from the uterus before it is capable of living independently, usually well before the twenty-eighth week of pregnancy. The body may prematurely expel the fetus for various reasons (spontaneous or habitual abortion), a physician may artificially induce expulsion on medical grounds (therapeutic abortion), or a woman may demand an abortion for an unplanned or unwanted pregnancy (such abortions were formerly outlawed and frequently obtained illegally or in other countries).

Abortions are not without complications, some of which can be serious (the mother's mortality rate has been estimated at 1 per every 100,000 abortions). The most common complications following an abortion are infection of the uterus or Fallopian tubes, which can cause fever, abdominal pain, and cramps; and incomplete abortion (the retention in the uterus of fetal or placental tissues), typically leading to excessive bleeding and painful cramps. To minimize the risk of such complications, it is essential to return to the physician or clinic for a follow-up examination.

The risk of abortion is much less if the pregnant woman makes an early decision and seeks prompt medical attention. An abortion is relatively safe if performed before the twelfth week of pregnancy and remains reasonably safe up to the sixteenth week. After this the risk increases rapidly. Abortions performed by unqualified people can be extremely dangerous and should not be considered. Abortion laws vary in different parts of the country; if a pregnant woman wants to explore all the alternatives, her best course is to see her physician, local health department, or Planned Parenthood without delay.

Abortion techniques depend largely on the length of pregnancy. Women who are between four and twelve weeks pregnant may qualify for an early vacuum abortion. This procedure is relatively safe and short (three to five minutes in most cases). The amniotic sac is removed by suction through a slender tube inserted into the uterus. Women who are between about thirteen and sixteen weeks pregnant may qualify for a technique known as dilation and evacuation (D and E), usually performed under general anesthesia. This procedure constitutes about 4 percent of all abortions and usually takes about half an hour; the neck (cervix) of the uterus is gently stretched (dilated) with surgical instruments to permit extraction of the amniotic sac by vacuum tube.

Women who are between fifteen

and twenty-four weeks pregnant may require an amniocentesis abortion. This involves the insertion of a hollow needle into the amniotic sac to withdraw amniotic fluid and inject a substance that will induce contractions of the uterus, thus causing the fetus to be expelled. The substances used include a strong salt (saline) solution, hormones including prostaglandins, or urea, a solution of concentrated nitrogen-containing waste material excreted by the kidneys.

abruptio placentae The premature separation or detachment of a normally placed placenta from the uterus. The condition is rare and its exact cause is unknown. In some cases it may be associated with high blood pressure (hypertension) of the mother or a temporary failure of her blood to clot normally.

As the placenta becomes detached from the wall of the uterus, bleeding occurs. The blood loss may be confined within this area (internal or concealed hemorrhage) or it may discharge through the vagina (external or revealed hemorrhage). The severity of the condition depends largely on the degree of separation of the placenta (in a few cases it may become entirely detached) and the amount of bleeding.

The condition may improve with bed rest, enabling a normal birth to occur. However, if the bleeding continues or worsens, it poses a direct threat to the life of both baby and mother. Prompt delivery is then essential.

SEE ALSO *placenta previa*

abscess A localized collection of pus in any part of the body, usually caused by bacterial infection. Pimples and boils are common examples of abscesses on the skin surface. They can develop following infection from a cut, minor scrape (abrasion), or infection of a skin gland (folliculitis). Small abscesses on the skin usually clear up within a short time with little or no treatment. Larger abscesses generally require medical attention.

When a skin abscess discharges its pus, it will heal quickly if the drainage is free and the area is kept dry. Plain dry dressings are used to cover a discharging abscess, and they are changed often.

An abscess deeper within the body can be caused by severe puncture wounds, accidental inhalation into the lungs of foreign material such as food particles, the spread of infection from the middle ear to the brain, or a ruptured appendix (pelvic abscess). All internal abscesses require prompt medical diagnosis and treatment.

acetaminophen The generic name of a synthetic drug, marketed under such trade names as Datril or Tylenol, available without a prescription and used to relieve minor pain and reduce fever. Unlike *aspirin*, acetaminophen cannot relieve inflammation. Products that contain acetaminophen are commonly recommended to people who are sensitive or allergic to aspirin.

An overdose of acetaminophen can cause potentially serious damage to the liver.

acetylsalicylic acid
SEE *aspirin*

Achilles tendon A thick band of connective tissue (tendon) that extends from the muscles of the calf to the heel bone. The contraction of the muscles attached to the Achilles tendon permits a person to stand on tiptoe. Excessive athletic activity or sudden strain on this tendon can cause it to tear (rupture).

At one time the Achilles tendon reflex was used by physicians to determine the normal or abnormal function of the *thyroid gland*. A sharp blow with a rubber mallet was given to the Achilles tendon, and the nature of the automatic leg-jerk response was thought to indicate the presence or absence of certain neurological (nerve) disorders. The specific diagnostic value of such relatively simplistic tests is now considered highly questionable.

achlorhydria The gross deficiency or absence of hydrochloric acid in the secretions of the stomach. If not treated, it can interfere with the absorption of iron from foods.

achondroplasia An abnormal *congenital* condition that primarily affects the growth of the long bones of the limbs. It is a form of dwarfism that leaves arms and legs short with a normal body (trunk). Sometimes the head may be slightly enlarged.

acidosis Excessive acidity of the body's fluids as the result of an abnormal accumulation of acids, as in some forms of kidney disease or diabetes mellitus. Mild forms of acidosis are characterized by nausea and vomiting; more severe forms may be accompanied by an increase in the depth and rate of breathing (hyperpnea) and circulatory *shock*. Correction of the condition is aimed at treating the underlying disease or disorder.
COMPARE *alkalosis*

acne A common skin disorder that can affect persons of all ages but is particularly prevalent during adolescence. Androgenic *hormones* are first secreted into the bloodstream during this period and cause greatly increased activity of the sebaceous glands in the skin. The sticky secretion of these glands, called sebum, sometimes fills and stretches the pores, resulting in blackheads. Blackheads block the pores and prevent the natural skin oils from reaching the surface; they collect beneath the skin and form tiny *cysts*. When the cysts break, harmful bacteria can enter the skin and cause infection and inflammation. Common acne (acne vulgaris) is the inflammation of the sebaceous glands, especially those on the face, chest, and back.

Treatment of acne depends on its severity. In simple cases it may be sufficient to wash the affected areas with a mild soap or antibacterial agent. Exposure to sunlight sometimes relieves the condition. The pimples that form around the pore openings should not be squeezed, as this may spread the infection to other areas or cause a secondary infection by bacteria under the nails or on the skin.

In severe cases of acne, the pimples become very large and may be filled with pus. It is best to consult a physician if this occurs; he or she may prescribe medicated ointments (often containing sulfur) or other preparations to help clear up the infection. In some cases small doses of tetracycline can be helpful.

Acne generally disappears by itself after the end of puberty.

acromegaly A slowly progressing disease, usually first noticed during middle age, in which the *pituitary gland* overproduces growth hormones. It is characterized by a gradual enlargement and thickening of the bones of the forehead, jaws (the lower jaw may protrude), feet, and hands. Skin covering the nose, lips, and other parts of the face may become thick and coarse. The skin typically becomes greasy due to the overactivity of the sebaceous glands, the tongue enlarges, and the voice deepens (particularly noticeable in women).

The increased secretion of growth hormone interferes with the action of insulin in approximately 25 percent of patients with acromegaly and may result in the further complication of *diabetes mellitus.*

Unless treated, acromegaly tends to worsen. Complications in addition to diabetes include visual disturbances, painful disorders of the bones and joints, high blood pressure (hypertension), and damage to the blood vessels (cerebrovascular disease).

Acromegaly can be diagnosed in several ways; the two most common procedures are laboratory tests that measure the amount of growth hormone in the blood, and x-rays of the skull. An x-ray may aid the diagnosis by revealing a characteristic thickening of the skull and an enlargement of the bony air spaces (sinuses) in the frontal bones. It could also reveal a change in the shape or size of the bony enclosure where the pituitary gland is normally confined. One cause of acromegaly is a tumor of the pituitary; a growing tumor may press against this enclosure or even break through and press against nearby tissues. Serious complications can occur if the growth presses against the optic nerves, including severe visual disturbances and total blindness.

ACTH

Treatment depends largely on the severity and rate of progression of the condition, and the patient's age. High voltage x-rays and heavy-particle irradiation have been used in the past with varying degrees of success. A widely used method of treatment is the surgical implantation of small amounts of radioactive yttrium or gold directly into the bony recess containing the pituitary gland. Other methods of treatment include cryosurgery (the selective destruction of a tumor by controlled freezing) and the surgical removal of part of the pituitary gland (hypophysectomy).

Research continues into possible methods of controlling acromegaly with drugs designed to suppress the excessive secretion of growth hormone by the pituitary gland or to interfere with its activity once released. At present, no such drug has been evaluated for its long-term effect.

COMPARE *gigantism*

ACTH Abbreviation for adrenocorticotropic *hormone*, secreted by the *pituitary gland;* it stimulates the cortex (outer layer) of the *adrenal glands*.

SEE *corticosteroid, cortisol*

actinomycosis A rare, chronic, and slowly progressive infectious disease caused by a species of fungus (*Actinomyces israelii*). It is most often seen in adult males. It affects the tissues of the mouth, lungs, and intestines, resulting in the formation of abscesses. In rare cases, it may spread to other areas of the body, such as the brain and heart. With early diagnosis and treatment, usually with antibiotics, recovery is common. Medical treatment may take several months and stubborn infections may also require surgery.

acupuncture A method of treating certain disorders and inducing anesthesia, originated by the Chinese. It consists of puncturing the skin with one or more long needles, which are then usually rotated back and forth by hand or given a mild electric charge. The needles are placed in position according to an ancient tradition that maps the nerves that supply various parts of the body. They apparently stimulate the appropriate nerves and result in healing or eliminating pain. Even the Chinese do not know exactly how acupuncture works.

acute A disease or disorder that appears suddenly and lasts for a relatively short time.

COMPARE *chronic*

addiction A compulsive physiological need for a habit-forming substance. In true addiction, the user typically begins to suffer severe *withdrawal symptoms* when the substance's effects wear off and no further doses are available. The terms *addiction* and *habituation* are commonly used to describe the long-term adverse effects of certain drugs on the body and mind. Traditionally, an addicting substance is capable of causing serious physiological changes that result in the user's becoming physically dependent. Typically, the addict requires increasingly large amounts to maintain a "normal" state. Once addiction has been established, failure to continue taking the drug may result in distressing withdrawal symptoms, including extreme anxiety, violent shivering, painful contractions of the stomach, forceful vomiting, and diarrhea. Habituation, by contrast, is thought of as a psychological addiction.

The continual use of some classes of drugs can lead not only to serious personality disruptions but also to irreversible physical disorders and death.

Addison's disease A disease caused by the inadequate secretion of hormones (mainly cortisol and aldosterone) from the cortex (outer surface) of the *adrenal glands*. The production of these essential hormones is interrupted by progressive wasting (atrophy) of the adrenal cortex (in about 70 percent of cases the cause of this wasting is unknown: idiopathic atrophy) or a slow destruction of the gland's surface by an infection, such as tuberculosis or various fungal diseases.

The early symptoms of Addison's disease (also called adrenocortical insufficiency) include weakness, fatigue, loss of energy, muscular aches, a gradual loss of sexual response, and loss of appetite, none of which is specific for this disease. One fairly common sign not always noticed by the patient is the development of patchy pigmentation of the skin, especially on the mucous membranes such as those of the lips and mouth. Other evidence of the disease typically includes low blood pressure (hypotension), weight loss (related to appetite loss), nausea, vomiting, diarrhea, increased sensitivity to cold, dizziness, and often behavior alterations that mimic neurosis.

The exact diagnosis of Addison's disease involves tests and procedures that are usually administered by an endocrinologist, a physician who specializes in disorders of the hormonal (endocrine) system. Treatment depends on the severity of the condition. In most cases replacement of the deficient hormones (substitution therapy) corrects the problem. These may be given orally or by injection and usually have to be continued for the rest of the patient's life. With early diagnosis and treatment, the person can live a normal life.

Addison's disease is named after the English physician Thomas Addison (1793–1860), who first described it.

adhesion An abnormal joining of adjacent surfaces or parts as a result of inflammation or injury. It sometimes occurs during the healing of a deep wound or surgical incision. In particularly severe cases,

adrenal glands

the adhesion may have to be corrected surgically, although there is no guarantee that a new adhesion will not thereby develop.

adrenal glands Two slightly flattened organs at the rear of the abdomen, one astride the top of each kidney; also called suprarenal glands. The cortex (outer layer) of the glands is yellow and the medulla (central portion) is dark red. Each part secretes entirely different hormones. The medulla secretes *epinephrine* (adrenaline) and *norepinephrine* (noradrenaline), together known as the catecholamines. These hormones are released in response to tension ("fright, flight, or fight" as physiologist Walter B. Cannon put it).

The cortex secretes the *corticosteroid* hormones, which have various functions. In general, they play an important role in sexual development, the maintenance of bodily strength, and metabolism. The two most important corticosteroid hormones are *cortisol* and aldosterone.

The adrenal glands and the major hormones that they secrete are essential to life. When these glands fail to function normally, potentially serious diseases may result.
SEE ALSO *Addison's disease, Cushing's syndrome, pheochromocytoma*

adrenaline Another name (especially in Britain) for *epinephrine;* the name Adrenalin is a trademark for a commercially available preparation of this hormone.
SEE *adrenal gland*

adrenogenital syndrome A rare condition also known as adrenal virilism, caused by the excessive secretion of male (androgenic) sex hormones by the *adrenal glands.* It is often congenital and affects males and females. In the congenital form, female infants may be temporarily mistaken for males and male infants may demonstrate accelerated body growth and abnormal enlargement of the penis. In the acquired forms of this disorder in adult women the cause may be a tumor of the adrenal glands or excessive growth of the normal cells of the adrenal glands (hyperplasia). The overproduction of male hormones in women can lead to the excessive growth of body hair (hirsutism), a deepening of the voice, the cessation of menstruation (amenorrhea), wasting of the uterus, an abnormal enlargement (hypertrophy) of the clitoris, a decrease in breast size, and an increase in general masculine characteristics such as facial hair. In mild cases the only sign may be an increase in body hair.

In severe and persistent cases —especially if a tumor is the cause—one or both adrenal glands may have to be surgically removed (adrenalectomy). Treatment of some forms of this condition may lead to a gradual disappearance of the signs and symptoms of masculinity (virilism) in women although the voice may remain deep.

afibrogenemia   A very rare condition involving a deficiency or absence of *fibrinogen*, a protein essential to the normal clotting process in the circulating blood. Unlike a person with *hemophilia*, who lacks a minor factor in the blood-clotting process, those with afibrogenemia are missing a major link in the blood's chemical chain to stop bleeding. There is no known cure.

afterbirth SEE *placenta*

agglutination test   A test designed to aid in identifying specific bacteria or viruses in the blood serum of infected persons. The principle of the test is the agglutination (clumping together) of cells, bacteria, or other particles in the presence of a specific *antibody*. The technique is also used to determine a person's blood group.

agranulocytosis   A serious and potentially fatal disorder characterized by a sharp decrease or absence of granulocytes (specific types of leukocytes or white blood cells) in the circulating blood. The condition typically begins with a high fever, severe sore throat, and ulcerlike sores in both the throat and other mucous membranes, such as the rectum and vagina. In some cases the cause is unknown; in others, it may be associated with the use of certain prescription drugs or exposure to x-rays or other radiation. The exact diagnosis involves specific blood tests to determine the number and type of leukocytes in the circulating blood.

Certain potent prescription drugs carry a risk of damaging the bone marrow, where blood cells are manufactured. When physicians prescribe these drugs they are strongly urged by the manufacturers to perform periodic blood tests—often as frequently as once a week—during therapy. Such tests should reveal early adverse changes in the ability of the bone marrow to manufacture blood cells.

albino   A person born with the partial or total inability to synthesize melanin, the brown pigment found in the skin, hair, and eyes; the condition is called albinism. Although this rare disorder is not harmful, an albino may experience *astigmatism*, *photophobia*, and *nystagmus* because the structures of the eye are insufficiently protected from light as a result of lack of pigment.

albumin   Any of various complex proteins that form the main part of the tissues in animals and man. They are composed of carbon, hydrogen, nitrogen, oxygen, and sulfur. The presence of albumin in the urine *(albuminuria)* can be a sign of kidney disease.

albuminuria   The abnormal presence of *albumin* in the urine; also called proteinuria. It is usually a sign of some kidney disorder,

alcoholism

although it may be found in some healthy persons as a result of extensive exercise.

alcoholism A chronic, progressive, and sometimes fatal disease caused by the repeated or constant drinking of alcoholic beverages. The term implies varying degrees of psychological dependence or physical *addiction*.

Alcohol (ethanol or ethyl alcohol) when used in moderation is perhaps the only example of a potentially addicting drug that has wide social approval in most societies. The definition of a heavy drinker depends largely on the society or culture involved. The excessive or heavy drinker seems to regard intoxication as a major goal in life. The heavy drinker may or may not be an alcoholic in the strict medical sense of the word; that is, physiological dependence on alcohol may not have developed. Nevertheless, heavy and persistent drinking can cause extremely serious problems in addition to addiction. The liver can become damaged *(cirrhosis)*, the heart can be seriously affected (alcoholic cardiomyopathy), and compulsive abuse may cause profound psychological disturbances.

Chronically high levels of alcohol in the blood can produce a state of physical dependence on the drug. When the consumption of alcohol is suddenly stopped, withdrawal symptoms are usually seen within twelve to seventy-two hours. They may be mild or severe, ranging from muscular trembling to delirium tremens (DTs), involving visual and auditory hallucinations. In severe cases, the alcoholic may attempt suicide. Symptoms of alcohol withdrawal also include fever and exhaustion. Prolonged and excessive use of alcohol can lead to a dangerously weakened state of the heart and circulatory system. If the patient does not die, recovery usually follows within about a week.

Heavy or steady drinking can also cause loss of appetite, with the result that more and more alcohol is consumed on an empty stomach. This can cause not only inflammation of the stomach lining *(gastritis)* but may lead to the formation of stomach ulcers. Loss of appetite means that less food is eaten, which in severe cases leads to malnutrition and vitamin-deficiency diseases.

It has taken a long time to recognize that alcoholism is a disease and that an alcoholic should be treated as being ill. Modern medical treatment of alcoholics is much more sympathetic to this than it was a few years ago.

Alcoholics Anonymous (AA), an organization of alcoholics who have stopped drinking, offers sound advice and understanding to anyone with a serious drinking problem. It has been traditionally accepted that once alcoholism is confirmed as the diagnosis, a true cure is possible only if the patient never accepts another drink. As difficult as this sounds, it is much easier to accept than physical and psychological deterioration and, in some cases, death.

Some physicians recommend aversion therapy in which the taking of alcohol is associated with extremely unpleasant experiences. For example, the patient receives a controlled electric shock each time a sip of alcoholic beverage is taken. A more common method, however, is to prescribe the drug disulfiram (Antabuse) in conjunction with psychotherapy or other methods of treatment. If a person taking disulfiram drinks, it produces side effects such as severe headache, throbbing in the neck and head, flushing, difficulty breathing, nausea, vomiting, sweating, chest pain, an increase in the heartbeat (tachycardia), palpitations (a sensation of the heartbeat), blurred vision, a feeling of faintness, and confusion. The type and intensity of these side effects varies widely from patient to patient and depends on both the amount of disulfiram taken and the quantity of alcohol consumed. Disulfiram should be used with extreme caution (if at all) in patients with diabetes mellitus, an underactive thyroid (hypothyroidism), epilepsy, or diseases of the liver or kidneys; anyone taking disulfiram should be under strict medical supervision.

aldosterone A *hormone* secreted by the cortex of the *adrenal glands*. It plays a role in regulating the metabolism of sodium and potassium.
SEE *corticosteroid, cortisol*

alimentary canal SEE *digestive tract*

alkaline phosphatase An enzyme widely distributed throughout the body. Specific forms of it appear normally in blood plasma or serum, bone, kidneys, lungs, spleen, intestines, and the placenta. A test for abnormally high levels of alkaline phosphatase in the blood can provide a diagnostic clue for the possible presence of liver disease. A single blood test is rarely of significant diagnostic value; usually several such tests must be made.

The blood levels of alkaline phosphatase may rise during pregnancy or as the result of taking certain types of prescription drugs, including the antibiotics erythromycin and oxacillin, some major tranquilizers (such as chlorpromazine), oral antidiabetic drugs, and oral contraceptives; such increases have little or no medical significance.

alkalosis Excessive alkalinity of the body's fluids as the result of an abnormal accumulation of alkalies (such as bicarbonates) or a reduction of acids, as in some cases of *Cushing's syndrome* (hyperadrenocorticism), prolonged vomiting (resulting in a loss of acid-containing gastric juice), and the long-term use of *diuretics*, which can cause the excessive loss of

allergy

potassium and chloride through the kidneys (metabolic alkalosis). The most common symptoms of alkalosis are irritability and neuromuscular hyperexcitability; in severe cases it can also cause muscular weakness, impaired motility of the gastrointestinal tract, and *tetany*. Correction of the condition is aimed at treating the underlying disease or disorder.
COMPARE *acidosis*

allergy A condition in which the body becomes sensitive to a substance (called an allergen), which can be food, pollen, feathers, dust, animal hair, or a chemical. Examples of allergic reactions include *asthma* and other breathing difficulties, skin rashes and hay fever (allergic rhinitis).

An allergic reaction may be considered as a malfunction of the body's normal defense mechanism against disease, the *immune* reaction. The body of an allergic person treats the allergen as if it were a disease-causing invader, such as bacteria. In the case of a bacterial infection, the body responds by producing antibodies, protective substances that are released in the bloodstream and attack the bacteria. In many cases these antibodies remain in the body for years and provide total or partial immunity to further attacks of the same disease. The foreign substance that stimulates the production of antibodies is called an *antigen*.

An allergic reaction is a distortion of the normal production and use of antibodies. Specific bodily tissues usually become sensitized during an initial encounter with an allergen and produce antibodies against future attacks. Unlike regular antibodies, allergic antibodies do not circulate in the bloodstream but become attached to the tissues at the site of contact of the allergen. During future exposures to the same allergen, the affected tissues are loaded with allergic antibodies that cause fairly specific allergic reactions. The basic mechanism of all allergic reactions is the same.
SEE ALSO *anaphylactic reaction, antihistamine, histamine*

alopecia The loss of hair, especially on the head; baldness, either total or patchy.

As people get older they tend to lose some hair. The hair follicles become less active and some cease to function altogether. Age-dependent hair loss is due to the secretion of the male sex hormone in both men and women. There is apparently a genetic element in its onset and extent. Although people may think that baldness is related to some significant event in their lives or to the degree of hair greasiness, the extent of dandruff, types of haircut or hairdressing, and the wearing of tight hats, these have nothing whatever to do with the natural process of hair loss.

There is no effective treatment to reverse natural balding, even if it occurs early in life. But such is human ignorance, credulity, and vanity even in today's enlightened age that a huge industry of deception continues to thrive. A great deal of money can be spent on tablets, stimulant lotions, and treatment with electricity, light, and friction—with no effect. People who claim that their hair grew as a result of such spurious treatments either had great faith and have convinced themselves that their hair grew when in fact it did not, or their baldness or hair thinning was not of the "natural" type and regrew spontaneously.

Abnormal baldness does occur in a few people, in which case medical treatment may be of help. One cause of such baldness is an infection due to the ringworm fungus. This can spread rapidly and should be promptly treated. The baldness of the affected area is not complete because some broken off and lusterless hairs remain. The scalp may be red, scaly, and crusted. A physician may take a sample of hairs and scales from the scalp if a fungal infection is suspected; the fungus can be seen under a microscope. Treatment involves the use of specific antifungal drugs.

In a condition known as alopecia areata, hair is lost over a well-defined area of the scalp or beard area and there may be multiple patches of baldness. The skin of the bald area looks quite normal. Provided the loss does not become too extensive, hair almost always grows back within a year, and usually no medical treatment is required.

Localized baldness may also occur in some skin conditions. Skin disease of the scalp may damage hair follicles and thus cause hair loss. There is very little dermatologists can do to suppress these scalp problems.

alphafetoprotein A protein present in the blood serum of a developing fetus. It occurs normally before birth and usually disappears from the blood shortly after birth. Its reappearance in the blood later in life may indicate liver damage.

The finding of specified levels of alphafetoprotein in the fluid surrounding a fetus can be used to diagnose certain birth defects, including *spina bifida* and *anencephaly*. Physicians use amniocentesis to test for the abnormal presence of alphafetoprotein.

alveoli The tiny air sacs of the *lungs;* one of these sacs is called an alveolus.

Alzheimer's disease A condition also referred to as presenile dementia, similar to *senile dementia* but with an earlier onset, usually between the ages of forty and sixty. It affects women more often than men. It is characterized by progressive and irreversible memory loss, deterioration of intellectual function, disorientation, and apathy. It is typically associated with atrophy (wasting) of brain tissues, especially the frontal, temporal, and occipital lobes. No specific treatment exists.

The disease is named after the German neurologist Alois Alzheimer (1864-1915).

amblyopia Dim or indistinct vision, especially in the absence of any apparent eye disease.

amenorrhea The absence or suppression of menstruation; the most common causes are pregnancy and *menopause*. The period may also be temporarily suppressed by illness or unusual stress. In such cases the menstrual flow should return spontaneously within a few weeks. If at least three menstrual periods have been missed and pregnancy has been ruled out, it is important to seek prompt medical attention.

It is fairly common for menstruation to stop when the use of oral contraceptives is suddenly discontinued. If normal periods do not return after about three or four months, a physician should be consulted.

Scanty or infrequent periods may be caused by a problem with *ovulation*.

amino acid Any of the twenty or so simple compounds of carbon, hydrogen, oxygen, and nitrogen that form the basic building blocks of *proteins*. The body is able to manufacture (synthesize) about half of the amino acids it needs for good health; the rest, the so-called essential amino acids, must be supplied in the diet by such foods as milk, cheese, eggs, meat, fish, and poultry.

amnesia Loss of memory. It may be limited to the temporary or prolonged inability to recall specific names, dates, events, or experiences (partial amnesia), or it may involve an inability to recall most of what one has previously learned or experienced (general amnesia). The cause of amnesia may be a severe emotional shock, brain damage (as from a blow to the head), alcoholism, or other disease.

amniocentesis A diagnostic procedure in which a hollow needle is inserted through the abdominal wall of a pregnant woman into the fluid-filled amniotic sac surrounding the fetus. The procedure is used to obtain a sample of the amniotic fluid. The cells in this fluid can be examined for evidence of such genetic or developmental defects as *Down's syndrome* (mongolism), *spina bifida*, *anencephaly*, and *Tay-Sachs disease*. In addition, the sex of the fetus can be determined by examining the *chromosomes* of the cells in the amniotic fluid.

This technique is most often used with women who have previously given birth to a child with one of these disorders or with advanced maternal age—pregnant women over thirty-five are often encouraged by doctors to have amniocentesis so that a presence of ab-

normality in the fetus can be determined prior to birth.
SEE ALSO *alphafetoprotein*

amniocentesis abortion A method of *abortion* usually performed in cases where the woman is between fifteen and twenty-four weeks pregnant. It involves the insertion of a hollow needle into the amniotic sac and the injection of a substance that induces uterine contractions to expel the fetus.

amphetamines A group of drugs that stimulates the central nervous system. They are effective in keeping awake people who have an abnormal tendency to fall asleep *(narcolepsy)*. Known in slang as "speed," amphetamines were once widely prescribed to suppress the appetite of seriously overweight people and to treat depression. Because of the indiscriminate and often illegal use of this class of drugs, physicians generally prescribe other products that do not lend themselves so easily to abuse. Prolonged use of amphetamines can lead to drug dependence and toxicity.

amyloidosis A rare chronic disease resulting in the accumulation in the organs and tissues of amyloid, a fibrous protein. The disease exists in two forms. Primary amyloidosis occurs in the absence of an underlying disorder and most often affects the heart, tongue, nerves, and gastrointestinal tract; localized amyloid "tumors" are often found in the respiratory tract. The secondary form, usually a result of a severe infection, may involve the spleen, liver, kidney, adrenal glands, and lymph nodes; vascular involvement may be widespread.

Symptoms and signs of amyloidosis are not specific for this disease and usually originate in the organ or system affected. Treatment is aimed at the underlying problem.

analgesic Relieving pain; a drug that relieves pain without causing loss of consciousness.

Analgesics such as *aspirin* and *acetaminophen* are available over-the-counter; others such as codeine and *morphine* require a prescription.
COMPARE *anesthetic*

anaphylactic reaction The most serious form of allergic reaction. It is a sudden and often explosive reaction of the body of a previously sensitized person to a subsequent encounter with the same foreign substance. It can follow the injection of certain drugs or diagnostic agents or be triggered by the sting of a wasp or bee. Certain foods, such as shellfish or strawberries, may also trigger this potentially life-threatening reaction.

The signs and symptoms of an anaphylactic reaction (anaphylactic shock) may occur almost immediately after the introduction into the body of the offending substance or, more commonly, within the first fifteen minutes. A typical reaction includes severe interference with breathing (due to spasm of the tiny air passages of the lungs or swelling of the throat), critical loss of blood pressure (hypotension), and sometimes convulsions, loss of consciousness, and death. Fortunately, physicians are fully prepared to deal with this dramatic emergency, which is relatively rare.

Anyone sensitive to a drug (such as penicillin) or any other substance (such as iodine or egg white) should make sure to tell a new physician before any drug or agent is prescribed, so that necessary precautions can be taken. In the case of sensitivity to insect stings, it is essential to avoid areas where wasps and bees are known to nest and flourish.

Emergency treatment of an anaphylactic reaction includes the injection of specific drugs and possibly immediate replacement of lost blood volume with intravenous infusions of a saline (salt) solution. An intravenous injection of *epinephrine* to constrict (narrow) the smaller blood vessels and thereby reestablish normal blood pressure in the major blood vessels may also be necessary.
SEE ALSO *allergy*

anastomosis The surgical connection of two hollow structures, as in the connecting of two healthy pieces of intestine after surgical removal of a diseased section.

The term is also used to indicate the natural communication between two hollow structures or vessels, either directly or by means of connecting channels.

anemia Any of various conditions characterized by a reduction in the total number of circulating red blood cells *(erythrocytes)* or impairment of their ability to transport oxygen.

The most common and generally the most easily corrected form of this disorder is iron-deficiency anemia. Blood loss during heavy menstrual periods is one cause. Poor dietary habits may also lead to iron deficiency in the absence of blood loss; it is common in infants who are weaned late from a milk diet, which is naturally deficient in iron. It may also occur in older children when rapid growth and a corresponding increase in blood volume results in a need for more dietary iron. In old age a combination of poverty, poor general health, isolation, or apathy may lead to a diet that lacks the iron naturally found in meat, liver, and other animal products. Both bread and vegetables, however, provide useful amounts of dietary iron.

Poor absorption of iron occurs in patients with certain intestinal disorders and following specific types of surgical operations on the gastrointestinal tract. Iron is rarely the only substance not absorbed, and in these cases multiple deficiencies are common. Fortunately, the treatment of iron-deficiency anemia is very easy, inexpensive, and successful. Foods naturally rich in iron or iron-supplement capsules quickly correct this condition.

All anemias are the result of one or more of the following: excessive loss or destruction of red blood cells; a shortage of the raw materials for the production of red cells; a failure of the bone marrow to produce sufficient red cells.

Continuous blood loss in any form will cause anemia, either through the actual loss of red cells or the depletion of the body's reserves of iron for the formation of *hemoglobin*. Red cells normally remain in the circulation for 120 days. Any increase in the rate of their destruction tends to produce anemia if the rate of destruction exceeds the ability of the bone marrow to replace them. This condition is described as hemolytic anemia. Many hemolytic anemias are the result of inherited defects in the red cells themselves. Some of these conditions are found in all populations, while others are more or less strictly confined to certain ethnic groups.

Sickle-cell anemia, an inherited abnormality of the red cells in which they become crescent shaped at low oxygen levels, is wide-spread in tropical Africa. *Thalassemia*, a similar defect resulting in thin and fragile red cells, is found in many millions of people in the Mediterranean, Middle East, and Far East.

Other hemolytic anemias are due to excessive destruction of normal red cells by agents acting on the cells from outside the body. In some cases the patient produces antibodies capable of destroying his or her own red cells, whereas in others toxic chemicals or drugs damage the red cells and shorten their existence.

Failure of the bone marrow to produce red blood cells in adequate numbers—although the cells may be well supplied with iron, vitamin B_{12}, and folic acid—occurs in a number of disorders. Any serious or prolonged illness tends to result in the reduction of red-cell output. This is seen particularly in cases of arthritis, cancer, kidney failure, and chronic infections. The marrow may also be physically impaired by the presence within it of tumor or leukemia cells, or by diseases of the bone marrow itself.

Radiation, many chemical poisons, and some drugs are capable of depressing the function and activity of the bone marrow, occasionally to such a degree that recovery is uncertain and the production of all types of blood cells is impaired. Such a condition is referred to as aplastic anemia. In some cases a similar disorder may occur without obvious cause.

The treatment of any type of anemia depends on its cause. Iron supplements are usually of value only in cases of simple iron deficiency.

SEE ALSO *pernicious anemia*

anencephaly A rare congenital defect occurring during the growth of a fetus and characterized by the absence or gross underdevelopment of the cerebral hemispheres of the brain. The condition is fatal.

Women who have given birth to an anencephalic baby may avail themselves of *amniocentesis* and other diagnostic procedures during subsequent pregnancies to determine whether the fetus is suffering from the same defect.
SEE *alphafetoprotein, neural-tube defect*

anesthesia The partial or complete loss of bodily sensations, especially that of pain. This state can be induced by the injection or inhalation of a local or general *anesthetic*.

anesthetic Relating to or producing *anesthesia;* a drug or agent that produces partial or complete loss of bodily sensations, especially the sensation of pain.

Anesthetics deaden the body's response to the sensations of pain and touch. Some are injected directly into a vein or tissue, whereas others take the form of gaseous mixtures (including oxygen) inhaled through a mask placed over the nose and mouth.

Anesthetics are classified as local if they deaden sensitivity in a particular area of the body, as does the procaine (Novacain) injected by a dentist before drilling a tooth. General anesthetics work on the brain and cause unconsciousness with a consequent loss of sensation throughout the entire body. Most major surgery involves the use of general anesthesia.
COMPARE *analgesic*

aneurysm A localized bulging of a weakened arterial wall. It is especially dangerous when the *aorta* or arteries in the brain are involved. If the weakened arterial wall bursts under increased blood pressure, the resulting uncontrolled internal bleeding may prove fatal.

An aneurysm that develops in an artery near the surface of the body may be recognized by the pulsation of its blood-filled sac against the skin. A deeper aneurysm may be partly diagnosed by the various symptoms it produces, including pain, faintness, shortness of breath on exertion, and swelling of the neck, face, and upper extremities. However, such symptoms are not confined to one vascular disorder, and other diagnostic methods (such as *arteriography*) may be required.

In most cases the only treatment of an aneurysm is surgical. Balloon-shaped aneurysms may be treated by tying off the neck of the bulge. Those that extend along the wall of an artery, formed by blood being forced through the weakened inner lining of the vessel and bulging into the outer layers, are treated by sealing off the involved section. If the affected artery is relatively small, normal blood circulation to the area is usually maintained by other nearby arteries. In the case of an aneurysm in a major artery, it may be necessary to remove the damaged section and replace it with a graft.

angina pectoris A sudden pain in the chest, often spreading down the left arm, caused by a temporarily insufficient blood supply to the heart muscle *(myocardium)*.

Sometimes the pain spreads down the left arm to the elbow or wrist and is occasionally felt in the neck or shoulder. It is also called angina of effort, because attacks most commonly follow strenuous activity. Angina, however, may be triggered by an excited or emotional state or by eating a particularly heavy meal.

Most attacks last only a short time and can be relieved by resting for a few minutes and by taking *nitroglycerin* or similar drugs that have proven especially helpful in relieving anginal pain by dilating the narrowed blood vessels. With proper treatment, including adequate rest and avoidance of excitement, a person with angina pectoris can expect to live a useful and full life.
SEE ALSO *coronary artery disease*

angiography A diagnostic x-ray technique in which blood vessels are injected with an x-ray contrast or *radiopaque* medium, making them more easily identified on x-ray films. This permits the diagnosis of various abnormalities of the blood vessels or the presence of growths (tumors) in the areas that these blood vessels supply.

When the arteries are outlined, the procedure is known as arteriography. When veins are outlined, the procedure is known as venography or phlebography. If the lymphatic vessels are outlined, the procedure is known as lymphangiography.

The resulting x-ray film is known as an angiogram.

angioma A swelling formed by the excessive proliferation of blood vessels. An angioma near the surface of the skin is the cause of relatively common birthmarks. Angiomas are technically tumors, although they are usually benign (harmless).

Angiomas are present on the skin in approximately 30 percent of newborn infants. Some disappear within a short time after birth, although a few may persist for two or more years before they disappear. In a few cases a "port-wine stain" or "strawberry mark" may persist. Medical treatment is rarely necessary.
SEE *hemangioma*

ankylosing spondylitis An inflammatory disease of the vertebral column characterized by gradual limitation of spinal movement. In severe cases the spine may become totally rigid. Occasionally the disease affects other joints as well, such as the shoulder and hips.

The cause of ankylosing spondylitis is unknown; some researchers

19

believe that a genetic or hereditary factor is implicated. Nine out of ten people affected are males between the ages of fifteen and thirty-five.

The disease typically spreads upward from the sacroiliac (bones at the spinal base) to affect increasingly higher levels of the spine. The first signs and symptoms, often noticed early in the morning, include pain in the lower part of the back or hip and general back stiffness. As the disease progresses there is a feeling of aching and various degrees of limitation of spinal movement, especially noticeable when the person bends forward. Spinal stiffness is frequently related to a period of inactivity.

It is extremely important for anyone with this disease to maintain good posture. In severe cases the bones of the spine become fused together. If posture has previously been poor, the spine will fuse in a bent position and make normal movement more difficult. A firm bed with a board placed under the mattress for additional support should be used. It is also a good idea to sleep without a pillow so the body remains as straight as possible.

There is no specific medical treatment for this condition. Relief of painful symptoms is possible with the use of aspirin or another analgesic or with a prescription drug designed to reduce inflammation.

ankylosis Stiffness or abnormal immobility of a joint. The condition may be present from birth (congenital ankylosis) or be the result of a joint disease or injury.

anorexia Loss of appetite. Appetite loss may be associated with the onset of a fever, general illness or debility, specific disorders of the stomach or intestinal tract, depression, the overuse of alcohol or certain drugs (including amphetamines and cocaine), or as a *side effect* of many different types of prescription drugs. Drugs designed to suppress appetite are known as anorexiants or anorectics.

Uncomplicated and temporary loss of appetite has nothing to do with the potentially more serious disorder known as *anorexia nervosa.*

anorexia nervosa A potentially serious disorder characterized by an abnormal and prolonged appetite loss leading to excessive weight loss. It mainly affects adolescent girls and in most cases is related to overemphasis on body image and an irrational fear of obesity, even if no overweight condition exists. It is not associated with any underlying physical disease.

If anorexia nervosa is not recognized early and treated with both medical attention and psychiatric counseling, it can lead to severe nutritional deficiencies and even death by starvation. Relapses may occur after physical health has been restored because of a failure of the patient to resolve the underlying

psychological compulsion to avoid food.
COMPARE *bulimia*

antacid A substance that reduces excess acid in the stomach juices and relieves mild forms of indigestion; most *over-the-counter* antacids contain a combination of aluminum hydroxide and magnesium hydroxide.

antibacterial Any drug used to treat a bacterial infection; also referred to as antimicrobials. Chemicals used to control bacterial infection outside the body are known as disinfectants or antiseptics.

Some antibacterials (such as *sulfonamides*) are developed in the laboratory; those that are originally derived from the natural substances produced by certain bacteria, molds, or other microorganisms are known as *antibiotics*.

antibiotic Any of various drugs including *penicillin, tetracycline*, and *erythromycin* that kill or prevent the growth and spread of microorganisms, especially bacteria. They were originally prepared from living organisms such as molds and bacteria, although some are now made synthetically.

The first antibiotic to be discovered was penicillin in 1928, although it was not until the 1940s that it began to be widely used to treat bacterial infections. New types of antibiotics are usually obtained from soil samples containing the appropriate microorganisms. Once the chemical structure of the natural substance is known, the drug can usually be produced in the laboratory. There is little practical difference between antibiotics that have a natural origin and those that are mass-produced synthetically.

As early as 500 B.C. the Chinese treated boils and other skin infections by applying the mold from soya beans to the affected area. They were thus probably the first to make use of the antibiotic properties of a specific mold.

Antibiotics either kill particular species of bacteria (bactericidal action) or inhibit the growth and multiplication of bacteria (bacteriostatic action). Narrow-spectrum antibiotics are effective against a limited range of bacteria whereas broad-spectrum antibiotics act against several types.

Bacteria may become resistant to a specific antibiotic. When this occurs, the physician chooses another antibiotic to control the infection. The choice of an antibiotic is also related to the fact that some people experience an unpleasant side effect from one type but not from another. For example, some people experience a severe allergic reaction to penicillin but can fully tolerate erythromycin.

A physician will normally prescribe the exact amount of an antibiotic to complete what is known as a full therapeutic course. If patients stop taking the antibiotic when they begin to feel better, instead of continuing to take it as

antibody

directed, the infection may flare up again. This is because some of the bacteria may not have been killed and those that survive are likely to start multiplying again rapidly. Worse still, the healthy survivors may have been subjected to just enough of the antibiotic to make them resistant to its bactericidal effect. These resistant bacteria could then cause a new infection—or be passed to someone else—and so begin the spread of a disease no longer capable of being controlled by the original antibiotic. In such cases an otherwise effective drug is rendered useless against that bacterial species.

If patients take more of an antibiotic than the physician prescribes or take it more frequently than instructed, annoying or even dangerous side effects can result. The physician's instructions should be followed to the letter if the treatment is to be effective.

SEE ALSO *antibacterial, sulfonamides*

antibody Any one of tens of thousands of proteins in the circulating blood that are produced by the body as a direct defense against the invasion of specific bacteria, viruses, or other foreign material *(antigens)*. Antibodies combine chemically with specific antigens to render them harmless.

Following many common infectious diseases, the body produces enough specific antibodies against them to provide lifetime protection *(immunity)* against future attacks of the same diseases.

SEE ALSO *allergy, gamma globulin, immunization, immunology, immunosuppressive, immunotherapy*

anticoagulant Preventing or delaying the coagulation (clotting) of blood; any drug or agent that provides protection against abnormal clotting.

Anticoagulants are prescribed to minimize the risk of blood clots forming and blocking important arteries, especially if the blood vessels are abnormally narrowed by a disease such as *atherosclerosis*.

SEE ALSO *embolism, embolus, thrombosis, thrombus*

antigen Any substance introduced into the body or formed within the body that stimulates the production of *antibodies*.

SEE ALSO *allergy, immunity*

antihistamine Any drug or agent that counteracts the effects of *histamine* in the body. It is used to provide relief of the symptoms associated with common *allergies* such as hay fever (allergic rhinitis).

Drowsiness is a frequent side effect of antihistamines, which are therefore also used in many over-the-counter sleep aids and motion-sickness remedies.

antipyretic Reducing *fever;* any drug or agent such as *aspirin* or *acetaminophen* that reduces fever.

SEE ALSO *hyperpyrexia*

antisepsis The process of destroying harmful microorganisms, such as bacteria, or preventing their growth and multiplication; any chemical or agent capable of establishing antisepsis is known as an antiseptic. The earliest antiseptic was carbolic acid (phenol); others include chlorine, hydrogen peroxide, and various preparations of mercury.

In general, antiseptics are used to disinfect objects and are not taken internally.

antitoxin A substance produced by the body in response to the presence of poisons (toxins) released by some species of bacteria. Antitoxins are special types of *antibodies* and can be prepared for injection to treat or prevent various diseases.

antitussive Preventing or relieving coughing; any drug or agent that prevents or relieves coughing, such as codeine or (in over-the-counter products) dextromethorphan hydrobromide.

anuria The absence or severe impairment of the flow of urine from the kidneys or urinary tract typically caused by a disease or disorder affecting these structures.

In a few cases the problem may be associated with mechanical obstruction, which is relatively easy to correct. Potentially more serious causes include acute *kidney failure* or a chronic and progressive kidney disease.

aorta The largest *artery* of the body. It receives oxygen-rich blood directly from the left ventricle of the heart.

At its origin in the upper surface of the left ventricle, it is approximately 1.2 inches (3 cm) in diameter. Blood pumped out of the heart through the aorta is conveyed to increasingly smaller arteries, which supply all the organs and tissues of the body.

aphasia A defect in or loss of language function as a result of damage or injury to the brain, characterized by impaired comprehension and usage of words or their nonverbal equivalents.

aplastic anemia
SEE *anemia*

apoplexy
SEE *stroke*

appendicitis Acute inflammation of the appendix, a small tube closed at its free end and attached at its other end to the cecum, the pouch that forms the beginning of the large intestine. It is called the vermiform (worm-like) appendix because early anatomists thought that it resembled a worm. The appendix has no known function in humans.

The appendix is about the length and half the diameter of the little finger and usually hangs freely within the abdominal cavity. The interior of the appendix is very narrow and sometimes hard pieces of waste matter or foreign bodies

arrhythmia

become trapped within it and cause an obstruction that leads to severe inflammation. It can also become inflamed as the result of a general infection or an abscess that spreads from a nearby area.

In an acute attack of appendicitis, the blood supply to the appendix becomes interrupted, which in turn leads to the death of part of its tissues *(gangrene)*. The inflamed appendix may then rupture; the infection spreads to other areas of the abdomen, leading to *peritonitis*.

Symptoms and signs of appendicitis vary from one person to another, but they usually include sharp pain that begins in the middle and moves to the lower right side of the abdomen (which feels tender), nausea and vomiting, diarrhea, and a fever of up to 102°F (39°C). In children the temperature may reach 104°F (40°C).

A physician must be consulted at the first suspicion of appendicitis. Any delay may result in a ruptured appendix, which is a potentially life-threatening complication. Laxatives must not be used as they may hasten rupture.

Treatment of acute appendicitis is surgical removal of the appendix (appendectomy). This is a relatively simple operation requiring only a short hospital stay. During other types of abdominal surgery, a healthy appendix may be removed as a preventive measure.

arrhythmia Any abnormal rhythm or disturbance of a natural rhythm, especially of the heartbeat. Some children have a harmless condition known as sinus arrhythmia, in which the pulse rate increases when they inhale and decreases when they exhale. It sometimes occurs in adults as well and in both cases is rarely associated with any other symptoms.

A potentially dangerous disturbance in the rhythm of the heartbeat (cardiac arrhythmia) can usually be diagnosed by a thorough physical examination or, more specifically, from the result of an *electrocardiogram*.
SEE ALSO *tachycardia*

arteriography A diagnostic technique or procedure in which x-rays are taken of arteries following the injection of a *radiopaque* or x-ray contrast medium that renders them opaque to x-rays. It is used in the diagnosis of various abnormalities of the arteries or the tissues and organs they supply.

The x-ray film obtained with this procedure is known as an arteriogram.
SEE ALSO *angiography*

arteriole The smallest vessel of the *arterial* system. Arterioles form a link with the *capillaries*.
COMPARE *venule*

arteriosclerosis A general term for any condition in which the walls of the arteries become thickened, inelastic, and hard. The condition can affect people at any age, but it is much more common among the late middle aged and the elderly. Arteriosclerosis may be particularly severe in people with diabetes or with an underactive thyroid gland. In a few cases there is a suspected inherited tendency toward the disease.

Arteriosclerosis is popularly known as hardening of the arteries. A potentially serious form of arteriosclerosis is *atherosclerosis.*

artery Any blood vessel that carries oxygen-rich blood away from the heart to all the organs and tissues of the body (with the exception of the pulmonary artery, which carries oxygen-depleted blood from the heart to the lungs to receive a fresh supply of oxygen).

Arteries generally have thicker walls than *veins* because they must withstand the forceful surge of blood from each heartbeat. Blood is pumped out of the heart into the arteries and returns to the heart through the veins.
SEE *aorta*

arthritis Inflammation of the joints.
SEE *osteoarthritis, rheumatoid arthritis*

artificial insemination The *fertilization* of a female sex cell (ovum) by a male sex cell (spermatozoon) other than by sexual intercourse. The technique usually involves the introduction of sperm cells into the vagina near the neck (cervix) of the uterus with a syringe.
COMPARE *in vitro fertilization*

artificial respiration
SEE *cardiopulmonary resuscitation*

asbestosis A disease of the *lungs* caused by inhaling tiny particles of asbestos. The first signs are usually shortness of breath and a dry cough. The disease, a form of *pneumoconiosis,* most frequently affects those who breathe asbestos dust while working in factories where asbestos is processed. It has been shown to be one cause of lung cancer.

Exposure to even small amounts of asbestos dust can cause potentially serious problems. Lung disorders can occur even with a single exposure to asbestos dust, although symptoms may not emerge for twenty or thirty years. Those who smoke cigarettes and have been exposed to asbestos dust run a greatly increased risk of lung cancer.

aspirin A white powder, usually in the form of a pressed tablet, used to reduce fever (antipyretic effect), relieve minor pain (analgesic effect), and reduce swelling and inflammation (antiinflammatory effect).

Aspirin is freely available without a prescription and is used throughout the world to relieve headaches, toothaches, muscular aches and pains, and symptoms of a wide range of other troublesome conditions from the common cold to rheumatoid arthritis.

Aspirin is acetylsalicylic acid, a member of a class of related drugs

aspirin

known as the salicylates. Salicylic acid was originally obtained from willow bark, a traditional home remedy for fevers. In 1875, a related aspirin compound, sodium salicylate, was used successfully to reduce high body temperature and relieve painful and swollen joints. The tablet form of aspirin became available in 1899.

Aspirin's analgesic effect is not as great as that of narcotic analgesics such as *morphine*. Aspirin is used mainly to relieve pain of mild or moderate intensity and has no effect on such deep-seated pain as that coming from the abdominal organs (visceral pain).

Aspirin can reduce body temperature only when it is above normal; it has no effect in the absence of fever. Taken in the correct dosage (as instructed on the label), it usually provides effective relief within a few minutes. When taken in massive doses, however, it can actually increase body temperature and cause a condition known as drug-induced fever, which is occasionally seen with a wide variety of other drugs.

Some people are sensitive to aspirin. One of its most common side effects is minor bleeding from the stomach and intestines. In an otherwise healthy person, this may go unrecognized; in fact, it has been estimated that some degree of gastrointestinal blood loss occurs in about 70 percent of people who frequently take aspirin. Sensitivity to aspirin is potentially much more serious in people with peptic ulcers. Massive bleeding from the stomach or intestines has occurred in such patients shortly after aspirin has been taken. Some physicians recommend that aspirin tablets should either be crushed or dissolved in water because evidence suggests less bleeding occurs when aspirin is taken in this manner.

Some aspirin products also contain buffering agents (alkaline substances such as aluminum hydroxide and magnesium hydroxide). Despite its manufacturers' claims, there is absolutely no scientific evidence that buffered aspirin provides a more rapid onset of action or a greater degree of pain relief than aspirin. Aspirin with buffering does tend to dissolve in the stomach more quickly and be absorbed into the bloodstream more quickly, which may reduce the possibility of stomach irritation: the shorter the time undissolved aspirin particles remain in the stomach, the less the chance of irritation and consequent bleeding.

Large doses of aspirin not only produce such unpleasant side effects as headache, nausea, visual disturbances, and ringing in the ears, but in the very young can be fatal. The combined effects of alcoholic beverages and aspirin can add to the danger of gastrointestinal irritation and bleeding.

Aspirin has a tendency to thin the blood. Thus, patients taking *an-*

ticoagulant drugs should not take aspirin or products that contain aspirin without a physician's approval. Diabetics taking medication to control the level of blood sugar should not take aspirin at the same time without medical advice because aspirin has been strongly implicated in lowering blood-sugar levels. Finally, patients taking prescription drugs to relieve the painful symptoms of arthritis and other inflammatory diseases should not take aspirin without the advice of their physician because the combined effects could result in severe gastrointestinal irritation or the development of ulcers.

Recent clinical studies have suggested that prescribed amounts of aspirin in patients who have suffered a heart attack *(myocardial infarction)* may reduce the likelihood of future attacks.

In the early 1980s aspirin was implicated as a possible contributing factor in the incidence of *Reye's syndrome*, when given to children during the fever stages of viral infections such as influenza or chickenpox. However, more extensive studies must be conducted to learn about this possible association.

SEE ALSO *acetaminophen*

asthma A disorder of the *lungs* that causes the bronchi (smaller air passages) suddenly to spasm and thus impede the supply of air to the lungs. In addition, the lining of the bronchial tubes swells and exudes a thick, sticky mucus. This results in recurring attacks of breathlessness (dyspnea) and wheezing. Exhaling becomes difficult and exhausting, and inhaling occurs in short gasps. In order to get enough air, the sufferer usually has to sit upright and forcibly lift and drop the chest and shoulders.

Many factors can cause asthma. Three major contributors are *allergy*, emotional stress, and infection. Asthma can start at any age, and although there is no general rule, when it begins early in life it is most commonly caused by an allergy.

Asthma often occurs in episodes, between which the patient appears quite normal. It can, however, also be a chronic condition where the sudden attacks are less severe but where there is always a wheeze. The attacks may last from a few minutes to several hours. The longer the attack, the more potentially dangerous the condition may be and the more important it is for the asthmatic to be under close medical supervision. The physician generally prescribes drugs (bronchodilators) to relieve or sometimes prevent asthmatic attacks. For many asthma sufferers it is essential to have these drugs always at hand in the form of tablets, sprays, or inhalers, to take at the beginning of an attack; they relieve the spasm in the air passages and in most cases are sufficient to stop the attack.

When the disease starts in

children or young adults it often appears spontaneously and, after a variable period, may not cause future problems. In chronic, severe sufferers, however, the outlook is less promising and a physician should be consulted at regular intervals to monitor and treat the disease.

Asthma of allergic origin is usually caused by sensitivity to inhaled pollen, dust, molds, or other allergens (less commonly it may be triggered by a reaction to certain foods and drugs). This causes a release of *histamine* from the cells that make up the smaller bronchi and the bronchioles. As a result, the mucous membrane that lines the bronchi swells and the muscles tighten and constrict the tubes. In addition, thick sticky mucus is secreted into the air passages, further blocking the constricted channels and making breathing even more difficult. Allergic asthma may be seasonal (especially if caused by a reaction to pollen) or occur any time of the year.

In severe cases, an asthmatic attack can be extremely frightening to both the patient and his or her family. The victim often believes that suffocation is taking place, and this fear only serves to intensify the attack.

astigmatism An eye disorder in which images do not focus properly on the *retina* because the *cornea*, and sometimes the lens, has an uneven curvature. This results in images being distorted or fuzzy; a circle may appear to be an oval, or a vertical line may be seen less clearly than a horizontal line. The problem may exist at birth (congenital astigmatism) or be acquired later, following a gradual change in the curvature of the cornea or lens.

An ophthalmologist determines the degree of astigmatism from the number of lines on a test chart that appear blurred or distorted and how out of focus they are. This information, together with the results of other eye tests, enables the eye specialist to prescribe eyeglasses to correct the distortion.

Astigmatism of some degree is often present in the elderly and in most people who wear corrective lenses. Older persons should have their eyes examined every two years. Uncorrected astigmatism can result in the eyes becoming fatigued.

ataxia Loss of muscular coordination and control, characterized by jerky movements of the arms and legs, especially during walking. It is usually caused by a disorder of the nervous system. One form, locomotor ataxia or *tabes dorsalis*, is slowly progressive and is caused by infection with the bacteria of *syphilis*, which gradually destroy the nerve fibers in the spinal cord. Temporary ataxia is sometimes experienced as a *side effect* of a prescription drug.

atelectasis A condition in which the lungs of a baby partially or totally fail to expand with air at birth. The term is also used to identify a condition in which part of a lung or an entire lung becomes airless and collapses. This can be caused by compression from outside the lung or by an obstruction of the bronchial tubes (air passages).

atheroma A fatty deposit on the inner lining of an artery, often leading to a thickening or degeneration of the arterial wall *(atherosclerosis)* and increased resistance to the flow of blood.
SEE ALSO *cholesterol*

atherosclerosis A potentially serious condition in which fatty deposits *(atheromas)* form on the inner lining of an artery. Although all arteries may be affected, the condition is most serious when it involves the arteries that supply the heart muscle *(myocardium)*, brain, and limbs, or the *aorta*, the main artery of the body.

As the fatty deposits build up inside an artery they cause a narrowing of its diameter. For a time the heart can compensate by pumping harder against the increased resistance. But when the deposits become excessive they may cause a serious interruption of the blood flow to a vital organ.

The deposits can lead to patchy roughening and damage to the arterial walls. This increases the likelihood that blood will stick to that part of the vessel lining and clot, further reducing the blood flow past that point. In severe cases the artery may become blocked. This can cause a *stroke*, some form of heart disorder, (such as *angina pectoris* or *myocardial infarction*), extreme pain and swelling in the lower limbs, or other potentially serious complications.

The exact cause of atherosclerosis is uncertain, but there are several possible contributing factors. Among these are eating foods rich in animal (saturated) fats (which contain the fatlike substance *cholesterol*), ingesting too much refined sugar, overeating, lack of sufficient exercise, and smoking.

If the fatty deposits are gradual and generalized there may be few or no symptoms for many years. In the elderly, the progressive loss of an adequate blood supply to the brain may result in the onset of confusion, forgetfulness, and other changes in personality associated with *senile dementia*.
SEE ALSO *arteriosclerosis*

athlete's foot
SEE *tinea*

atrophy The shrinking or reduction ("wasting") in size of all or part of an organ or body structure. It is usually associated with a chronic debilitating illness or occurs when a patient is otherwise confined to bed for prolonged periods. The process can frequently be controlled or reversed with special exercises and well-balanced meals.

Localized atrophy (as of an arm

auscultation

or leg) can be caused by prolonged disuse of a group of muscles following injury or because of nerve damage.

COMPARE *hyperplasia*, *hypertrophy*

auscultation The technique or procedure of diagnosis by listening to and interpreting the sounds that arise from the heart, lungs, and various other organs, especially through a *stethoscope.*

autism A severe disorder of communication and behavior usually affecting infants and children (also known as infantile autism) characterized by profound withdrawal, constant rocking movements, head banging, violent tantrums, and a marked delay in the development of or the virtual absence of speech. The autistic child usually fails to maintain eye contact and is indifferent to repeated attempts to be engaged in social interaction.

The cause is unknown. There is no evidence to suggest that the condition is associated with parental rejection. No specific treatment exists, although in severe cases, institutional care may be necessary.

autoimmune disease Any disease in which the body fails to distinguish between a foreign invader (such as a microorganism) and its own tissues as the result of a disorder in the body's defense system *(immunity).* Autoimmune diseases such as *rheumatoid arthritis,* hemolytic *anemia,* and *myasthenia gravis* are characterized by the formation of *antibodies* against parts of the body to such an extent that tissues are injured.

autopsy Medical examination of the body after death, also called necropsy and postmortem examination. It is usually performed to ascertain the cause of death, as in cases of suspected contagious disease or criminal circumstances. An autopsy also adds to general medical knowledge about the causes and processes of disease.

B

Babinski reflex An abnormal reaction (except in babies) in which the large toe extends upward and the other toes fan out when the sole of the foot is stroked. It is a sign of a disorder of the central nervous system (brain and spinal cord). The normal reaction (except in babies and the very young, whose nervous systems are not yet fully developed) is for the large toe to curl downward.

This routine diagnostic test is named after the French neurologist who discovered it, Joseph Babinski (1857–1932).

bacteria A large group of single-celled microorganisms technically classified as belonging to the plant kingdom. They are so small that over a million could easily fit on the head of a pin. They generally reproduce by splitting into two identical cells. In a suitable environment (such as an open wound) a small number of bacteria can multiply into several million within a relatively short time.

Some bacteria are able to form a thick wall around themselves (forming a cyst or spore), making them resistant to heat, drying, or toxic chemicals—thus, the need for very high temperatures when sterilizing surgical or dental instruments.

Bacteria are classified in several ways. One is by general shape: round (coccus), rodlike (bacillus), and spiral (spirillum). Another method of classification is whether or not they retain a special laboratory stain called the Gram stain. Bacteria that retain the stain are referred to as Gram positive; those that do not are Gram negative. (This method was developed by the Danish physician Hans C. J. Gram, 1853–1938.) This classification helps to indicate which of various *antibiotics* are appropriate in treating specific infections.

Some bacteria require oxygen in order to live (aerobic bacteria); others cannot survive in oxygen (anaerobic bacteria).

Only a few of the known types of

bacteria cause disease (pathogenic bacteria). Most are harmless and quite a few provide essential services in breaking down dead plant and animal tissues into simpler compounds that can be used as food for plants. They also act on milk to produce cheese, yogurt, and other dairy products, and even convert sewage into nutrients for soil. Some bacteria are sources of antibiotics.

Bacteria are found all over the world, from the edges of active volcanoes to the ice caps of the Antarctic. They exist naturally in the soil, in fresh water, and in the sea. They live and thrive in the mouth, in the digestive tract, and on the skin, usually without causing any problem at all.
SEE ALSO *rickettsia, virus*

baldness
SEE *alopecia*

ballistocardiography A diagnostic technique or procedure in which an electrically amplified graphic record (ballistocardiogram) is made of the tiny vibrations set up in the body by the heartbeat. Although the procedure is primarily used in research, it may provide diagnostic information about the condition of the *aorta*, largest artery of the body. Trained cardiologists observe characteristic waves that suggest a reduction in the normal elasticity of the aorta, as from the formation of fatty deposits *(atheromas)* on its inner surface.

barbiturates A group of drugs with *sedative* effects; they induce sleep. Popularly known as sleeping pills or "downs," barbiturates are capable of causing intoxicating effects similar to alcohol: slurred speech, inability to walk straight, poor judgment, and confusion. Barbiturates are sometimes illegally used to counteract the nervous effects of a stimulating drug, such as cocaine or *amphetamines*. Large doses of barbiturates can be fatal, especially when taken with alcohol.
SEE *addiction, hypnotic drugs*

barium sulfate A chemical that is opaque to x-rays. It is used in a mixture that is either swallowed (barium meal) or inserted rectally into the large intestine under pressure (barium enema). The barium provides contrast on x-ray films and permits the radiologist to observe an outline of the digestive tract. The presence of such abnormalities as growths or tumors will appear as a "filling defect" on the x-ray film or fluoroscope screen.
SEE ALSO *radiopaque*

bed sore An open sore, also known as a pressure sore or decubitus ulcer, on a part of the skin that is under constant and prolonged pressure when a patient lies in bed in one position. It commonly occurs on the buttocks, shoulders, elbows, heels, and ankles, where the flesh is pressed against an underlying bone. Bed sores can be prevented by regular changes in the person's position and by observing the rules of hygiene.

Bell's palsy A neurological (nerve) disorder that affects only one nerve and its branches—the facial (VII cranial) nerve that supplies the facial muscles. The cause is unknown, but it is thought that the facial nerve becomes swollen and compressed; this can happen relatively easily, since it passes through a narrow bony tunnel on its way to the facial muscles.

The onset is sudden; in most cases the full signs of facial paralysis occur within a single day. Some patients occasionally experience pain behind the ear before the facial muscles become incapable of movement. The abrupt onset is important in diagnosis, since other forms of facial paralysis may appear similar but be the result of a different disorder.

The classical signs of Bell's palsy involve only one side of the face, although rarely both sides are involved. One corner of the mouth droops, the furrows or wrinkles of the skin over the forehead relax (it is impossible to scowl) and it may not be possible to close the eye on the affected side. The face feels heavy and numb and saliva may dribble from the affected corner of the mouth. The patient is unable to blow out the cheeks or whistle. A few people also experience a partial loss of taste.

Recovery is less common in the elderly than in younger patients, although if some improvement is noticed within a few weeks of the onset of paralysis the outlook is favorable, and total recovery may occur. Prompt medical attention is important, including protection of the exposed eye (especially during sleep). The earlier treatment is begun, the better the chances of recovery.

The condition is named after the Scottish physiologist and surgeon Sir Charles Bell (1774–1842).

bends A painful condition (also known as decompression sickness or caisson disease) of the limbs and abdomen caused by bubbles of nitrogen in the blood and tissues as a result of a rapid reduction of air pressure; it affects divers and others who spend time in high-pressure environments.

benign Any condition that is not life-threatening, recurrent, or progressive; especially applied to a growth or tumor that is not cancerous.
COMPARE *malignant*

beriberi A disease caused by a deficiency of thiamine (vitamin B_1). It is characterized by a painful inflammation of the nerves, anemia, and generalized swelling (edema) caused by an abnormal accumulation of body fluids in the tissues. The disease is now uncommon except in those parts of the world where the diet consists mainly of polished (husked) rice.

beta blockers Drugs that block the heart's response to stimulation by the sympathetic nervous system, that part of the nervous system that acts to increase heartbeat, narrow the inner diameter of blood vessels, and increase blood pressure. Beta blockers include the prescription drugs propranolol (Inderal) and metoprolol (Lopressor). Also called beta-adrenergic blocking agents, they reduce the heart's workload and thus lower the coronary arteries' demand for blood. They are used to treat *angina pectoris, hypertension,* and cardiac *arrhythmia.*

b.i.d. Abbreviation for the Latin phrase *bis in die* ("twice a day"). It is commonly used in *prescriptions.*

bile A thick brown or greenish yellow fluid produced in the *liver,* stored in the *gallbladder,* and emptied by means of ducts into the duodenum, the first part of the small intestine. It aids in the digestion of fatty foods.

bilharziasis
SEE *schistosomiasis*

bilirubinemia The presence of bilirubin, an orange pigment found in *bile,* in the circulating blood. Although bilirubin is normally present in the blood in small amounts, the occurrence of excessive amounts (hyperbilirubinemia) can lead to *jaundice* and is a diagnostic sign of various disorders of the *liver* or associated structures.

biopsy The removal and microscopic examination of a small piece of living tissue to establish a diagnosis, particularly to determine if a growth is benign (harmless) or malignant (cancerous).

Biopsy specimens may be taken from organs that have a natural opening onto the body surface, such as the intestines or bladder, without major surgery. A slender illuminated instrument (fiberoptic endoscope) is inserted into the natural opening until it reaches the desired site and a tiny sample of tissue is removed.

Biopsies of internal organs such as the liver or kidneys are usually performed by needle biopsy, the insertion of a hollow needle into the organ through the skin surface.

The results of most biopsies are available within a day. However, during some surgical operations a frozen-section biopsy may be requested and the operation is temporarily interrupted (for example, before the surgical removal of an organ or part suspected of being cancerous) while the specimen is sent quickly to the pathology lab, frozen, sliced into extremely thin sections, and examined under a microscope. The pathologist then advises the surgeon of the presence or absence of suspected disease so that appropriate decisions can be made on the spot.

SEE ALSO *bronchoscopy, cytoscopy, endoscopy, gastroscopy*

birthmark
SEE *angioma, nevus*

birth control
SEE *contraception*

bladder The distensible muscular sac, also called the urinary bladder, in which *urine* is temporarily stored prior to its elimination from the body. In older children and adults the emptying of the bladder is under conscious control, making it possible to delay urination for a time even though nerve impulses indicate that the bladder is full.
SEE *cystitis, ureter, urethra*

blinking
SEE *cornea*

blood cell
SEE *erythrocyte, leukocyte, platelet*

blood poisoning
SEE *septicemia, uremia*

blood pressure
SEE *diastolic, hypertension, hypotension, systolic*

blood test Any one of many specific tests performed on a blood sample for such purposes as determining blood type or parentage; detecting the presence of infection, anemia, or diseases of the bone marrow (where blood cells are manufactured); and measuring the amounts of various chemicals in the blood.

The blood sample may be obtained by pricking the finger, earlobe, or (in infants) the heel. If a larger blood sample is required, it is removed by means of a hypodermic needle (syringe), usually inserted into a vein near the inner surface of the elbow. This procedure is relatively painless.

The range of tests that can be performed on a sample of blood is enormous. A very common test is known as a complete blood count (CBC). This involves measuring the amount of *hemoglobin* as an index of anemia and counting the numbers of red and white blood cells. A stained film of the blood is often examined as well to study the nature of the cells under a miscroscope. Apart from the diagnosis of anemia and other specific hematological (blood) disorders, a CBC is a commonly requested test in a patient whose diagnosis is still uncertain, since many diseases produce characteristic changes in the blood count.

A test that frequently accompanies a CBC is the rate at which red blood cells *(erythrocytes)* settle at the bottom of a long narrow tube *(erythrocyte sedimentation rate)*. In general, a normal sedimentation rate is a good indication that certain diseases can be eliminated. An increased rate of sedimentation provides evidence that a thorough search should be made for the responsible underlying disease.

Laboratories also perform a wide range of tests on blood samples in which the concentration of many chemical constituents of the blood is measured. In most cases, specific measurements are made to detect characteristic alterations in the chemical composition of the blood that are associated with particular diseases. One example is the measurement of the level of glucose (sugar) in the blood as an indication of diabetes.

Blood tests are frequently performed on healthy subjects during a complete medical examination as a screening procedure designed to detect early evidence of a potentially serious disease.

Blood tests are also used in the diagnosis of infectious diseases. Such tests as the *Wassermann test* involve the detection in the patient's blood of characteristic antibodies that have formed as the result of a specific bacterial or viral infection.
SEE ALSO *hematocrit*

boil
SEE *furuncle*

bone marrow The soft red or yellow tissue that fills the interior cavities of bones. Red marrow is found especially in the breastbone (sternum), pelvic bones (pelvis), ribs, and vertebrae (bones of the spinal column). Red marrow is the site of production of red blood cells *(erythrocytes)*, white blood cells *(leukocytes)*, and *platelets*.

Yellow marrow is found in the central cavities of long bones, which consist of a shaft and two extremities (such as the bones that form the skeleton of the arms and legs). Yellow marrow consists largely of fat and plays no role in the production of blood cells and platelets.

A *biopsy* is sometimes made of a tiny sample of red bone marrow to determine the presence or absence of a disease that interferes with the production of blood cells. The specimen is usually obtained by needle biopsy, the insertion of a hollow needle into the breastbone or pelvis.

botulism A rare but potentially fatal form of *food poisoning* caused by contamination of improperly canned or preserved food with the toxin (poison) produced by the anaerobic bacteria *Clostridium botulinum*. The toxin affects the central nervous system (brain and spinal cord) and may cause paralysis of the muscles of the respiratory system or heart. Other symptoms may include double vision, difficulty in speaking clearly, difficulty swallowing (dysphagia), constipation, and dryness of the eyes and mouth.

Spores of the bacteria are rarely destroyed by cooking the contaminated food. Approximately four out of five victims of botulism recover, although some symptoms may persist for a year or more. Home-canned foods, particularly vegetables, pose the greatest risk. In the supermarket, never buy cans that are dented or exhibit a prominent bulge, which could be evidence of bacterial contamination.
SEE ALSO *salmonellosis*

bowel
SEE *large intestine*

bradycardia An abnormally slow heartbeat and a consequently slow pulse rate. Bradycardia may occur in healthy persons at times, especially in athletes or the young. It can also occur in patients with jaundice and those recovering from an infectious disease.

If bradycardia is suspected, a physician should be consulted to rule out the possibility of any underlying physical disorder. Associated feelings of faintness or dizziness can usually be relieved by lying down.
COMPARE *tachycardia*

brain The major center for coordination and regulation of all bodily activities. It is composed of three major structures: the *cerebrum*, *cerebellum*, and *brain stem*. The human brain is a soft mass of jellylike tissue that weighs an average of about 3 pounds (1.3 kilograms). Together with the *spinal cord* it forms the *central nervous system*.

brain death A condition characterized by irreversible *coma* (unconsciousness), failure of the brain to show evidence of electrical activity as measured by an *electroencephalogram*, lack of any response to external stimuli, absence of spontaneous breathing, fixed pupils, and other evidence that the brain has been irreparably damaged. The cause is usually a severe head injury or massive and uncontrollable bleeding within the brain (cerebral hemorrhage).

When the brain dies the individual is in no traditional sense alive, even if breathing and blood circulation are maintained by artificial means (life-support systems). It is nevertheless a very painful decision for relatives and physicians to give permission to withdraw these external means once the brain has ceased to function.
SEE ALSO *death*

brain scan A diagnostic technique used to detect any of various abnormalities within the brain, such as a tumor or structural damage. The first step is injection, usually into a vein in the arm, of a *radioactive isotope* or a tracer, such as technetium. A scintillation scanner is then used to detect the tiny emissions of radioactivity as the tracer flows through the blood vessels of the brain.

If blood vessels in the brain are damaged, some of the radioactive tracer will leak out and collect in nearby areas of brain tissue. This can be picked up by the scanner as a "hot spot" that often has a characteristic shape, depending on the nature of the underlying problem. The radioactivity of the tracer does not last long and the procedure is normally quite safe.
COMPARE *computerized axial tomography*
SEE ALSO *nuclear medicine*

brain stem All the parts of the *brain* except the *cerebrum* and *cerebellum;* its main anatomical divisions are the pons, *medulla oblongata,* and midbrain. The lower end of the brain stem extends to the opening at the base of the skull known as the foramen magnum and is continuous with the *spinal cord.* The brain stem contains a diffuse network of nerve cells and fibers called the reticular formation or *reticular activating system* that plays an important role in wakefulness, alertness, and sleep.

breast cancer The most common form of *cancer* among women. The number of newly diagnosed cases per year has been rising steadily since 1935, but the rate of deaths has remained constant. This suggests that progress is slowly being made in this disease, which claims more female victims between the ages of forty and forty-four than any other disease. Modern methods of diagnosis and examination, plus women's growing awareness of breast self-examination, have helped considerably in the fight against breast cancer.

Several factors have been identified that influence a woman's chances of developing breast cancer. The two factors that have proved most significant are a family history of breast cancer and previous cancer of the breast.

Daughters and sisters of women who have had breast cancer are more likely to suffer the disease than those who have no family history of it. This is not because cancer is inherited (which has not been proven); it may be that a predisposition to tumors is inherited. Women who are treated for breast cancer in one breast run a high risk of developing it in the other breast.

Breast cancer under the age of thirty is rare; over thirty, its incidence rises sharply with age. It is therefore very important that women examine themselves each month for changes in the general shape and feel of their breasts. Many developing lumps are not cancerous but are small cysts or other relatively harmless disorders.

Nearly all women with breast cancer can first detect some breast abnormality themselves. The signs and symptoms may include a lump, stabbing or aching pain in the breast, retraction of the nipple (it turns inward), a discharge from the nipple, or areas of redness on the breast.

One of the most important factors in the early diagnosis of breast cancer is the interval between the woman's first noticing some breast abnormality and her seeking medical attention. The earlier the diagnosis is made, the greater the chance of halting the progress of the disease. After a careful examination, the physician will want to have additional diagnostic information, which can be obtained only from one or more special tests or procedures.

Mammography is a commonly

used technique where x-rays are used to detect areas of breast tissue that are denser than usual. If this technique is performed correctly, it can detect breast cancer up to about two years before any suspicious lump is felt by the hands.

Thermography is a diagnostic procedure based on the detection and measurement of minute changes in temperature in the skin of the breast. It is thought that a cancerous lump may be one or two degrees warmer than tissue around it. Some nonmalignant conditions may also give rise to increased skin temperatures, but when a *biopsy* is performed it will confirm the presence or absence of breast cancer.

Treatment generally is surgical. The most limited operation, *lumpectomy*, involves the removal of the primary tumor and a small amount of the breast tissue immediately surrounding it. Frequently, only a dimple in the normal breast shape remains. *Mastectomy* is the surgical removal of the breast. A simple mastectomy involves the removal of the breast tissue, but the underlying chest muscles remain untouched and there is no surgery in the armpit (axillary nodes). Many women who have had a mastectomy are fitted with a padded bra (prosthesis).

To help minimize the possibility of recurrence, *cytotoxic drugs* may be prescribed two to four weeks following mastectomy. One or a combination of cytotoxic drugs may be administered to destroy any remaining cancer cells. The results have been encouraging.

breathlessness
SEE *dyspnea*

Bright's disease An inflammatory or degenerative disease of the kidneys; nephritis. It is named after the British physician Richard Bright (1789-1858).
SEE *glomerulonephritis*

bronchi The two large tubular branches of the *trachea* leading to the *lungs* and composed of rings of cartilage; the major air passages, each of which is called a bronchus.

bronchiectasis A chronic condition of the *lungs* in which the bronchi (air passages) are abnormally and sometimes permanently dilated (widened). There are three major causes: infection, physical injury, and congenital defects.

Bronchiectasis may occur after chronic bronchitis, emphysema, or a severe lung infection such as pneumonia. The bronchial walls can be damaged by the infection and resultant severe coughing and lose their natural resilience.

Any obstruction of a bronchus or bronchiole (one of the many smaller bronchi) can result in dilation of its walls beyond the site of the obstruction. This may be caused by thick mucus, an inhaled foreign body, or an abnormal growth (tumor). A chest wound can cause the lung tissues to become fibrous, with subsequent development of bronchiectasis.

bronchitis

In some cases a child may be born with bronchiectasis due to a failure of the lungs or related organs to develop normally.

The symptoms of bronchiectasis are usually mild at first and become more noticeable with time. Fits of coughing typically occur, producing occasional sputum (phlegm) that is foul smelling from accumulation in the dilated air passages. Later, the amount of sputum coughed up will increase and both it and the breath will give off a strong unpleasant smell. Coughing up small amounts of blood is common and occasionally may even be the first sign of the disorder. In some cases the patient may also have a fever.

With early diagnosis and treatment with antibiotics to control any infection, many of the troublesome symptoms of bronchiectasis can be greatly relieved. In addition, most patients are instructed in the technique of "postural drainage"—they lie with the head inclined downward below the affected lung area, thus permitting any secretions of sticky mucus or pus to drain out of the air passages by means of gravity.

bronchitis Inflammation of the bronchi, the air passages of the *lungs*. Bronchitis may be acute or chronic.

Acute bronchitis is common in damp and foggy climates and occurs more often in young children and the elderly. It can be caused by a bacterial or viral infection or be a complication of other illnesses, such as whooping cough or measles. Many cases are the result of inhaling irritating substances such as smoke, dust particles, and some gases. A few cases may also be related to a specific *allergy*.

Acute bronchitis may be triggered by exhaustion, lack of proper food, or exposure to a cold or wet environment. In the beginning the patient feels ill, with aches and perhaps a slight fever. There may be some discomfort in the chest, particularly behind the breastbone (sternum). This soon becomes a feeling of tightness accompanied by a dry, irritating cough, which will generally loosen up after a few hours. The amount of sputum (phlegm) coughed up increases over a period of a few days and then is gradually reduced; coughing up of yellowish sputum is generally a sign of infection.

Acute bronchitis is usually a mild disorder of short duration. Antibiotics are used to control any associated bacterial infection; however, they have no effect against viral infections. Patients should avoid fatigue and eat well-balanced meals. Although attacks of acute bronchitis ordinarily last less than two weeks, repeated attacks can lead to the potentially more serious chronic form.

Chronic bronchitis is an inflammation of the bronchi that develops slowly and is generally more common among the middle aged and elderly. Like acute bronchitis, it can develop from the inhalation of irritating substances, including tobacco smoke. Chronic bronchitis is a gradually progressive disease that, unless controlled, can lead to serious lung problems. The condition is often associated with or accompanied by diseases such as *emphysema*, *bronchiectasis*, *pneumoconiosis*, and pulmonary *fibrosis* (in which the tissues of the lungs become fibrous and produce breathing problems that resemble chronic asthma).

Although the life expectancy of the patient with chronic bronchitis is shorter than normal, the progress of the disease can be considerably reduced by avoiding polluted atmospheres, including cigarette smoke. Bedrooms should be kept warm (but not stuffy) at night, obesity (which puts an extra burden on breathing) should be avoided, and clothing should be kept light but warm. Antibiotics are prescribed to control bacterial infection.

bronchography A relatively uncommon procedure occasionally used in the diagnosis of disorders involving the bronchi, the air passages of the lungs. Before x-rays are taken, a *radiopaque* or x-ray contrast medium is placed into the air passages by means of a catheter inserted into the trachea through the nose or mouth.
SEE ALSO *bronchiectasis*

bronchoscopy A technique or procedure for direct examination of the interior of the bronchi, the larger air passages of the *lungs*. It is performed by passing a slender rigid or flexible illuminated instrument known as a *bronchoscope* through the mouth and into the trachea until it reaches the appropriate site in one of the two main bronchial branches. Bronchoscopy may be performed under either local or general anesthesia.

The procedure can be used to diagnose suspected bronchial diseases or disorders and to remove tiny tissue specimens for *biopsy*, foreign bodies, or thickened secretions.
SEE ALSO *endoscopy*

bulimia An abnormal increase in the urge to eat. The condition is most common in females and is thought to be associated with various underlying psychological or sociological causes, which may demand professional help. In most cases the victim will gorge with food and then induce vomiting by sticking a finger down the throat.

The emotional causes of bulimia are not easily resolved, but if the motivation to stop overeating is sufficiently strong and the victim has the understanding of the immediate family, the outlook is promising.
COMPARE *anorexia nervosa*

bursitis Inflammation of a bursa, any of the approximately 140 small fluid-filled sacs located at points of continual friction or pressure, usually near the cavity of a movable joint. A bursa acts as a cushion between bones, muscles, and tendons; some are not essential and may be surgically removed if they become chronically inflamed.

The most common sites of bursitis involve the bursas in the shoulder, elbow, hip, knee ("housemaid's knee") and heel. The cause is unknown, although a sudden attack may follow a few hours or days after an injury to the affected joint. Bursitis of the shoulder is probably the most common form, resulting in severe pain that radiates down the arm or up to the neck. The bursa becomes swollen and tender and movement of the associated joint is extremely painful and limited.

An attack of bursitis may not last long and often does not recur for many months, if at all. Recurring attacks should receive medical attention, especially since the pain may be due not to bursitis but to some other joint disorder. Chronic bursitis may be related to repeated injury, infection, *gout*, or *rheumatoid arthritis*.

Treatment of bursitis may not be necessary in acute attacks that last only a few days. Relief may be obtained with aspirin or, in more severe cases, with antiinflammatory drugs. Restriction of movement in the affected joint and the application of hot packs and gentle massage also help relieve discomfort. In persistent cases a physician may inject a *corticosteroid* directly into the bursa.

It is important to exercise the affected joint as soon as relief of pain permits; otherwise, the joint may become stiff and the muscles may become flabby or start to atrophy.

bypass The construction of an alternate route (shunt) for the circulating blood to avoid a blocked or diseased section of a blood vessel, especially an artery.
SEE ALSO *coronary bypass*

C

calculus Any solidification or stone that forms in a body cavity. Calculi are usually formed by the gradual buildup of mineral salts in the *gallbladder* (gallstones) or *kidneys* (kidney stones).

Dental calculus describes the deposit on teeth of the minerals calcium phosphate and calcium carbonate and organic matter (cellular debris and various microorganisms), forming tartar or dental plaque.

SEE *cholelithiasis, nephrolithiasis*

cancer Any of various diseases characterized by an abnormal and uncontrolled growth of body cells. Cancer cells may remain in the original area where they were formed (resulting in the formation of a slowly growing malignant tumor) or they may enter the bloodstream or lymphatic system and be carried to other parts of the body *(metastasis)*. The latter condition is much more serious because localized treatment becomes impossible.

Specific names are given to the various types of cancer depending on the cells or tissues involved; these include *carcinoma, epithelioma, Hodgkin's disease, leukemia, lymphoma, melanoma,* and *sarcoma*. Although cancer is not contagious, there is some evidence to suggest that sexual transmission of the *herpes* virus (type II) may be implicated as a predisposing factor in the development of cancer of the *cervix*.

Cancer may affect almost any part of the body, although the most commonly involved sites are the large intestine (colon and rectum), lungs, reproductive system (uterus and cervix in women, *prostate gland* in men), breasts, bladder, bone marrow, skin, and the brain and spinal cord.

There is no one known cause of cancer. Statistical evidence is overwhelming that smoking can cause lung cancer (it has been demonstrated directly in laboratory animals); inhalation of coal and asbestos dust has also been implicated.

Among the predisposing factors

cancer

in some forms of cancer are exposure to radiation (including x-rays and the sun's ultraviolet light), viruses, and prolonged exposure to various chemicals or physical agents.

The major signs and symptoms of cancer are not specific. However, it is essential to seek immediate medical attention if one or more of the following signs or symptoms appear: unusual bleeding or discharge from any site, including the vagina; a change in the shape, size, or appearance of a wart or mole; unexplained weight loss; difficulty in swallowing (dysphagia); persistent coughing or hoarseness; any sore that refuses to heal, including those in the mouth or throat; any change in regular bowel or bladder habits; and the development of a lump or thickening of tissue in any area, particularly the breast. Pain is not a reliable sign.

If cancer is suspected, a biopsy may be performed. This is the removal of a small piece of tissue, which is examined carefully under a microscope. A biopsy is the only sure method of correctly diagnosing cancer.

Once the diagnosis of cancer has been confirmed, the patient will be carefully examined to make sure that the disease has not spread to other parts of the body and to ensure that appropriate treatment may be given. Early detection and early treatment are major factors in preventing metastasis and secondary growths elsewhere in the body.

The two main factors that determine the general treatment of cancer in most patients are the stage of the disease and the patient's age. Patients whose diagnosis indicates that the cancer has remained in one place and has not spread will be candidates for surgery: the removal of the tumor and whatever surrounding tissues may be affected.

Radiation therapy (treatment with x-rays) has been used as an important method of treatment both alone and before and after surgery. Radiotherapy before surgery tends to prevent the spread of cancer cells that may be freed during the operation, thus minimizing the possibility that they will spread to other parts of the body and cause secondary cancers. Radiation therapy has been used extensively following *mastectomies*.

Sometimes radioactive elements such as radium are surgically implanted in the cancerous tissue.

Hormone treatment is normally reserved for patients in advanced stages of breast cancer when it is not usual to perform surgery. Many advanced cancers, especially of the sex organs, respond to changes in hormone levels in the body.

Certain medications are also used to treat cancer. Drugs designed to attack and destroy cancer cells are called cytotoxic drugs and the technique of using them is called *chemotherapy*.

Regular medical checkups can often reveal cancer at an early stage, when successful treatment is much more likely. Women over the age of thirty should have a *cervical smear* (Pap test) at regular intervals to detect possible early signs of cervical and uterine cancer.

Cancer is the second leading cause of death (after heart disease) in the United States, where it claims approximately 390,000 victims each year. It is estimated that more than 115,000 of these deaths could have been prevented by early diagnosis and treatment.

SEE ALSO *asbestosis, breast cancer, in situ, lumpectomy*

candidiasis A common and usually mild infection caused by a specific type of yeastlike fungus, *Candida albicans;* formerly known as moniliasis. When the membrane that lines the mouth is affected, the condition is called *thrush.* When the vagina is infected, the microorganisms cause inflammation of the vaginal walls *(vaginitis).* A creamy white discharge may be produced and intense itching experienced; white patches may be seen on the labia, the fleshy folds at the entrance to the vagina.

Candidiasis may occur as a result of a lowering of body resistance during the course of another disease, or it may represent a *superinfection* following the destruction of normal protective bacteria in the digestive tract by antibiotics. Debilitation or prolonged antibiotic therapy may permit the fungus to grow and multiply at an abnormal rate. When this occurs the signs and symptoms of candidiasis are seen.

Treatment involves the administration of an antifungal drug, such as nystatin (Mycolog), miconazole (Monistat), or clotrimazole (Lotrimin).

capillary Any one of the smallest blood vessels, forming the connecting links between the *arteries* and *veins.* Capillaries are visible only under a microscope. Their walls are formed of a single layer of thin flattened cells (endothelial cells) of the same type that line all body cavities.

Capillaries form a dense network throughout all body tissues but are thickest in those tissues, such as active muscles, that require the greatest amount of blood. In the capillary "bed," oxygen and essential nutrients pass through the single-celled capillary walls to the tissues. Waste material such as carbon dioxide diffuses back through the capillary walls to be transported by veins to the heart and then, via the pulmonary arteries, to the lungs for elimination from the body during breathing.

carbohydrate One of the three general classes of nutrients (along with *protein* and *fat)* essential for health. Carbohydrates are composed only of carbon, hydrogen, and oxygen, and include *glucose* and other sugars, *glycogen,* dextrins, and starches (cellulose is also a carbohydrate but it provides no nutrient value in humans). The breakdown of carbohydrates provides most of the body's heat and energy.

The excessive intake of carbohydrates in the diet can lead to obesity and tooth cavities (dental caries). Those with *diabetes mellitus* must be especially cautious in controlling carbohydrate intake.

carbon dioxide A colorless, odorless, and incombustible gas, CO_2, produced in the body tissues as a waste product of *metabolism* and transported in the venous blood to the lungs to be expelled during breathing.

carbon monoxide A colorless, odorless, and poisonous gas, CO, produced by the incomplete combustion of carbon or materials that contain carbon. It is present in the exhaust fumes of cars and other motor vehicles, in coal gas, and in the fumes of fires stoked with coal, wood, coke, and kerosene space heaters. Proper ventilation is essential to prevent carbon monoxide poisoning, which may result in severe brain damage and death.

carcinogen Any substance or agent that can cause *cancer* or is strongly implicated in causing cancer.

carcinoma Any *malignant* (cancerous) growth or tumor originating in cells of the *epithelium*, the tissue that lines and covers all body cavities and surfaces. Carcinomas tend to spread *(metastasize)* to surrounding healthy tissues and may lead to *cancer* in other parts of the body if carried in the blood or lymphatic vessels.
COMPARE *sarcoma*

cardiac Relating to the *heart*.

cardiac arrest A sudden stopping of the heartbeat or a spontaneous and uncoordinated twitching of the heart's largest chambers *(ventricular fibrillation)* resulting in a dramatic interruption of blood flow through the heart. The signs of this condition are loss of consciousness and the absence of pulse. It is a medical emergency requiring immediate attention.
SEE ALSO *cardiopulmonary resuscitation, myocardial infarction*

cardiac catheterization A diagnostic technique or procedure in which a *catheter* is inserted into a vein, usually in the arm, leg, or neck, and slowly passed through the blood vessels until it reaches one of the hollow chambers of the heart. The procedure is performed with the help of a fluoroscope.

Once the tip of the catheter is in the appropriate position it is possible to obtain a sample of blood from within any area of the heart, measure the blood pressure within each chamber, and help determine the presence of any physical deformities or defects in the heart valves.
SEE ALSO *catheterization*

cardiology The branch of medical science concerned with the diagnosis and treatment of diseases of the heart and associated blood vessels. Physicians who practice this specialty are known as cardiologists.

cardiomyopathy Any of various diseases and disorders that directly affect the heart muscle *(myocardium)*, especially one in which the cause is obscure or difficult to diagnose. Used alone, it is a general or tentative diagnostic term without specific significance.

cardiopulmonary resuscitation (CPR) A potentially lifesaving technique or procedure for reviving a person whose heartbeat and breathing have suddenly stopped *(cardiac arrest)*. It basically involves both mouth-to-mouth artificial respiration and compression of the heart muscle through the chest wall by exerting rhythmic pressure on the breastbone (sternum).

The correct technique cannot be learned from books; it requires personal instruction from an expert. Hundreds of special CPR courses are conducted regularly throughout the United States.

CPR must never be performed on a victim who is unconscious (in a faint or coma) but whose heart is still beating. If the heart has stopped, no pulse will be felt at the victim's wrist. Without a thorough knowledge of CPR technique, potentially serious damage can be done to the victim, including fractured ribs, punctured lungs, and injury to the heart itself.

SEE ALSO *Heimlich maneuver*

cardiovascular Relating to the heart and blood vessels.

carotid artery The large artery on each side of the neck (left and right common carotid arteries) formed from branches of the body's largest artery, the *aorta*.

carrier Any person who harbors potentially harmful microorganisms or defective genes without displaying any signs or symptoms. Such people are said to carry the causative agent of such diseases as hemophilia and typhoid fever and can unknowingly pass it to others.

cartilage The white elastic substance attached to the surfaces of the bones of a joint. Cartilage is a dense connective tissue that in the fetus forms the major part of the developing skeleton; most but not all of it becomes bone. In adults it forms the separation between the nostrils (nasal septum), the outer parts of the ears, and the disklike pads (intervertebral disks) between the vertebrae.

cataract The partial or total clouding of the lens of the eye resulting in various degrees of defective eyesight. In severe cases a cataract can lead to total blindness. The lens normally loses some of its transparency as a person grows older and it is not surprising that the most common cause of cataracts is old age. Other possible causes include inherited or congenital defects in the lens, infection, injury, radiation, or diseases such as *diabetes mellitus*.

The first symptom of a cataract is usually a gradual and painless dimming of vision. The nature of the visual defect depends on the site of the opacity (clouding) and the area of the lens affected. In older persons both eyes are usually involved, although the first disturbance in vision may be experienced in one eye. Vision may remain slightly impaired for several years before any serious change is noted or the lens may become almost totally opaque within a relatively short time. Ophthalmologists have classified nearly one hundred types of cataracts according to their size, shape, involvement, and cause.

Treatment of cataracts depends largely on the extent of defective eyesight and whether or not both eyes are affected. The use of glasses, with periodic changing of the prescription, will help maintain useful vision for several years in most uncomplicated cases. When vision is seriously impaired it may be necessary to remove the defective lens surgically; this operation has proven most successful. Contact lenses or eyeglasses can then be worn to restore vision. Research continues on the long-term effectiveness of the surgical implantation of artificial lenses.

catheter A tubular instrument passed into and along a body channel such as a blood vessel or the urethra to remove or introduce fluids. Catheters are available in a variety of lengths and diameters depending on their intended use and may be made of metal, rubber, plastic, or other materials.
SEE *catheterization*

catheterization The technique or procedure of passing a *catheter* into a body cavity or channel. Frequently, catheterization involves the bladder; a catheter is passed through the urethra to the bladder to obtain a urine sample or allow elimination of urine.
SEE ALSO *cardiac catheterization*

CAT scan
SEE *computerized axial tomography*

celiac disease A relatively uncommon condition characterized by an intolerance of the digestive system to gluten, a component of wheat and other grains. It can affect both children and adults. Hereditary factors have been implicated as a possible underlying cause of celiac disease (also known as nontropical *sprue*). There is a strong tendency for the disorder to run in families, and the age at onset can be as young as six months.

Untreated celiac disease during childhood is typically marked by swelling of the abdomen, pale fatty stools, atrophy (wasting) of muscles, loss of appetite, severe diarrhea, lack of growth, and general listlessness. It is rare in developed countries for the disease to progress to this stage because of early diagnosis and treatment. The treatment is simple: elimination of gluten from the diet. The results are often dramatic.

cellulitis Any spreading inflammation of cellular or connective tissues. The term is usually used to refer to an inflammation of the tissues immediately below the skin, but it can also refer to an inflammation of deeper structures, such as the connective tissues surrounding the uterus (pelvic cellulitis). Cellulitis is usually caused by an infection, although it may also follow an injury to the affected area or be associated with some failure of the immune system.

The signs and symptoms of cellulitis include fever, chills, headache, and a general feeling of being unwell (malaise). The affected area is typically red, swollen, warm, and painful. In addition to the use of antibiotics, the involved part should be rested and, if possible, elevated above the head. Bed rest and the local application of heat or wet dressings may be helpful, although it is important not to permit the area to remain moist (macerated).

central nervous system (CNS) The *brain* and *spinal cord*.

cerebellum The second largest anatomical division of the *brain*, situated toward the back of the *cerebrum* under the *occipital lobes*. It consists of two equal halves, the cerebellar hemispheres, joined in the middle by a connecting lobe (vermis). The main function of the cerebellum is the coordination of muscular movements; severe damage to this part of the brain can result in jerky, inaccurate movements, although the basic ability to move is not affected (that is, there is no paralysis or other loss of muscular function).

A part of each cerebellar hemisphere has nerve connections with the inner ear and plays an important role in maintaining balance.

cerebral cortex The surface of the *cerebrum*, consisting of gray matter formed mainly by closely packed nerve cells that provide the characteristic color. The cortex is very thin (about 1/8 inch/3 mm) compared to the cerebrum's underlying parts, which appear much lighter in color as the result of millions of insulated nerve cells. The nerve cells in the cortex are arranged in six distinct layers or zones, each containing cells predominantly of one type and density.

Various areas of the cerebral cortex are specialized for specific sensory or motor functions. The strip of cortex just in front of the large central fissure, forming the boundary of the frontal and parietal lobes, is known as the motor area; it is here that voluntary movements are controlled. Directly opposite the motor area on the other side of the central fissure is the sensory area. Despite the term, the sensory area receives only sensations of touch; it is also known as the somatic sensory area.

cerebral hemorrhage The escape of blood from a ruptured blood vessel into brain tissues, often as a consequence of prolonged high blood pressure or *arteriosclerosis*. The severity of the condition depends largely on the site and extent of the damage. Immediate signs include low pulse, paralysis of the side of the body opposite that of the ruptured vessel, unconsciousness, and uncontrollable movements of the eyes and tongue. Death may follow.
SEE ALSO *stroke*

cerebral palsy A condition usually caused by damage to the *brain* before or at birth, characterized by various degrees of muscular weakness, spasm, lack of coordination, and speech difficulties. About 70 percent of children affected appear to be mentally retarded, although in many cases this is due to their physical handicap, which makes them react more slowly than normal.
SEE *spastic*

cerebrospinal fluid The clear fluid produced in the hollow cavities (lateral ventricles) of each half of the brain that bathes the surface of the brain and spinal cord. It constantly circulates around the outer surfaces of the brain and spinal cord, where it acts as a protective cushion of water. While older fluid is absorbed back into the blood, new fluid is slowly secreted from the choroid plexus, an area deep within the brain. Under normal circumstances, a perfect balance of output and return of this fluid is maintained.

The cerebrospinal fluid normally contains slight traces of proteins, glucose (sugar), and some cells. If any part of the brain or spinal cord or their protective membranes becomes infected, the fluid may show evidence of the disease by containing an increased quantity of cells and proteins.

Other disorders may be first detected or confirmed by the presence of small amounts of blood or pus in the fluid. The normal amount of glucose in the fluid may be reduced in some forms of *meningitis* (inflammation of the membranes that surround the brain and spinal cord) or raised in diabetes.
SEE ALSO *hydrocephalus*, *lumbar puncture*

cerebrum The largest part of the human *brain*, consisting of two halves, the right and left cerebral hemispheres, divided by a deep central cleft and joined at the bottom by a wide band of fibers (corpus callosum). The surface of the cerebrum, the *cerebral cortex*, is compressed into numerous folds called convolutions or gyri; deep fissures form anatomical boundaries between the gyri and divide the cerebrum into four major lobes

in each cerebral hemisphere: frontal, parietal, temporal, and occipital. A fifth lobe, called the island of Reil or the insula, sits beneath the surface of each cerebral hemisphere. Each cerebral hemisphere controls the actions and sensations of the opposite side of the body; for example, when a right-handed person writes, the hand receives instructions from the left side of the cerebral cortex, and vice versa.
SEE *hypothalamus, thalamus*

cervical smear Also called *Pap test*, a routine test for *cancer* of the *cervix* (neck of the uterus), a common form of cancer in women. Cervical cancer is one of the easiest types of cancer to detect and treat in its early stages.

The cervical smear is a simple technique in which a few cells are scraped from the cervix. When these are spread on a slide and examined under a microscope, it is possible for medical experts to recognize the possible development of cancer at a time when it can be easily treated and eradicated. The procedure is performed quickly and painlessly.

Although the possible causes of cervical cancer are not clearly understood, evidence points toward an increased incidence of this disease in women who have not had children and those who regularly have sexual intercourse with several partners.

The danger of undetected cervical cancer is that it may spread to other parts of the body faster than standard treatment can be effective. Regular cervical smears should therefore be standard policy for all women over the age of thirty.

cervix The neck of the *uterus*. It is a shiny and smooth dome-shaped structure, forming the narrowest part of the uterus and extending downward into the back part of the vagina. The cervix can be felt as a rubbery bump at the upper part of the vagina.

In the center of the cervix is a dimple-shaped opening; in women who have given birth, the opening may be slightly enlarged. It is through this opening, normally closed by a plug of mucus, that sperm cells enter the uterus on their way to the ovum in the *Fallopian tube*.

During childbirth the cervix, which has gradually become softer and larger during pregnancy, easily expands to permit passage of the baby. The normally small opening of the cervix can also be gently expanded by a physician to permit examination of the interior of the uterus.

Cesarean section The removal of a fetus from the uterus by means of a surgical incision through the abdominal wall and into the uterus. Several valid medical reasons exist for choosing this method over vaginal delivery. These include an abnormally narrow pelvic opening

51

chancre

or a disproportionately large baby (head and shoulders) in relation to the mother's pelvic bones, severe forms of *placenta previa*, severe forms of *abruptio placentae*, certain cases of *preeclampsia*, and all other cases when the life of the mother or baby is at risk if vaginal delivery is permitted.

The cesarean section is one of the oldest known surgical operations, its origin lost in antiquity and ancient mythology (Julius Caesar was allegedly born this way, hence the name). It was not until the middle part of the twentieth century that the procedure became relatively safe for the mother; this is largely the result of improved surgical techniques and the advent of antibiotics to prevent or control any associated infections.

Controversy exists over the accusation that cesarean sections are often performed when no clear danger exists to the mother or child. Some critics have even suggested that the operation may occasionally be performed for its economic benefit to the obstetrician rather than the health or well-being of the mother. Proper medical judgment should not permit this potentially dangerous procedure to be used for trivial reasons or when there is only marginal evidence prior to labor that some obstetrical abnormality may interfere with vaginal delivery. Moreover, there is no valid medical reason in the absence of a clear need to repeat a cesarean section in future pregnancies.

chancre A hard open sore that often occurs at the primary site of infection with *syphilis*.

chancroid A soft open sore caused by bacterial infection. It is highly *infectious*, usually occurs in the area of the genitals, and is not related to infection with syphilis.
COMPARE *chancre*

chemotherapy The use of drugs or chemical agents to treat disease. The term is often limited to the use of various potent drugs (*cytotoxic* agents) intended to destroy cancer cells.

chickenpox A common and usually mild infectious childhood disease caused by a virus. Known medically as varicella, chickenpox is spread by close contact with an infected person or by airborne droplets. The incubation period is about fourteen days, after which separate spots begin to appear all over the body, concentrated mostly on the trunk and upper thighs. Some can occasionally be seen inside the cheeks, on the roof of the mouth, or on the scalp.

The spots appear in crops and begin as small pink marks. These turn into tiny blisters within a few hours and look like drops of water resting on the skin, varying in size from a pinhead to a split pea. The blisters then cloud over and crust up, and about ten to twenty days after the spots appear the crusty scabs fall away, leaving pink marks that eventually disappear. At any one time during the course of the illness the patient will have crops of spots in all stages of development.

Rarely will the child feel ill enough to remain in bed more than four or five days. Just before the spots appear the child may have a slight fever that usually lasts a short time. The main discomfort comes from itching, which can be partially relieved by calamine lotion or some other substance prescribed by a physician. The child should not scratch or pick at the scabs; the hands should be kept clean and the nails clipped to reduce the chance of bacterial infection.

When the rash first appears, a physician should be consulted to confirm the diagnosis. He or she will probably recommend that the child be kept isolated about a week or two to prevent the child from infecting others.

Although it is possible to catch the disease at any age, chickenpox is fairly common in children between the ages of five and ten. One attack generally provides *immunity* for life. The chickenpox virus is thought to be identical with the one that causes *herpes zoster* (shingles) in adults.

chiropractic A system of health care based on the belief that disease is caused by an abnormal function of the nervous system, which can be restored by spinal manipulation.
COMPARE *naturopathy*

cholangiography An x-ray technique for examining the *bile* ducts, which move bile from the *gallbladder* to the first part of the small intestine. It is most commonly performed by first injecting a contrast or *radiopaque* fluid into a vein; the fluid eventually enters the bile ducts and permits them to be clearly outlined on x-ray film.

cholecystectomy Surgical removal of the *gallbladder*. The operation is usually performed to relieve the painful symptoms of gallbladder inflammation associated with the presence of gallstones.
SEE *cholecystitis, cholelithiasis*

cholecystitis Acute or chronic inflammation of the *gallbladder*. The symptoms of an acute attack, which is most often associated with the presence of gallstones, include sudden pain in the upper part of the abdomen, nausea, vomiting, and fever. Some patients may also experience pain in the back or the right shoulder.

Chronic cholecystitis may occur with or without gallstones and the symptoms are less severe than those of an acute attack. Not all cases of inflamed gallbladder are associated with gallstones.

Treatment depends largely on the severity of the condition. The acute

cholelithiasis

form of the disorder may require surgical removal of the gallbladder (cholecystectomy), as may the chronic form if gallstones are present.

SEE ALSO *cholelithiasis*

cholelithiasis The presence or formation of stones *(calculi)* in the *gallbladder* called gallstones.

Gallstones may cause no problems, or they may be associated with painful attacks when the gallbladder becomes inflamed *(cholecystitis)*. The diagnosis can be made based on typical symptoms in acute attacks and may also involve x-rays of the gallbladder and bile ducts. The presence of bile in the blood may help establish the diagnosis.

If symptoms are severe, especially in the presence of a blockage of the bile ducts, the gallbladder may have to be surgically removed *(cholecystectomy)*.

SEE ALSO *bilirubinemia, cholangiography*

cholera An acute infectious bacterial disease caused by curved microorganisms known as *Vibrio cholerae* or *Vibrio comma* (their shape resembles a comma). Spread of the disease occurs if the infected feces contaminate water or food. It is thus a disease more common in areas of the world with inadequate hygiene and sanitation, particularly sewage disposal. Sudden outbreaks of cholera occur regularly in parts of Asia and occasional epidemics precede the rainy season in India and Pakistan. The incubation period varies from about one to six days.

The onset of the disease is abrupt, characterized by vomiting, abdominal pain, and profuse colorless and watery diarrhea. The extensive loss of body fluids in the watery stools can lead to serious *dehydration* associated with intense thirst, muscular cramps, and general weakness. The eyes may appear deeply sunken and the skin abnormally wrinkled and inelastic. In a few patients, however, the disease runs its course within a few days without complications; in such cases the patient recovers completely without medical treatment.

The diagnosis of cholera involves obtaining samples of fresh stools from which bacterial cultures are grown; the cultures are then tested to identify the causative microorganisms. Treatment is primarily aimed at replacing the lost fluids and essential electrolytes (salts). Death occurs in more than 50 percent of untreated patients. Tetracycline has been useful in dramatically limiting the duration and volume of diarrhea. Preventive measures include the purification of public water supplies and improved sewage disposal.

cholesterol A fatlike substance (sterol) found in animal fats and oils, nerve tissue, bile, blood, and egg yolks. It can also be synthesized (manufactured) in the liver and is a normal constituent of bile. An excessive amount in the circulating blood has been implicated as a contributing factor in hardening of the arteries *(arteriosclerosis* and *atherosclerosis)* and *coronary artery disease.*

The formation of some gallstones *(cholelithiasis)* can be associated with an excessive amount of cholesterol in the bile.

chorea A nervous condition characterized by involuntary muscular twitching of the limbs or facial muscles. Two basic forms exist: Sydenham's chorea (St. Vitus's dance), which is not hereditary and is usually seen as a complication of some bacterial infection, most commonly rheumatic fever; and *Huntington's chorea,* a rare hereditary disease not usually noticed until early adult life or middle age.

Sydenham's chorea is a temporary condition usually affecting children between the ages of about five and fifteen; it responds to medical treatment, rarely lasts more than a few months at most, and has no effect on the mind (unlike Huntington's chorea).

chromosome A microscopic elongated body present in all living cells, containing *genes,* the particles responsible for determining hereditary characteristics. The normal number of chromosomes in each human cell is forty-six, arranged in twenty-three pairs. The exceptions are the sex cells *(spermatozoa* and *ova),* each of which contains half this number: twenty-two (eleven pairs) plus one sex chromosome *(X chromosome* or *Y chromosome).*

chronic Relating to a disease or disorder that persists for a long time or tends to recur repeatedly.
COMPARE *acute*

circulatory system The system that supplies blood to all organs and tissues of the body, consisting of the *heart* and blood vessels (arteries, arterioles, capillaries, venules, and veins); the *cardiovascular* system.

circumcision Surgical removal of the foreskin (prepuce) of the penis, typically performed for religious or hygienic reasons. Circumcision does not affect sensitivity during sexual intercourse. Some physicians believe that routine circumcision is unnecessary and that apart from religious considerations, the operation should be performed only in cases of *phimosis.*

Some researchers believe that cancer of the penis (an extremely rare disease) is less frequent in males who were circumcised at birth. Evidence also exists that wives of circumcised men have a reduced incidence of uterine and cervical cancer. However, the reason has not been proven.

cirrhosis A disease of the *liver* characterized by degenerative changes, including the gradual formation of dense fibrous tissues that interrupt the organ's normal functioning. The liver tissue typically undergoes fatty changes and becomes fibrous and scarred, often with the formation of hundreds of firm nodules.

The most common cause of cirrhosis is chronic *alcoholism* or prolonged heavy drinking combined with malnutrition. During its early stages, the patient may appear relatively healthy and experience no symptoms. As the liver's functions are progressively impaired, symptoms can include abdominal discomfort, nausea, vomiting, weight loss, general weakness, and loss of sexual drive. If the blood flow through the liver becomes obstructed, portal hypertension (an abnormal increase in blood pressure within the liver) can result.

In advanced cases of cirrhosis, the formation in the liver of substances affecting the clotting of blood is reduced, and this may result in a tendency to bleed. Other complications of cirrhosis include liver failure, *jaundice*, and hepatic (liver-induced) coma. The massive loss of liver cells in advanced cirrhosis interferes with the liver's detoxifying function, thus allowing harmful chemicals to accumulate and pass into the bloodstream, leading to impairment of the central nervous system. Hepatic coma or death may follow.

Treatment of cirrhosis basically involves rest, total abstinence from alcohol, and a well-balanced diet. Hospitalization may be required in severe cases.

clitoris The most responsive of the external female genital organs. Composed of erectile tissue and located at the front of the *vulva*, it enlarges slightly when a woman is sexually aroused. Its only function is to intensify sexual excitement, which may lead to *orgasm*.

clotting The ability of the blood to form a jellylike substance called a blood clot, especially at the site of a wound or injury to a blood vessel.
SEE *embolism, fibrin, hemophilia, platelets, thrombosis*

clubfoot A deformity of the foot, known medically as talipes, that occurs in several varieties named according to the direction or severity of the twist. The condition is usually present at birth (congenital clubfoot) but may be associated with an infection or injury.

Early treatment with splints and bandages is often successful, but in severe cases and those not treated during infancy the only means of correction is surgery. In some cases, special footwear may be required to give support to the ankle and make walking more comfortable.

codeine A *narcotic* drug often prescribed alone or in combination with other pharmaceuticals to suppress coughs and relieve pain. Prolonged use can lead to *addiction*.

colic Severe pain caused by involuntary spasm or obstruction of a tube or duct. Biliary colic is caused by a gallstone in the bile duct, renal colic is caused by a stone in the ureter (the tube that carries urine from the kidney to the bladder), and intestinal colic may be caused by obstruction of the intestines or be associated with food poisoning.

Colic also describes a condition often seen in babies and characterized by crying and irritability. It may be caused by an intestinal allergy, overfeeding, swallowing of air, or emotional factors.

colitis Inflammation of the colon (large intestine).
SEE *ulcerative colitis*

collagen A fibrous insoluble protein found in connective tissue such as ligaments and cartilage, representing approximately 30 percent of the total body protein.
SEE *collagen diseases*

collagen diseases Any of various diseases, such as *lupus erythematosus*, whose only common feature is that they involve the body's connective tissue (collagen). Collagen diseases are characterized by a general inflammation of connective tissue and blood vessels and share basic anatomical and pathological features.

colostomy The surgical formation of an opening from the large intestine (colon) through the abdominal wall, creating an artificial passage for solid waste to the outside of the body. It may be temporary (as part of the treatment of an intestinal obstruction) or permanent (as in the removal of a cancerous section of bowel). Permanent colostomies require the surgical fitting to the opening of a colostomy bag, for the collection and disposal of waste.

Although the condition requires initial training in the care and hygiene of the colostomy opening and some changes in diet, most patients lead normal lives.
SEE *ileostomy*

coma Unconsciousness from which a person cannot be aroused. Over half of the cases are the result of disease or injury involving the brain or its blood vessels. Coma is sometimes seen in patients with *diabetes mellitus* (diabetic coma or hypoglycemic coma).
COMPARE *brain death*

communicable Relating to any disease that is transmitted directly or indirectly from one person to another or to humans from animals.
SEE ALSO *contagious, infectious*

complete blood count (CBC)
SEE *blood test*

computerized axial tomography (CAT) A computer-aided x-ray system (known as a CAT scanner) that provides highly detailed and accurate pictures of the brain, lungs, pancreas, kidneys, and other

concussion

organs and tissues where traditional x-ray examination has been difficult or inconclusive.

A CAT scan involves a series of hundreds of thin beams of x-rays that pass at a slightly different angle through the appropriate area of the body. The rays are focused at a predetermined level and provide a complete picture of a cross section of the patient's body (or a specific organ). Each section is about 1 cm thick and can be scanned in only twenty seconds. A minicomputer in the scanner analyzes the x-rays and processes the high-definition pictures within a few minutes.

A CAT scan is quick, effective, and safe. The patient is exposed to no more radiation than from a single conventional chest x-ray. Soft tissues of the body are easily visible along with bone without the inconvenience and potential dangers of injecting or swallowing an x-ray contrast *(radiopaque)* medium. The avoidance of such invasive techniques is one of the most important diagnostic features of the CAT scanner, although in some cases, an x-ray contrast medium may be used during a CAT scan to enhance visualization.

concussion A violent jarring of the brain (cerebral concussion) caused by a blow to the head or a fall and marked by temporary or prolonged unconsciousness. Return of consciousness is usually gradual. Signs and symptoms following a concussion include vomiting, short-term amnesia, severe headaches, dizziness, and unusual behavior. Some symptoms may persist for weeks after the injury. Prompt medical attention is essential in the case of any head injury.

congenital Relating to any condition that is present at birth, either because of hereditary factors or prenatal events.

conjunctivitis Inflammation of the conjunctiva, the membrane that lines the eyelid and covers the white of the eye; popularly known as pink eye. It can be caused by specks of dirt or other foreign bodies in the eye or under the eyelid or, more commonly, by bacterial or viral infection. Some infectious forms of conjunctivitis are highly contagious and seem to appear in epidemics.

The first sign of conjunctivitis is usually a burning or smarting of the eyelids, accompanied by intense itching. The white of the eye becomes bright red or pink and the eye waters excessively. The watery discharge may change to a sticky secretion containing pus, which causes the eyelashes and eyelids to stick together. The lids often become swollen. In severe forms, both eyes are involved.

Mild forms of conjunctivitis usually clear up within a few days; more severe or persistent cases require medical attention, such as antibiotic eyedrops or ointments.

contagious Relating to any disease that is transmitted directly by contact with an infected person, by touching contaminated secretions, or by handling contaminated objects.
SEE ALSO *communicable, infectious*

contraception Any process, device, or method that prevents the fertilization of an ovum by sperm cells; also called birth control and family planning. With the exception of the condom or prophylactic sheath, withdrawal, and *vasectomy* contraceptive methods currently available place responsibility with the woman. She must therefore decide, with the help of her physician, which method is best for her. The most reliable methods, the *oral contraceptive* and *intrauterine device*, are the most common and are easy to use, but they do pose some risks. Neither method requires preparation before sexual intercourse.

The diaphragm or cap, a rubber cup with a metal spring around the edge, is a popular method that was extensively used before the development of oral contraceptives; it works by covering the cervix, thus preventing sperm from entering the uterus. The diaphragm is smeared with spermicidal jelly before it is inserted, which can be up to two hours before intercourse; it must be kept in place for at least six hours afterward. It is initially fitted by a nurse or physician, who makes sure that the diaphragm is the correct size. A new diaphragm must be fitted after the birth of each child or following a large weight loss or gain. When used in conjunction with a spermicide, it is about 95 percent effective.

Chemical contraceptives available as creams, jellies, foams, and vaginal tablets are only moderately effective when used alone. They must be inserted not more than half an hour before intercourse.

contraindication Any condition or factor that makes the use of a specific drug or other form of therapy potentially dangerous to the extent that proper medical practice forbids it. Many prescription drugs are contraindicated for use in patients with severe diseases of the liver or kidneys; other drugs are contraindicated for children under the age of twelve.
COMPARE *indication*

Cooley's anemia
SEE *anemia, thalassemia*

convulsion A strong involuntary muscular contraction. The muscles may remain rigidly contracted for some time (tonic convulsion) or they may alternately contract and relax in rapid succession (clonic convulsion). Convulsions generally affect major muscle groups resulting in rapid and uncontrollable movements of the body or limbs. In adults the cause is usually *epilepsy*, but convulsions in young children are most often the result of a high fever or infection. In many cases the child loses consciousness for a short time, during which the spasms continue.

In children under five, the nervous system is not yet fully developed. During a fever or other infectious illness, the nerve centers that control bodily movements may become disturbed, causing a rapid twitching of an arm, leg, or other part. A physician should be consulted immediately, even if the convulsions stop after a short time (as they generally do). He or she will determine the exact cause and eliminate the possibility of serious illness, such as *meningitis* or, in newborn babies, some form of brain damage.

cornea The transparent outer covering of the eyeball that bends incoming light into a narrow cone and directs it to the *lens*. The cornea contains no blood vessels but is extremely sensitive because of its rich supply of nerves, which are responsible for triggering the protective reflex action of blinking.

If the cornea is injured, its delicate tissues become susceptible to infection from bacteria and other microorganisms. Unless injuries and infections receive prompt medical treatment, serious damage may occur to the cornea and the underlying structures of the *eye*. An untreated corneal infection can cause localized destruction of the surface tissues, or corneal ulcer.

The first signs of a corneal ulcer are usually intense pain, watering of the eye, and sensitivity to light. The affected area can often be seen as a dull grayish spot or speck. The ulcer may penetrate deeply into the cornea or spread to involve the greater part of its surface. A deep ulcer may result in the formation of pus in the aqueous humor, the watery chamber between the cornea and the *iris*. When such ulcers heal they sometimes leave scars that affect vision.

A corneal ulcer demands prompt medical attention to avoid partial or total loss of sight. A physician will prescribe an appropriate antibiotic in the form of eyedrops or ointments; an oral antibiotic or a *corticosteroid* may also be prescribed.

In some cases it is necessary to perform a corneal graft, a surgical procedure in which a damaged cornea is replaced by a healthy one removed from the eye of a deceased donor within six hours after death.

coronary Relating to the arteries that supply blood to the heart. The word is often short for *coronary occlusion* or *coronary thrombosis* (heart attack).

coronary artery disease Any disease of the coronary arteries, the vessels that supply blood to the *heart*. There are two main coronary arteries, one on each side of the heart, that gradually branch out into smaller blood vessels. These arteries may become abnormally narrowed by deposits of fatty material on their inner walls *(atherosclerosis)* or become hardened and inelastic with advancing years. When this occurs they may be unable to supply the heart muscle with an adequate supply of blood during moments of stress or exertion. This insufficient blood supply (coronary insufficiency) results in the typical pain of *angina pectoris*.

During a heart attack *(coronary occlusion, coronary thrombosis, myocardial infarction)*, the coronary arteries are suddenly blocked. This usually causes intense pain in the chest (described as a constricting, crushing, or squeezing sensation behind the sternum that is not relieved by resting. The victim often turns pale and begins to sweat.

In most cases the victim of a heart attack is able to resume mild activity after a sufficient period of bed rest, perhaps as little as three weeks. During this time the heart muscle is given a chance to repair any damage, although full healing may take several months.

coronary bypass A major surgical procedure used to provide an adequate supply of blood to the heart when the coronary arteries are blocked with fatty deposits *(atheromas)*. The blocked coronary artery is bypassed with a section of vein taken from the patient's leg and grafted into position. More than one such graft may have to be made.

It is estimated that in 1980 more than 110,000 patients underwent coronary bypass surgery. Such open-heart operations are not without potentially serious complications, including death in approximately 2 to 5 percent of cases.
SEE ALSO *bypass, coronary artery disease*

coronary occlusion The complete blockage of one of the coronary arteries usually as a result of severe and progressive *atherosclerosis*. Popularly referred to as heart attack, it is a leading cause of death.
SEE ALSO *coronary artery disease, coronary thrombosis, myocardial infarction*

coronary thrombosis The complete blockage of one of the coronary arteries by a blood clot *(thrombus)*. This form of *coronary occlusion*, popularly called heart attack, is a leading cause of death.
SEE ALSO *coronary artery disease, myocardial infarction, thrombosis*

cortex The outer layer of an organ, as distinguished from its inner portion *(medulla)*.
SEE *adrenal cortex, cerebral cortex*

corticosteroid Any of various *hormones* produced by the cortex (outer part) of the *adrenal gland* or prepared synthetically. They are classified according to their basic biological activity: glucocorticoids mainly influence the metabolism of carbohydrate, fat, and protein; mineral corticoids play an important role in regulating the body's mineral, salt, and water balance.

Corticosteroid drugs are used

61

cortisol

therapeutically in hormone-replacement therapy (when natural hormones are deficient), in the treatment of various inflammatory diseases (including rheumatoid arthritis), and as part of the treatment of certain severe allergies.

Corticosteroids belong to a larger family of substances known as steroids. Corticosteroids are also known as adrenocortical hormones or corticoids.

cortisol A *corticosteroid* hormone secreted by the *adrenal glands;* its synthetic form is called *hydrocortisone.* Cortisol plays an important role in the metabolism of fats, carbohydrates, sodium, potassium, and proteins and promotes the conversion of proteins to carbohydrates (which are stored in the liver as glycogen).

CPR
SEE *cardiopulmonary resuscitation*

cranium The part of the *skull* that encloses the *brain;* loosely, the entire skull, including the bones of the mandible (lower jaw).

cretinism A congenital disorder characterized by dwarfism, retarded mental development, rough dry skin, coarse brittle hair, a large protruding tongue, abdominal distension, and irregular spacing of the teeth. It is caused by a deficiency of hormone secretions from the *thyroid gland.* If recognized and treated early with therapeutic doses of thyroid hormone, the condition may improve slightly or be arrested.
SEE ALSO *hypothyroidism*

Crohn's disease An inflammatory disease of the intestinal tract named after the American gastroenterologist Burrill B. Crohn (born 1884). It is also known as regional *ileitis* and regional *enteritis.*

crib death
See sudden infant death syndrome (SIDS)

cryosurgery A technique or procedure in which tissues are exposed to extreme cold, usually below 0°F (−20°C) to destroy tumors, control pain and bleeding, and treat some forms of intracranial (within the brain) and cutaneous (skin) lesions. It is typically accomplished by use of a probe that contains liquid nitrogen.

curettage The scraping of foreign matter, small growths such as polyps, and cellular debris from a body cavity with a small spoon-shaped instrument (curette).
SEE ALSO *dilation and curettage*

Cushing's syndrome A condition associated with overproduction of the hormone *cortisol* by the cortex of the *adrenal glands.* It is characterized by obesity of the trunk, a round ("moon") face, muscular weakness, fatigue, menstrual irregularity, and often emotional disturbances. The cause may be a tumor of the adrenal glands or an excessive stimulation of the adrenal cortex by a disorder of the *pituitary gland.* If the pituitary secretes an excessive amount of ACTH (adrenocorticotrophic hormone), the adrenal glands are overstimulated.

Several tests are available to help confirm the diagnosis of Cushing's syndrome. Treatment is directed at correcting the underlying problem; when the primary cause of the disorder is oversecretion of ACTH by the pituitary gland, it is fairly common to treat severe cases by surgical removal of one or both adrenal glands.

The outlook is extremely favorable if treated early. Following surgery, replacement hormones are usually given.

cyst An enclosed space within an organ or tissue that forms a sac or capsule, usually filled with fluid or semisolid material. Cysts most commonly occur in the skin and ovaries. SEE ALSO *cystitis*

cystic fibrosis A rare inherited disease of *exocrine* glands affecting the *pancreas*, respiratory system, and sweat glands; also called mucoviscidosis. It usually begins during infancy and is characterized by chronic respiratory infection, pancreatic insufficiency and intolerance to heat. The first sign of the disease in infants is usually obstruction of the *small intestine* with meconium—greenish black to light brown tarlike stools (meconium ileus)—and a delay in normal weight gain.

By the age of about one year approximately 80 percent of children with cystic fibrosis experience disturbances in breathing or digestion. Cough is the most troublesome complaint during the early stages of the disease and may be mistaken at first for whooping cough; episodes of vomiting also occur. Older patients typically sweat excessively, and this may lead to a severe loss of essential body fluids and salts (electrolytes); unless treated, the patient may suffer *dehydration* and circulatory failure.

The cause of cystic fibrosis is unknown. The immediate cause of symptoms involves increased viscosity of bronchial, pancreatic, and other mucous gland secretions with a consequent obstruction of glandular ducts.

The incidence of cystic fibrosis is highest (about 1 in 2,000 live births) among Caucasians. The underlying biochemical defect is thought to reflect an abnormal alteration in a protein or enzyme and accounts for nearly all cases of pancreatic enzyme deficiency in children. Cystic fibrosis is the most common fatal genetic disease of Caucasian children; although some victims survive to thirty and above, about 50 percent of children afflicted die during their late teenage years.

There is no cure for cystic fibrosis. Treatment is aimed at relieving symptoms and helping the child lead as normal a life as possible. Additional information and support for the patient and family can be ob-

cystitis

tained from the Cystic Fibrosis Foundation.

cystitis Inflammation of the urinary bladder, usually caused by a bacterial infection. It is much more common in women than men, because the urethra (the passage leading from the bladder to the outside of the body) in women is more accessible to infections. The disease may be acute or chronic.

Acute cystitis is typically characterized by painful urination and the frequent urge to urinate, even though the bladder may be empty. Freshly passed urine is clouded by the presence of pus and often has a characteristic fishy odor. A steady dull aching pain may also be experienced in the lower part of the abdomen and the region may be extremely tender to the slightest pressure. In severe forms of the disease the patient may have a high fever and sweat profusely.

The diagnosis is made by the presence of typical symptoms and by laboratory tests of a urine sample. In order to confirm the diagnosis it may be necessary in some cases for a urologist to examine the inside of the urethra and bladder (cystoscopy). X-rays may also be taken of the urinary system to make sure that the infection is not related to a structural defect or obstruction of the urinary tract.

The successful treatment of cystitis involves the early administration of an appropriate antibiotic, the intake of ample amounts of fluids, and the restriction of alcohol and highly spiced foods that might irritate the bladder after their filtration into the urine.

Cystitis in women is a condition that may have a tendency to recur. Symptoms should be promptly reported to a physician.

cystoscopy The examination of the inside of the bladder with a cytoscope, a slender illuminated instrument.

cytotoxic drug Any one of various chemical compounds used to destroy *cancer* cells or prevent their multiplication. The ideal cytotoxic (cell-destroying) agent would eliminate fast-growing cancer cells without damaging normal body cells. In practice this is not yet possible. Potentially severe side effects often occur with the use of these drugs during the course of *chemotherapy* (cancer treatment with drugs).

Representative cytotoxic drugs currently used include (by brand name) Adriamycin, Blenoxane, Cytoxan, Fluoroplex, Matulane, and Myleran.

D

D and C
See *dilation and curettage*

death The cessation of life. The entire body does not die in a single instant. Even after the death of the individual, some organs and tissues remain alive for several days. Nerve cells die within a few minutes following the interruption of the blood circulation.

The medical and legal definitions of death are complex and subject to interpretation, especially since the development of modern medical techniques and equipment that can maintain the circulation of blood throughout the body after the heart stops. This permits oxygen to reach organs and tissues by means of artificial respiration (heart-lung machine).

Basic body functions can often be supported with mechanical aids even after the apparent death of the brain. There is general agreement in the medical profession that *brain death* is the ultimate criterion of the individual's death.

When the brain fails to show any signs of electrical activity for a prolonged period and the patient has remained in a state of deep unconsciousness without signs of neurological activity (no response to painful stimuli, fixed pupils, absence of spontaneous breathing, for example) all that remains of the individual is a vegetative existence.

In extremely rare cases some of these negative signs are the result of a critically lowered body temperature (hypothermia) or the effects of massive doses of barbiturates or other drugs that depress the activity of the central nervous system. Fewer than one in a million survive the effects of this deathlike state without a significant loss of essential brain cells.

decompression sickness
See *bends*

decubitus ulcer The medical term for *bed sore*.

Delaney clause A clause that appears in the 1958 amendments of the Food, Drug, and Cosmetic Act of

dermatitis

1938. Sponsored by congressman James J. Delaney of New York, the amendment states that no food additive be approved for human use if it is found to induce *cancer* when ingested by man or animal.

dermatitis Inflammation of the skin. Dermatitis varies greatly in severity but is typically characterized by redness, irritation, itching, swelling, and sometimes the formation of tiny blisters in the affected area.

Contact dermatitis is caused by contact with a substance to which one is allergic or sensitive, such as plants, fruits, chemicals, therapeautic agents, cosmetics, clothing, soap, and animal hair and feathers. The inflammation may be limited to the site of contact or may spread over a large area of the body. In troublesome cases a dermatologist may suggest a *patch test* to determine the exact cause.

Dermatitis is an outward sign of a problem rather than a disease or disorder in itself. The cause is often simple and easy to treat—usually the avoidance of the offending substance or material.
SEE *allergy*

dermatology The branch of medical science concerned with the study of the skin and the diagnosis and treatment of diseases that affect it. A specialist in this field is known as a dermatologist.

dermis The thick layer of *skin* that lies just below the *epidermis* (outer skin). It contains the hair follicles, sebaceous glands, sweat glands, blood vessels and various specialized nerve endings.

desensitization The process or technique by which a specific allergic sensitivity to a particular offending substance (allergen) is reduced or removed. It involves giving the patient frequent, gradually increasing small doses of the allergen until the body becomes adjusted to it and does not respond with an allergic reaction. Desensitization has had varying degrees of success.
SEE *allergy*

detached retina A separation of part of the retina, the light-sensitive portion of the eye, from the underlying tissues of the eyeball. It may be the result of an injury to the eye or it may occur spontaneously for no apparent reason or as a result of aging.

The first symptoms of a detached retina are usually the sensation of flashes or sparks of light or of a curtain moving down across the eye. The extent of impaired vision depends on the site of detachment. The area of the retina responsible for sharpest vision, the fovea centralis, is a small depression in the retinal lining slightly to one side of the exit of the optic nerve. If the retina becomes detached over this area, central vision may be permanently lost.

If the condition is diagnosed early, retinal detachment can usually be repaired successfully in areas other than the fovea centralis. The affected area can easily be seen by an ophthalmologist with the aid of an *ophthalmoscope.*

Any hole, tear, or other separation of the retina must be sealed against the underlying tissues. This can be done with an operation using an intense beam of light (not necessarily a laser) that is directed into a pinpoint and focused for a split second on the separated part of the retina. This produces an inflamed reaction in the underlying tissues and causes them to fuse with the retina. The operation is usually performed in a hospital under a local anesthetic and in most cases can prevent further damage to the retina.

In some cases following repair the retina may again become detached or detach in other places. Immediate treatment is essential. If surgical repair of a detached retina is delayed too long, the condition may progressively worsen and result in permanent loss of vision.

diabetes insipidus A relatively rare disease usually caused by a chronic disorder of the *pituitary gland* in which it fails to secrete sufficient quantities of antidiuretic hormone (ADH), which controls urine secretion. The condition is characterized by the passing of abnormally large amounts of pale urine and an excessive thirst. An adequate fluid intake must be maintained to prevent dehydration. In some cases the physician will prescribe hormone-replacement therapy. The onset of the disorder may be abrupt or develop slowly and can occur at any age.

A less common form of the disease is known as nephrogenic diabetes insipidus and is caused by a failure of the *kidneys* to respond to a normal output of antidiuretic hormone. It is a genetic disorder and is typically first noted soon after birth. Early diagnosis and treatment are essential to prevent dehydration of the infant, which could lead to fever, vomiting, and convulsions.

Unless the lost water is replaced, the condition can lead to brain damage and subsequent mental retardation.

Diabetes insipidus has nothing whatever to do with *diabetes mellitus.*

diabetes mellitus An extremely common disease caused by a failure of the body to control the amount of sugar in the blood because of insufficient secretion of the hormone *insulin* by the pancreas or (less commonly) a failure of the body to make normal use of the insulin secreted.

The symptoms of diabetes depend largely on the age of the patient at onset. In children and young adults they may be abrupt whereas in older persons they may be preceded by years of what is known as a developing or prediabetic condition.

The first evidence of diabetes in older patients may be an associated complication, such as recurring skin

diabetes mellitus

infections or impaired vision. In general the early signs of diabetes in all age groups include the frequent passing of urine, persistent thirst, itching, dry skin, hunger, weakness, and weight loss (despite the fact that obesity is thought to play a role in the development of diabetes in many cases).

When the disease is seen in children it tends to be more severe. The urine contains abnormally large amounts of sugar (glycosuria) and the breath and urine may smell unusually sweet. This is caused by the accumulation in the body of chemicals known as ketones, a condition known as ketosis.

As the first step in diagnosing the severity of diabetes and determining the treatment required, the patient undergoes tests to reveal the concentration of glucose (sugar) in the blood or urine. The physician may first perform a simple test on a urine sample, the results of which are generally available immediately. Another means of diagnosing diabetes is the oral *glucose tolerance test* (GTT) in which blood samples are taken to determine the sugar level.

If a severe case of diabetes is left untreated or if the patient fails to observe the dietary restrictions imposed by the physician, the consequences can be extremely serious. The gradual accumulation of sugar in the blood in the absence of sufficient amounts of insulin may result in a diabetic coma. In such a state the patient loses consciousness; without prompt medical attention or first aid, the condition is a threat to life. The patient may have the following warning signs of an impending coma: nausea (often followed by vomiting), drowsiness, dry mouth, and deepened breathing. The treatment is the administration of insulin.

A diabetic coma caused by too much sugar in the blood can be confused with loss of consciousness brought on by too low a level of blood sugar *(hypoglycemia)* or because of an overdosage of insulin (insulin shock) that abnormally reduces the blood-sugar levels. Low blood sugar is a much more common cause of loss of consciousness than high blood sugar.

Most diabetic patients carry an emergency supply of sugar to take when they sense that their blood-sugar level is falling. Symptoms of hypoglycemia include restlessness, confusion, faintness, cold perspiration, hunger, and muscular unsteadiness. If the patient recognizes these symptoms in time, the coma may be prevented by eating sugar or an item rich in sugar such as a candy bar.

It is impossible to cure diabetes although the condition can be kept under control in most cases by the use of oral hypoglycemic drugs and careful attention to the diet to restrict the intake of sugars, starches, and other carbohydrates. Other diabetic patients require the regular injection of insulin. They are given instructions on the proper method of self-injection of daily insulin doses and shown how to perform a simple test on their urine so they can adjust their daily doses of insulin if the need arises.

With proper attention to dietary restrictions, exercise, personal hygiene, and the use of either oral hypoglycemic drugs or insulin injections, patients with diabetes can enjoy long and productive lives with a minimum of inconvenience.
COMPARE *diabetes insipidus*
SEE *diabetic retinopathy*

diabetic retinopathy A disorder of the retina, the light-sensitive portion of the eye, associated with *diabetes mellitus*. It is characterized by the formation of tiny bulges (microaneurysms) in the retinal blood vessels, bleeding into the eye, edema (swelling) of the retinal tissues, and progressive loss of vision. It is a major cause of blindness. The condition can affect anyone with diabetes, although it may be particularly severe in diabetic children (juvenile-onset diabetes). The progress of diabetic retinopathy can be hastened by the presence of high blood pressure (hypertension).

Treatment of the disorder involves control of both diabetes and high blood pressure. At one time many patients with diabetic retinopathy were treated by the surgical removal of part of the pituitary gland; this is becoming less common because not all patients are ideal candidates for the operation and major deficiencies of lost pituitary hormones involve lifelong replacement. Some patients with diabetic retinopathy may experience a *detached retina*, which must be repaired as soon as possible.

diagnosis The art or process of identifying the nature of a particular disease or disorder. To diagnose means to distinguish, discern, perceive, or decide. When a physician makes a diagnosis he or she tries to recognize a specific disease or disorder. Outward evidence (*signs* such as skin rash, lump, or swelling) and the patient's own feelings and reactions (*symptoms* such as headache, dizziness, or muscular aches and pains) must be distinguished from all other evidence and a likely cause identified; this process is called differential diagnosis.

Sometimes the diagnosis is obvious to a physician as soon as the patient is seen; at other times it may require simple diagnostic procedures such as measuring the heartbeat, blood pressure, and temperature or extensive laboratory tests. If the diagnosis remains in doubt or if expert treatment is necessary, the general practitioner may refer the patient to an appropriate specialist.

Making an accurate diagnosis is essential; if the initial diagnosis is incorrect, the chances are that the treatment will also be incorrect. Time wasted with ineffective treatment because of a faulty diagnosis can mean that the patient's condition may worsen.

Many problems are fairly obvious to any physician. Examples are the common diseases of childhood, for example, measles, chickenpox, and mumps. But many medical problems are not easily recognized, and how soon they are recognized depends to some extent on the physician's experience and training and whether or not he or she keeps up to date with current trends in medical research.

Almost all physicians approach a difficult diagnostic problem through a process of selective elimination, going from the likely cause to the rare. Medical students are taught that "If you hear the sound of hoofbeats, think first of a horse, not a zebra." No competent physician would first consider a diagnosis of a rare tropical disease—even though the initial signs and symptoms suggest it—if the patient had never left St. Louis.

One point must be made clear: not all patients with a particular disease or disorder will exhibit the "classic" or "textbook" signs and symptoms of the disease. This makes a definitive diagnosis more difficult for both the family physician and any specialist.
SEE ALSO *auscultation, blood test, computerized axial tomography, electrocardiogram, stethoscope, syndrome, urinalysis*

dialysis A process used to separate or extract certain substances in solution by diffusion through a porous membrane. When this procedure is used to purify the blood of patients with *kidney failure*, it is known as *hemodialysis*

diaphragm The dome-shaped muscular membrane that separates the abdomen from the chest and is the chief muscle of breathing. The term is also for a cuplike device of thin rubber or plastic shaped to fit over the cervix and used as a method of *contraception.*

diastolic Relating to blood pressure when the chambers of the heart are in their brief period of relaxation (diastole) between beats. The diastolic pressure is given after the *systolic* pressure when a measurement is made. Normal diastolic pressure in a young person is about eighty.
SEE *hypertension*

diarrhea The passing of excessively loose or watery stools. It is a symptom of many disorders of the digestive system and is a fairly common occurrence in babies and very young children. The condition is generally the result of an irritation or inflammation of the lining of the intestinal tract, which causes an abnormal forward movement of the intestinal contents. Thus, stools do not have time to have water absorbed from them in the *large intestine*.

One of the most common causes of diarrhea is a minor intestinal infection; the underlying disease is usually brief and the diarrhea may even help the *digestive tract* to dispose of the infecting microorganisms. Some infections, however, are serious and demand prompt medical attention.

Diarrhea is especially dangerous in babies because of the excessive loss of body fluids *(dehydration)* and salts, which can be very weakening and even life threatening.

digestive tract The hollow tube extending from the mouth to the anus, consisting of the *esophagus, stomach, duodenum, jejunum, ileum, large intestine,* and *rectum;* also called the alimentary canal.

digitalis A group of powerful stimulants obtained from the dried leaves of the common foxglove *(Digitalis purpurea)* used to treat some heart diseases by strengthening the heartbeat while enabling the *ventricles* to beat more slowly. Digitalis and the related drugs digitoxin and digoxin are available orally.

dilation and curettage (D and C) A diagnostic and therapeutic procedure in which the neck (cervix) of the uterus is gently dilated (widened) to permit access to the uterine lining, which is then scraped with a spoon-shaped instrument called a curette. The technique, popularly called D AND C, is used to obtain tissue samples from the uterus, remove abnormal growths or cellular debris, or insure that all of the placenta is removed from the uterus following childbirth or *abortion.*
SEE *dilation and evacuation*

dilation and evacuation A technique often used for the termination of pregnancy in women who are between about thirteen and sixteen weeks pregnant. It involves dilating (stretching) the neck *(cervix)* of the uterus and extracting the amniotic sac with a vacuum tube.
SEE *abortion*

diphtheria A serious contagious bacterial disease, once common during childhood, caused by infection of the nose and throat and spread by coughing, sneezing, or the breath of an infected person. The incubation period is from two to four days. During the first part of the twentieth century diphtheria was a common cause of death among babies and very young children. Since the introduction of a protective *vaccine* it is extremely rare.

The first signs of diphtheria are often a sore throat, fever, and symptoms resembling a common cold. As the bacteria multiply in the body they release a toxin (poison) that may affect the entire body and make a child extremely weak and ill. Swallowing may become difficult and painful due to infection and swelling of the throat. The most typical finding is the formation of a glistening white or grayish membrane across the air passages. This often interferes with breathing, and in extreme or emergency cases it is necessary for a physician to perform a *tracheostomy* to permit respiration.

After one attack of the disease the individual is usually protected for life; the Schick test determines *immunity* to diphtheria.

diplopia A visual disorder in which an object is seen as two; double vision.

diuretic Any drug or agent that acts to increase the secretion of urine, either unintentionally as with caffeine or as a therapeutic measure (sometimes called a water pill). Diuretics act on the cells of the *kidneys* to increase urine output.

Some diseases or disorders are associated with an abnormal accumulation of fluid in the body, causing *edema* (swelling of tissues). Diuretic drugs are prescribed to rid the body of the excess fluid.

Edema fluid is concentrated not within the cells but in the areas between them (extracellular spaces). Thus, in cases of high blood pressure or congestive heart failure, this fluid can exert pressure on nearby organs and possibly damage them. To prevent this, physicians prescribe diuretics. In addition to their direct effect on the kidneys, they also withdraw water from the tissues by creating a "negative extracellular fluid balance."

Several types of diuretics are available; the one prescribed depends largely on the nature and severity of the edema. Various diuretics have slightly different methods of action in addition to differing degrees of potency. One group, the thiazide diuretics, are commonly used to treat high blood pressure (hypertension) by increasing the output of urine (thus reducing edema) and inhibiting the reabsorption into the kidneys of sodium and potassium salts. If the body's potassium becomes depleted by thiazide diuretics, dietary supplements of potassium may be prescribed during therapy.

diverticulitis A condition in which tiny sacs or pouches (diverticula) form in the walls of the large intestine and become inflamed. If the pouches do not become inflamed, the condition is known as diverticulosis.

With advancing age, part of the muscular wall of the large intestine may become weakened. When this occurs, the pressure within the bowel may cause the weakened wall to bulge outward, thus creating a small pouch or sac. The pouches are nearly round and are connected to the intestinal wall by narrow necks. They often cause no problem at all.

Sometimes the necks of these pouches become blocked by swelling or waste matter. This encourages the growth and multiplication of bacteria within the sealed areas. The pouches then become infected and inflamed. Sometimes the inflamed pouches heal spontaneously, but in severe cases the inflammation may spread and affect adjacent areas of the bowel and lead to the formation of abscesses. Swelling and spasm of the affected section may result in intestinal obstruction or the pouch may rupture and cause a generalized infection.

The signs and symptoms of acute diverticulitis include abdominal swelling and severe pain (usually on the lower left side), nausea and vomiting, and sometimes alternating constipation and diarrhea with traces of blood in the stools. Severe infection is typically accompanied by fever, chills, and a general feeling of being unwell (malaise). Prompt medical attention is essential, especially in the presence of severe bleeding or other signs of acute abdominal distress. In some cases surgical treatment may be required.

In milder forms of diverticulitis the physician may recommend bed rest, the intake of clear liquids, and a change in the diet to include more roughage (dietary fiber) to enhance healing of the diverticula and help prevent more from forming. Antibiotics may also be prescribed to control bacterial infection.

dosage The determination and regulation of the appropriate amount (strength), frequency of administration, and number of *doses* of a drug or radiation.

dose The amount or strength of a drug or radiation to be administered at one time. In the case of drugs, the total daily dose is the combined amount of medication prescribed each day.
SEE *loading dose*

Down's syndrome An abnormal condition also known as mongolism in which a child is born with a small and slightly flattened head, eyes that are narrow and slanted, a large tongue that typically protrudes from the mouth, and mental deficiency. Fifty percent of such children are born to women over the age of thirty-five. The condition occurs in approximately 45 per 1,000 live births in women over the age of forty. The congenital abnormality is caused by the presence of an extra *chromosome*, referred to as chromosome 21.

The life expectancy of children with Down's syndrome may be decreased by the general tendency for them to develop acute leukemia or heart disease. Many victims do survive to adulthood in the absence of heart disease; a few even reach old age.

The condition is named after the

DPT

British physician J. Langdon Down (1828–1896).
SEE ALSO *amniocentesis*

DPT Abbreviation for *diphtheria, pertussis,* and *tetanus;* a triple *vaccine* used for the *immunization* of children.

duodenum The first part of the *small intestine,* situated between the *stomach* and the *jejunum.*

dysentery Inflammation of the *large intestine* accompanied by diarrhea and abdominal pain. The two most common causes are infection with *bacteria* (bacillary dysentery) or *protozoa* (amebic dysentery or amebiasis). Effective treatment depends on an accurate diagnosis of the cause by laboratory examination of a stool sample.

dysmenorrhea Painful menstrual periods. The causes are varied and may be both physical and psychological.

Physicians typically refer to two types of dysmenorrhea: primary and secondary. Primary dysmenorrhea is very common, usually occurring shortly after menstruation begins and disappearing as the woman grows older. No underlying cause is known, although several possibilities have been suggested, including a high level of *prostaglandin* hormones, which are thought to cause excessive muscular activity or uterine contractions.

Secondary dysmenorrhea may typically occur in older women who have had years of painless menstruation. It is usually associated with an underlying problem in the pelvic area, such as inflammation of the pelvis, tumors (such as *fibroids*), or *endometriosis.* Any woman who develops painful periods should see her physician to discover any possible underlying problem.

The symptoms of primary dysmenorrhea often disappear after pregnancy. In addition, reassurance by the physician and an analgesic such as aspirin or codeine may provide relief of symptoms. Oral contraceptives provide relief of dysmenorrhea by suppressing ovulation.

The symptoms of secondary dysmenorrhea usually demand correction of the underlying problem. Dilation of the cervix may also provide relief for up to several months in some patients.
SEE ALSO *premenstrual tension*

dyspareunia Pain experienced during sexual intercourse. Dyspareunia may be primary, in which case there is no organic cause, or secondary, the result of infection of the penis, vagina, or nearby tissues, which results in the sensation of burning or itching. Pain may also be experienced by a woman whose vaginal secretions are insufficient. In such cases an artificial lubrication such as petroleum jelly can be used to reduce friction.

An ovarian cyst or an infection of the uterus or Fallopian tubes are other possible causes of secondary dyspareunia. If the pain persists, it is important to consult a physician to discover and treat the underlying cause.

dyspepsia Imperfect digestion (indigestion) characterized by abdominal discomfort or pain, a feeling of fullness shortly after eating, flatulence (gastrointestinal wind or gas formation), and occasionally nausea and vomiting. The cause is usually overindulgence in food or drink, although it may be early evidence of *peptic ulcer*. In most cases the symptoms can be relieved by an *antacid*.

dysphagia Difficulty in swallowing or the inability to swallow, caused by an abnormal narrowing of the esophagus or pharynx, spasm of the muscles of the throat or esophagus, or emotional upset (a feeling of having a "lump in the throat") without any physical obstruction. Treatment is aimed at the underlying cause.

dyspnea Difficult or labored breathing; breathlessness; shortness of breath. It is a common symptom of diseases or disorders of the lungs or heart, especially if it occurs when no exercise or physical stress is taking place.
SEE *asthma, bronchiectasis, bronchitis, emphysema, pneumoconiosis.*

dysuria Difficulty in urination often accompanied by a painful or burning sensation. It is usually a symptom of infection of the urinary tract particularly in the neck of the bladder and its outlet, the urethra.

E

eardrum
SEE *tympanum*

ecchymosis A bruise caused by the escape of blood from blood vessels (especially capillaries) into tissues, resulting in a characteristic discoloration. A black eye is an example of ecchymosis.
COMPARE *extravasation*

ECG Abbreviation for *electrocardiogram*.

echocardiography The diagnostic use of high-frequency sound to visualize the heart's internal structure, including valves and hollow chambers.
SEE ALSO *ultrasonography*

eclampsia A serious complication of pregnancy, typically occurring in a very few women during the last three months of pregnancy, during the second stage of labor, or during the first few hours following delivery. Its cause is not known. It is marked by high blood pressure, convulsions, and coma. The condition, which is usually preceded by characteristic warning signs known as *preeclampsia*, demands immediate medical attention to maintain life.

With regular medical examinations during the prenatal period, early signs of the condition can be recognized by the physician and treatment started at once. For this reason, eclampsia is becoming very rare.

ectopic pregnancy An abnormal condition in which the fertilized ovum remains in the *Fallopian tubes* and develops outside the uterus.

Ectopic pregnancy is not a common condition but it is serious when it occurs. In normal conception, sperm travel up through the cervix into the uterus and then up the Fallopian tubes, usually fertilizing the ovum while it is traveling down the tube. The fertilized ovum begins to develop while it is still in the tube, and its passage down the tube to the uterus often takes several days. Occasionally the passage is obstructed and the ovum is unable to reach the uterine wall. It then continues to develop in the tube, which stretches further and further until it ruptures. This rupture generally occurs within the first months of pregnancy.

This condition is often difficult to diagnose and may be mistaken for appendicitis or miscarriage. Usually the first indication of an ectopic pregnancy is that a woman who has missed a period develops pain in the lower part of the abdomen, often in the groin. The pain may develop gradually or suddenly, and may take some time to build up in severity. Following the pain, she may start bleeding from the vagina, the blood flow often being darker than the usual menstrual flow.

If the physician suspects an ectopic pregnancy, he or she will advise immediate hospitalization; an operation may be required if the diagnosis is confirmed. It is almost always necessary to remove the damaged Fallopian tube and sometimes the ovary as well, although pregnancy through the other tube and ovary should still be possible.

Ectopic pregnancy is particularly likely to occur if the Fallopian tube has been damaged by a previous infection or injury, and it may occur more readily while a woman is wearing an intrauterine contraceptive device.

eczema An imprecise term no longer considered a medically acceptable diagnosis for various forms of *dermatitis*. The term was formerly used to describe chronic skin inflammations characterized by patches of red and scaly skin often covered with crusts or scabs that itch intensely.

edema An abnormal accumulation of fluid in the tissues, characterized by puffiness or swelling. It may be localized in a specific part of the body (such as the ankles or legs) as the result of an obstruction of the veins or lymphatic vessels, or it may be generalized as the result of congestive heart failure or kidney disease.

When edema becomes a problem that interferes with the body's normal functioning, *diuretics* may be prescribed to aid in the elimination of excess fluid from the tissues.

EEG Abbreviation for *electroencephalogram*.

EKG Abbreviation for *electrocardiogram*.

electrocardiogram A graphic record or tracing of the electrical activity of the *heart*, often referred to by the abbreviations ECG or EKG. When any muscle contracts it creates a very weak electric current. By examining the ECG, a cardiologist can usually tell if the heart seems normal or diseased.

The record is made by placing small metal disks (electrodes) on the chest over the heart. (This is absolutely painless and a normal pro-

electroencephalogram

cedure in a thorough medical examination.) The electrodes may be placed nearly anywhere on the body, but for practical reasons the connections are usually made to both arms and a leg in addition to the chest. They are attached to wires from an electrocardiograph, an instrument which picks up the electrical impulses, amplifies them, and charts them on a moving graph paper. (No electrical shock is possible during the procedure: the patient's own electricity goes into the instrument, not the instrument's electricity into the patient.) These records are then carefully analyzed by the cardiologist for evidence of abnormality.

The electrocardiogram is an extremely useful and important diagnostic aid. It can provide information about the heart's ability to conduct the normal electrical impulses that maintain its rhythm, whether or not any areas of the heart contain dead tissue as the result of a previous heart attack *(myocardial infarction)*, the position of the heart in the chest cavity, and the possible presence of an abnormal muscular enlargement of the heart.

electroencephalogram A record or tracing (often referred to by its abbreviation: EEG) of the electrical activity of the brain. It can be used for various purposes, including the diagnosis of brain tumors and other disorders and research into sleep and dream patterns.

Nerve cells have the ability to generate and transmit a very small electric current. The electrical activity of the outer surface of the brain (cerebral cortex) can be measured indirectly with the aid of a delicate instrument, the electroencephalograph. By means of several flat electrodes attached to the scalp or of minute needlelike electrodes inserted into the skull itself, this instrument can record the "brain waves" produced by the synchronized electric discharge of millions of nerve cells in the cerebral cortex.

The electrical signals are picked up, amplified, and made to activate an array of tracing pens. These movements are recorded on a moving strip of paper, which constitutes the electroencephalogram. When the EEG is analyzed it can reveal information about the location of a brain tumor or help to locate the site of some other brain malfunction.

The EEG picks up three main frequency bands in normal subjects, representing fairly distinct types of brain waves. These are called alpha rhythms (eight to ten cycles per second), beta rhythms (fifteen to sixty cycles per second), and delta rhythms (fewer than five cycles per second). In cases where brain damage proceeds rapidly, as in a fast-growing tumor or acute abscess of the cerebrum, changes in the patterns of brain waves can provide valuable clues that contribute to the diagnosis.

electrolytes Any of various chemicals which, when dissolved in water, can conduct an electric current. Electrolytes in the body, including the salts of sodium, potassium, calcium, magnesium, and chloride, play an important role in the normal functioning of cells, maintenance of fluid balance, and transmission of nerve impulses.

electromyography A diagnostic technique or procedure for recording the electrical activity of selected muscle groups at rest and during voluntary contraction. It involves the use of a needle electrode inserted into a muscle and is used to diagnose various muscle disorders such as *myotonia*.

embolism The blocking of a blood vessel by an *embolus*. The symptoms and severity of the condition depend on the size and location of the blocked vessel.

embolus A blood clot, clump of cellular debris, air bubble (air embolus), or foreign body that is carried in the bloodstream until it reaches and lodges in a vessel too small in diameter to permit it to pass.
COMPARE *hematoma, thrombus*

embryo The stage of development within the uterus of a human offspring from the moment the ovum is fertilized by a sperm cell until the end of the eighth week, when it is called a *fetus*.

emesis The medical term for *vomiting*.
SEE ALSO *emetic*

emetic Any drug or agent that induces *vomiting* (emesis), such as *ipecac syrup*. Emetics are used in the emergency treatment of known or suspected cases of poisoning and drug overdosage.

An emetic must never be given to an unconscious person. If possible, a physician, hospital emergency room, or poison control center should be contacted for advice before an emetic is given.

emphysema A chronic disease of the *lungs* characterized by excessive stretching or distension of the alveoli (air sacs). This can occur for several reasons. Obstruction of the bronchi (major air passages) with mucus, inflammation, or swelling can cause the air sacs to become inflated with trapped air. Damage by infections such as *tuberculosis* and *bronchiectasis*, or contamination as in *pneumoconiosis* or chronic *bronchitis*, may cause the air sacs to lose their elasticity and become distended. Smoking is also implicated. Occasionally some of the air sacs burst. This is generally not serious and is usually the result of violent efforts to expel air from the lungs, as may occur in cases of whooping cough.

Emphysema mainly affects persons during middle or late adult life. It may be related to an inherited weakness of the lung tissues,

empyema

polluted atmospheres, cigarette smoke, or infection. The diagnosis can be difficult to make since the most common first symptom is slight lack of breath (dyspnea) after mild exertion, which is also a symptom of many other lung disorders, of which emphysema may or may not be a complication.

The breathlessness of emphysema is normally mild and may remain so for a long time, slowly worsening over a period of many years. As it does, the chest becomes enlarged because of long and continued efforts to inhale sufficient air. Also, the extent to which the victim is capable of expanding the chest during inhaling is reduced.

Emphysema is a progressive disease. Unless the cause can be discovered and treated in some way, the disease will shorten life. In addition to the treatment recommended by a physician, it may also be beneficial for the patient to move to an area that is not heavily polluted; daily walks in fresh country air can be of considerable benefit.

empyema The presence of pus in the cavity between the lungs and the ribs (pleural space), occurring most often as a complication of pneumonia or tuberculosis. Empyema is treated by antibiotics and the removal of pus with a hollow needle and the surgical opening of a drainage outlet.

encephalitis Any inflammation of the brain. It can follow as a complication of illnesses such as influenza, measles, German measles, chickenpox, or other viral infections.
SEE ALSO *meningitis*

encephalopathy Any disease or disorder of the brain.

endarterectomy The surgical removal of the diseased inner lining of an artery, usually one that has become blocked with fatty deposits *(atheromas)*.

endemic Relating to a disease that commonly occurs in a given region or is peculiar to a certain group of people.
COMPARE *epidemic, pandemic*

endocarditis Inflammation of the lining of the heart (endocardium), especially around the valves.

The heart and its internal and surrounding structures may become infected. If the involved parts are congenitally deformed or have been previously weakened or damaged by disease (such as *rheumatic fever*), the resulting inflammation may lead to some form of heart disease. Endocarditis is the most serious of these infections if not diagnosed and treated at a relatively early stage.

Bacteria may enter the blood in various ways and become trapped around the valves that control the flow of blood through the heart's hollow chambers. Treatment with antibiotics and bed rest until the infection has cleared up are important to minimize further complications.

endocrine glands The ductless glands that secrete *hormones* directly into the bloodstream. Endocrine glands include the *pituitary gland, adrenal glands, thyroid gland, parathyroid glands, ovaries,* and *testicles.* The *pancreas* also secretes the hormone *insulin* in an area known as the islets of Langerhans.
COMPARE *exocrine glands*
SEE ALSO *endocrinology*

endocrinology The branch of science concerned with the study and function of the *endocrine* glands and with the physiological effects of the *hormones* they secrete. A specialist in this field is known as an endocrinologist.

endometriosis A condition in which the same type of *mucous membrane* that makes up the uterine lining (endometrium) is found growing in other sites, such as the surface of an ovary, various tissues of the pelvis, or in vaginal and abdominal scars. In a few cases these abnormally placed fragments are affected by the menstrual cycle. The woman may experience swelling and pain in the lower part of the abdomen prior to each period, when the fragments swell and bleed in response to hormones released to induce menstruation.

Treatment depends largely on the severity of the symptoms—menstrual pain *(dysmenorrhea)* and pain during sexual intercourse *(dyspareunia)*—and the age of the patient. Surgical removal of the ovaries is effective in women past childbearing age. In many cases the condition can be treated by administering the sex hormones naturally secreted by the ovaries.

endometritis Inflammation of the endometrium, the *mucous membrane* that lines the *uterus,* caused by bacterial infection.

endoscopy The technique or procedure used to examine the interior of various hollow organs such as the bladder and body cavities by means of an illuminated tubular instrument (endoscope) equipped with lenses and various attachments.

endotoxin A poison (toxin) released by some bacteria when their cell walls are broken down.

enteritis Inflammation of the intestines, especially the small intestine.

Regional enteritis is a disorder of uncertain origin in which the lining of the small intestine becomes inflamed, thickened, and inelastic. Sometimes the disease may spread to affect the large intestine and the stomach.

Signs and symptoms of regional enteritis (also known as regional *ileitis* and *Crohn's disease)* include chronic diarrhea, recurrent pain in the abdomen, weight loss, and sometimes the presence of a hard mass in the abdomen. Many patients, however, have only sharp cramps or pains in the abdomen

enterobiasis

before the disease is diagnosed. In some cases the pains may mimic the symptoms of acute *appendicitis*. A definite diagnosis involves x-rays of the digestive tract after the patient swallows a barium solution. This is opaque to x-rays and its progress through the intestinal tract can easily be followed.

In some forms of regional enteritis there may be very little inflammation of the bowel but a striking increase in the thickness of the alimentary canal in the affected area. It may be so great as to cause intestinal obstruction; if the obstruction is severe it may be necessary to remove the diseased section. Some patients with the disease develop abscesses in the affected area, especially following the walling off of a perforated section of bowel. This rarely may lead to the creation of a *fistula*, an abnormal passage between one section of the intestine and another or between the intestine and structures outside it.

Although the exact cause of regional enteritis is not known, there is some evidence to suggest that emotional stress plays a part. In some cases a single attack of the disease will be followed by total recovery and the patient may remain without further symptoms for life. More commonly, however, there will be recurring periods extended over many years during which the characteristic signs and symptoms persist.

enterobiasis
SEE *oxyuriasis*

enuresis Involuntary urination, especially at night during sleep (nocturnal enuresis or popularly, bed-wetting). Although this is a common phase of childhood, especially in boys, persistent urinary *incontinence* may require medical evaluation. Most children outgrow the problem without special treatment. When involuntary urination occurs during the day (diurnal enuresis), it may be a sign of physical disorder of the urinary tract.

enzyme Any one of the various complex proteins produced by living cells that act to induce or speed up chemical reactions in other substances without themselves being altered in the process. Enzymes are present in abundance in the digestive juices and play an important role in breaking down food particles into simpler compounds that can be absorbed by the body.

epidemic An outbreak of an infectious disease or condition that affects many people in a particular geographical area at the same time. An example is influenza, which can spread rapidly throughout an entire country. If such a disease continues uncontrolled, it can affect millions of people worldwide.

Among the other infectious diseases that may reach epidemic proportions are cholera, yellow fever, typhoid fever, typhus, and plague. The greatest recorded epidemic was the outbreak of bubonic plague that killed nearly half the population of Europe during the late fourteenth century.

Many diseases that were once of epidemic proportions have been largely brought under control, as the combined result of modern medical care, effective drugs, education in personal hygiene, and stringent public-health measures.

After it was discovered that certain species of mosquitoes, rats, snails, and other animals were carriers of disease-producing (pathogenic) organisms, it was much easier to control the spread of a particular epidemic by eradicating the intermediate hosts or their breeding grounds. The introduction of modern plumbing and sewage-disposal systems has had perhaps an even greater beneficial effect on controlling the spread of many types of infectious diseases.

Control of an epidemic includes vaccination against the infecting microorganisms in those who do not yet have the disease and prompt medical treatment (with antibiotics or other drugs) in those who have been infected.

COMPARE *endemic*, *pandemic*

epidemiology The branch of medical science concerned with the study of the incidence, distribution, and types of diseases and the various environmental influences that favor their spread. An expert in this field is known as an epidemiologist.

epidermis The outermost layer of the *skin;* the cuticle. It contains no blood vessels and is made up almost entirely of dead skin cells that have been pushed outward by newly formed cells. The dead cells are constantly cast off from the skin surface and replaced with new ones. Beneath the epidermis is the so-called true skin, the *dermis*.

epididymis A coiled tube forming part of the seminal duct, situated at the top rear portion of the *testicle*. Sperm cells *(spermatozoa)* pass from each testicle into the epididymis, which acts as a storehouse in the system of ducts that transport the spermatozoa from the testicle.

The epididymis is about as thick as a piece of thread, and if straightened out would measure between eighteen and twenty feet. It is lined with hundreds of tiny waving hairs, which help move the sperm along into a duct known as the *vas deferens*.

SEE ALSO *epididymitis*, *vasectomy*

epididymitis Inflammation of the *epididymis,* usually as the result of a bacterial infection. It is commonly a consequence of an infection that spreads from another part of the urinary tract. The bacteria may reach the epididymis from the urine, seminal ducts, or the prostate gland.

epiglottis

Epididymitis can affect males at any age, although it is rare before puberty and usually occurs in men between the ages of forty and fifty. Either testicle may become infected; in rare cases both testicles may be involved, which can occasionally cause sterility if the infection is severe. The onset of the infection may be sudden or gradual. As it progresses, swelling appears and the region becomes tender, making it impossible to distinguish the epididymis from the testicle on examination.

Treatment of epididymitis includes bed rest, support for the scrotum, and an appropriate antibiotic.

epiglottis A thin elastic flap of cartilage covered with mucous membrane that forms a lid over the opening of the *trachea* during swallowing. It prevents food particles or fluid from being inhaled. COMPARE *glottis*

epilepsy A group of brain disorders characterized by recurring temporary attacks of impaired consciousness, with or without convulsions or loss of consciousness. It is triggered by sudden and uncontrolled electrical discharges in the cerebrum, the main part of the brain. In some cases the exaggerated electrical activity of the brain results in violent muscular convulsions (seizures) and loss of consciousness. In milder attacks consciousness is affected and there may be little or no outward evidence that an attack is taking place. The patient may experience only a brief period (ten to fifteen seconds) of mental blackout and immediately afterward regain normal composure.

Most epilepsy is *idiopathic* (causes unknown); among the known possible causes are a localized brain tumor, head injury, and disease of the blood vessels of the brain (especially in patients over the age of fifty).

As many as 1 person in every 200 is affected by some form of epilepsy. This makes it all the more surprising that many superstitions regarding this condition persist. One of the oldest is the belief that a person with epilepsy is possessed by the devil; oddly enough, another superstition claims that epilepsy is a manifestation of spiritual grace.

Epilepsy should not be regarded as a frightening disease but as a fairly common disorder of the brain's "wiring." The two representative forms of epilepsy are *grand mal* (major) and *petit mal* (minor).

Grand mal epileptic seizures are quite dramatic, in that the patient may have a brief mental warning of the impending attack and utter a sharp cry just before losing consciousness and falling. The muscles of the body go into violent contractive spasm for up to twenty to thirty seconds; this is followed immediately by violent jerky movements of the face, arms, and legs lasting

84

about thirty seconds, caused by rapidly alternating contraction and relaxation of major muscle groups.

Petit mal seizures are characterized by a very brief disruption of consciousness (a few seconds at most), and the attacks may recur several times daily. The temporary blackout is not accompanied by convulsions, although the arms may suddenly jerk a few times during an attack. This form of epilepsy usually begins in childhood and may not persist beyond puberty.

Treatment of epilepsy is aimed at removing the cause, if known. Should brain tumors be discovered to be the cause of the seizures (which is relatively rare), their successful removal by a neurosurgeon will usually end epilepsy. If no organic (physical) disease is the cause, the physician may prescribe one or more anticonvulsant drugs to keep the attacks under control. With appropriate treatment it is possible to go several years or forever without another seizure.

Epileptics are perfectly normal between attacks and can usually remember only their onset. If the seizures are not too frequent and severe most everyday activities can be carried on, except driving or operating dangerous machinery, where sudden loss of consciousness could be fatal.

Not all cases of convulsive seizures are the result of epilepsy. Only a thorough examination by a medical specialist can determine the cause of any such physical or mental disorder. After strokes, epilepsy is the most common disorder of the nervous system.

epinephrine A *hormone* also called adrenaline secreted by the medulla (inner part) of the *adrenal glands*. It acts to stimulate the activity of the autonomic nervous system, the part of the nervous system that is not ordinarily under conscious control and that affects or regulates heartbeat, breathing, and intestinal movement.

Synthetic epinephrine and that obtained from the adrenal glands of animals is sometimes used by physicians to treat cardiac arrest, asthma, and certain conditions caused by an allergic reaction.

episiotomy Surgical incision of the tissues at the entrance to the vagina (the *perineum*), frequently performed at childbirth to enlarge the opening of the birth passage and prevent tearing by the emergence of the baby's head.

epispadias A congenital defect in which the *urethra* of a baby boy fails to form properly during development in the uterus and opens on the underside of the penis instead of at the tip. Surgical correction of this defect is usually possible.

epistaxis The medical term for nosebleed. There are many possible causes of nosebleed, including injury, high blood pressure, arteriosclerosis, general bleeding

epithelioma

disorders (such as hemophilia), systemic infections, and local infections of the nasal passages. In most cases bleeding may be controlled by pinching the nostrils together for five to ten minutes. In more severe forms of nosebleed, it may be necessary for a physician to cauterize the bleeding point. The nasal passages may also be packed with a small cotton plug impregnated with a vasoconstrictor such as phenylephrine and a topical anesthetic such as tetracaine. More serious causes of nosebleeds, such as liver disease, demand treatment of the underlying condition.

epithelioma A *malignant* (cancerous) growth originating in the skin or in a *mucous membrane.*

epithelium The tissue that covers all the surface of the body and lines body cavities and channels. It consists of a single layer or multiple layers of closely packed cells.

erythema Redness of the skin that occurs in patches. Among the possible causes are inflammation of the skin, heat, sunlight, or exposure to cold.

erythrocyte Red blood cell. The red blood cells are very small and extremely numerous: one drop of blood contains about 500 million erythrocytes. They are produced in the *bone marrow;* all the bones in an infant's body are involved in this process but only the bones of the trunk are involved in an adult.

The rate of production of red bloods cells is well over 2 million cells per second. They have an average life of approximately 120 days, at which time they are removed from the circulation along with other waste products. Mature red cells lack the nucleus characteristic of other body cells; since they have no nucleus, they cannot carry out any cellular repair or regeneration and so gradually deteriorate.

When this deterioration exceeds a certain degree, the dying cell is removed from the circulation by scavenger cells in the *spleen* and other organs. Here it is broken down and iron from the *hemoglobin* pigment is carefully conserved for incorporation into the hemoglobin of a new generation of red cells.

The main role of erythrocytes is to carry oxygen from the lungs to all the organs and tissues of the body. The hemoglobin that erythrocytes contain is adapted to this purpose. SEE ALSO *leukocyte, platelet*

erythrocyte sedimentation rate A diagnostic procedure to determine the time it takes for red blood cells *(erythrocytes)* in a sample of blood to settle to the bottom of a vertical tube. This *blood test* is not specific for any particular disease, although it is frequently used as an early indicator of disease when other test results are normal. Should the result of this test be abnormal, the physician will usually request other

diagnostic procedures to determine the underlying problem.

erythrocytosis An abnormal increase in the number of red blood cells *(erythrocytes)*, usually as the result of an insufficient amount of oxygen in the blood circulation; this puts an extra demand on the *bone marrow* to manufacture more red cells. It is commonly caused by living at high altitudes.
SEE ALSO *polycythemia*

erythromycin An antibiotic mainly prescribed to treat relatively mild or moderate bacterial infections, especially when the bacteria are resistant to *penicillin*. It is not the drug of first choice to treat severe bacterial infections because it tends not to kill bacteria but to inhibit their growth and development. At the recommended dosage level most forms of erythromycin are relatively free from serious *side effects*.
COMPARE *tetracycline*

esophagus The long muscular tube that connects the *pharynx* (throat) with the *stomach;* popularly called the gullet.

estrogen Any of several female sex *hormones* (particularly estradiol and estrone) produced naturally by the *ovaries* or prepared artificially for hormone-replacement therapy or as an ingredient in oral contraceptives.

Estrogen is responsible for the secondary sexual characteristics of women, such as the particular distribution of body fat that gives rise to the typical female shape. It also influences the monthly cyclic changes in the lining of the vagina and uterus. A synthetic preparation of estrogen may be used to treat the symptoms of menopause.
SEE ALSO *progesterone*

etiology The cause of a disease or the study of the causes of disease.
SEE *diagnosis*

Eustachian tube The narrow canal that connects the middle ear to the upper part of the throat *(pharynx)* at the back of the nose. Its function is to equalize the air pressure on each side of the eardrum.

exocrine glands Glands such as sweat glands whose secretions reach the skin or a mucous membrane either directly or by means of a duct.
COMPARE *endocrine glands*

exophthalmos A condition in which the eyeballs appear to protrude from their sockets. Among the various causes (which include inflammation, swelling, tumors, and injuries of the socket) the most common is a disease or disorder of the *thyroid gland* resulting in an overproduction of thyroid hormone.
SEE ALSO *hyperthyroidism*

expectorant Any agent that facilitates the loosening of phlegm or mucus from the throat or lower air passages, thus permitting it to be more easily coughed up and expelled.

extravasation The escape of blood or other body fluids from vessels into the tissues. Injury to the bladder may result in the extravasation of urine into nearby tissues; injury to a blood vessel may result in the discharge of blood into the tissues, resulting in a bruise *(ecchymosis)* if the capillaries are involved or a blood clot *(hematoma)* if greater amounts of blood escape.

exudate The fluid that escapes through the walls of blood vessels into nearby tissues or cavities during inflammation. It usually contains large numbers of white blood cells *(leukocytes)* and other constituents of the circulating blood.

eye The organ of vision. The eye functions much like a camera: light entering the eye passes through the clear outer covering *(cornea)* and is focused by the *lens* onto the light-sensitive *retina* at the back of the eye.
SEE *amblyopia, astigmatism, cataract, conjunctivitis, detached retina, glaucoma, ophthalmoscope*

F

Fallopian tube The duct or tube that leads from each *ovary* to the *uterus*. It conveys the ovum from the ovary and is a passageway for spermatozoa.

The Fallopian tubes (also called uterine tubes or oviducts) are approximately 4 inches (10 cm) long. At its base, each Fallopian tube opens into the uterus, one on each side of the rear uterine wall.

A Fallopian tube is wider toward its far end, where it arches over the ovary. The end of the tube swells out into an irregular trumpet-shaped bell formed by a series of tiny tendrils (fimbriae), the longest of which is in contact with the ovary. In spite of this point of contact, a released ovum must pass over a gap between the two structures in order to reach the tube. Normal pregnancy has been shown to occur even if an ovary is missing on one side and a Fallopian tube is missing on the opposite side; the ovum can occasionally find its way across the abdominal cavity to the intact Fallopian tube on the other side.

SEE ALSO *ectopic pregnancy, salpingitis, tubal ligation*

familial Relating to diseases, disorders, and symptoms that tend to occur among people in the same family.
COMPARE *hereditary*

fat Any one of a group of organic compounds that form adipose (fatty) tissues. Animal fats provide an important source of energy in the diet—twice as much by weight than *carbohydrates* or *protein*.
SEE ALSO *atheroma, lipid*

febrile Related to, having, or characterized by a *fever*.

feces The waste matter formed in the *large intestine* and expelled through the anus; stools. It consists of indigestible food residues, unabsorbed food, bacteria, and various secretions of the digestive tract, such as *bile*.
SEE ALSO *constipation, diarrhea*

femur The thigh bone. It extends from the hip to the knee and is the

fertilization

longest and strongest bone in the body.

fertilization The point at which conception occurs; the penetration (impregnation) of the *ovum* by a *sperm cell*.
COMPARE *sterilization*

fetal monitoring An electronic method used to measure the heart rate and evaluate the general state of health of a *fetus* (most commonly during the first stage of labor or just before) and to determine the frequency of uterine contractions.

In external fetal monitoring, which presents no risk to the fetus, a device known as a transducer is placed on an appropriate area of the mother's abdomen. It picks up the fetal heartbeat and converts it to electrical signals, which are then amplified and recorded on a moving graph. A similar device is used to measure and record the frequency and strength of uterine contractions.

A less commonly performed procedure (used only during labor, mainly to help determine the need for performing an emergency *cesarean section*) is known as internal fetal monitoring. This involves the positioning of an electrode on the fetus's scalp to measure fetal heart rate. A fluid-filled catheter is inserted into the uterus to measure the frequency and pressure of uterine contractions after the amniotic sac has broken and delivery is at hand. Unlike external fetal monitoring, internal fetal monitoring poses a slight risk to both the mother and fetus. In a few cases internal fetal monitoring may inadvertently lead to perforation of the uterus, uterine infection, or an abscess or blood clot *(hematoma)* on the scalp of the fetus. In selected cases the information obtained is worth the risk.

fetus The stage of development within the uterus of a human infant from the beginning of the third month until birth.
COMPARE *embryo*
SEE ALSO *fetal monitoring*

fever An abnormally high body temperature. The normal body temperature is approximately 98.6°F (37°C), although it can vary slightly depending on such factors as time of day and activity level.

Fever may contribute to fighting an infection by accelerating all body processes. Aspirin or acetaminophen helps to reduce fever when taken as directed.
SEE ALSO *hyperpyrexia*

fibrillation Abnormally rapid, irregular, and uncoordinated contractions of muscle fibers, especially the chambers of the *heart*. It may primarily involve the upper chambers (atrial fibrillation) or the lower chambers (ventricular fibrillation). The diagnosis is confirmed by means of an electrocardiogram.

Atrial fibrillation is frequently the result of a heart disease such as *rheumatic fever* or *coronary artery disease*. It is commonly treated with the drug digoxin.

Ventricular fibrillation is a much more serious condition, requiring immediate medical attention to prevent death. The most effective means of stopping the ineffective pumping rhythms of ventricular fibrillation is use of a defibrillator, a machine which delivers short bursts of electric current to the chest wall. Ventricular fibrillation may occur in cases of a heart attack, drowning, severe electrical shock, overdose of digitalis, and in various heart diseases.

fibrin An insoluble protein in the blood, created by the body from *fibrinogen*. It forms the basis of a blood clot.

fibrinogen A clotting factor in solution in the blood from which *fibrin* is made.

fibroid Any fibrous tumor, especially one that develops in the smooth muscular wall of the *uterus*. Uterine fibroids (also known as fibromyomas or leiomyomas) are usually harmless growths that vary greatly in both size and number, from clusters of small nodules to large projecting masses. They may cause no symptoms at all and be discovered only as the result of a routine examination of the pelvis. When fibroids grow very large (some may be larger than a grapefruit) they may exert pressure on the bladder, resulting in a frequent need to urinate or interfering with the ability to become pregnant.

Fibroids are extremely common. It has been estimated that from 20 to 50 percent of all women over thirty have at least some evidence of fibroids.

Large fibroids may cause painful cramps and an increase in blood flow during menstruation and sometimes between periods. Other symptoms typically include pain or a feeling of pressure or fullness in the lower part of the abdomen. Normally a fibroid causes no pain unless some complication occurs. However, it may project so much from the uterine wall that it becomes attached to the uterus only by a stalk of tissue. If this stalk becomes twisted it can cause intense abdominal pain. Occasionally the center of the fibroid softens (degenerates) as the result of an inadequate blood supply and the whole tumor swells, becoming extremely painful and tender. Rarely does the tumor become *malignant*.

When fibroids cause trouble, surgical removal (myomectomy) is the usual form of treatment. If the growth is excessively large, it may be necessary to remove the entire uterus *(hysterectomy)*. Many smaller fibroids tend to shrink in size after menopause.

fibroma Any fibrous tumor of connective tissue, generally benign (harmless).

fibrosis The formation of tough, fibrous, scarlike tissue in place of normal tissue that has been injured, infected, or deprived of an adequate blood supply.

fibrositis A vague clinical condition caused by inflammation of fibrous connective tissues, characterized by pain, tenderness, and stiffness of the muscles. It is a form of muscular *rheumatism*.

fibula The bone that forms the lower part of the leg. It extends from the ankle almost to the knee and is one of the longest and thinnest bones in the body.
COMPARE *tibia*

fistula Any abnormal connecting passage, congenital or acquired, between two body surfaces or organs, or between a hollow organ and the exterior surface of the body. In many cases fistulas must be surgically repaired.

flu Short for *influenza*, the term is often applied loosely and incorrectly to various minor upsets of the gastrointestinal system.

fluoridation The addition of a fluorine compound (fluoride) to drinking water as a method of reducing the incidence of tooth decay (dental caries). Some public water supplies contain natural quantities of fluoride; other communities have found that tooth protection can be significantly enhanced by adding about one part fluoride to a million parts of water.

Although excessive amounts of fluoride in the water can cause discoloration of the teeth, with the currently recommended amount no problems have been encountered. The World Health Organization fully supports the convincing evidence that fluoridation of water is a safe method of controlling tooth decay in children.

fluoroscope A diagnostic device consisting of a screen covered with a crystalline substance that lights up when exposed to x-rays. When a patient stands between the x-ray beam and the fluorescent screen, a radiologist can observe the outline of the internal organs and note their movement.
SEE ALSO *barium sulfate, radiopaque*

folic acid One of the B vitamins, considered significant in the human diet. Good sources include liver, yeast, and green leafy vegetables. A gross deficiency of folic acid can result in *pernicious anemia*.

follicle Any of various tiny cavities, sacs, or glands of the body, some of which produce secretions.
SEE ALSO *Graafian follicle, hair follicle*

folliculitis Inflammation of one or more follicles, especially *hair follicles*, due to infection, friction, or irritation. It is characterized by the appearance of yellow pus spots with a surrounding red rim.

Folliculitis caused by infection

usually produces pain and swelling. If the top part of the hair follicle is involved, a pus spot appears. But if the infection is deep in the follicle, a nodule is produced which may discharge and bleed and leave a scar on healing. Should this occur in the scalp, some permanent damage to the hair follicles may follow, with hair loss or baldness *(alopecia)* in the affected area.

Folliculitis of the beard area in men, caused by infection, is fairly common and can be spread by shaving. This is often difficult to eradicate and may result in warty swellings of the skin surrounded by many small pus spots.

fontanell The soft spot or membrane-covered space between the yet unjoined separate bones of the skull in the fetus and infant. All the fontanels become ossified (turn to bone) by the age of eighteen months.

Food and Drug Administration (FDA) A federal agency of the United States government responsible for protecting the public health. It is headed by a commissioner and consists of six major divisions. One of these, the Bureau of Drugs, evaluates the safety and effectiveness of pharmaceutical products available with and without prescription.

food poisoning An acute illness caused by eating food that has been contaminated with bacteria or food that contains natural poisons, as do some mushrooms. The signs and symptoms usually occur within a few hours of eating and typically include nausea, vomiting, diarrhea, fever, and, in severe cases, collapse.

Diarrhea and vomiting may drain the body of fluids and essential mineral salts, which must be replaced by drinking meat or vegetable extracts or citrus fruit juices.
SEE *botulism, salmonellosis*

forceps Any of various types and sizes of surgical instruments used to grasp or hold tissues, parts, needles, suture material or to assist in childbirth (obstetrical forceps).

forensic medicine The branch of medical science concerned with the legal aspects of medicine, such as determining criminal involvement in suspected unnatural deaths (poisoning or other concealed forms of murder). Forensic scientists, who need not be physicians although they must be highly qualified and experienced in one or more biomedical fields, are also called upon to analyze and identify samples of body tissues, fluids, bloodstains, and hairs.

frostbite Damage to the skin caused by exposure to extreme cold; it mainly affects the extremities: nose, fingers, and toes.
SEE *gangrene*

fulminating Occurring suddenly and with great intensity; rapid. The word is used to describe the onset or course of a disease or its symptoms,

functional disease

indicating a severe worsening or deterioration in the patient's condition.

functional disease Any disease or disorder in which the function of an organ or part is disrupted but in which no physical (organic) damage can be observed; inorganic disease. COMPARE *organic disease*

fungus A primitive and simple form of vegetable life that includes molds, mushrooms, yeasts, and mildews. Not all are harmful to the body and only a few are capable of infecting the skin. The parasitic fungi most often responsible for skin disorders are those that cause *ringworm (tinea)*, a general term that includes fungus infections of the feet (athlete's foot), hands, nails, scalp, and groin.

Ringworm infections are caused by several types of parasitic fungi that are spread by contact with an infected person or contaminated objects (it has nothing at all to do with worms). Itching and redness (inflammation) are the most common first signs.

Early treatment, which includes medical preparations and washing of the affected area, will usually clear up the infection within two to four weeks. Medicated powders or ointments are available without a prescription; these may help relieve the itching and keep the area dry. If the symptoms persist a physician should be consulted so that more effective treatment can be prescribed. SEE ALSO *actinomycosis*

furuncle A boil. Bacteria that invade the protective barrier of the skin through a break in the surface can cause a wide range of skin disorders. Some bacteria attack the hair follicles or oil-secreting glands and cause a localized infection that becomes red, tender, and filled with pus. Such furuncles are normally not serious and in most cases disappear spontaneously after a short time.

If a furuncle persists or becomes larger it is best to have a physician pierce it to release the pus and apply a dressing. Furuncles should never be picked at, squeezed, or pierced at home; this may result in spreading the bacteria to other sites, including the bloodstream, and could lead to blood poisoning.

Such infections are less likely to occur if proper hygiene is maintained.

furunculosis A bacterial infection of the skin characterized by the outbreak of boils *(furuncles)*.

G

gallbladder The organ attached beneath the *liver* that stores *bile* before its release into the first part of the small intestine (duodenum).

The gallbladder is a pearshaped sac approximately 3 inches (7.6 cm) long situated under the right lobe of the liver. It acts as a reservoir for bile, a thick brown or greenish yellow fluid produced by the liver. Bile aids in the digestion of fatty foods by breaking up the fat into tiny droplets.

Bile is forced out of the gallbladder as the sac contracts in response to the stimulus of food in the duodenum. It travels through the narrow neck of the sac (cystic duct) and joins other ducts from the liver (hepatic ducts) to form the common bile duct.

The gallbladder is not essential for life. Even without it (as in surgical removal) bile finds its way into the small intestine, although not as efficiently. The gallbladder stores and concentrates bile; it does not produce it.

SEE ALSO *cholecystectomy, cholecystitis, cholelithiasis*

gallstones *Calculi* in the *gallbladder.*
SEE *cholelithiasis*

gamma globulin A general term for any of various proteins produced in the *lymphatic system, bone marrow,* and *spleen,* associated with the formation of *antibodies.* Gamma globulins circulate in the blood and are important in the body's ability to resist infection.

gangrene Death of tissue in a circumscribed area, usually as the result of an inadequate blood supply. Gangrene involves the death of a relatively large area of tissue—enough to be clearly visible—and is accompanied by degenerative changes and decay caused by *bacteria* in the affected part. It can be caused by a severe injury, frostbite, burns or caustic chemicals, certain forms of poisoning, kidney disease, diabetes mellitus, or various diseases of the blood vessels. Gangrene is seen in two basic forms, dry and moist; the moist form is by far the more serious.

Dry gangrene occurs if the dead area of tissue is dry or is kept dry, in which case there may be no spread beyond the immediate area. A sharp line of demarcation appears between it and the healthy tissue, which continues to receive an adequate blood supply. The area of dead tissue is separated from the healthy tissue by a red ring of inflammation. In many cases the dead part becomes "mummified" and eventually drops off or separates from the healthy tissues. Dry gangrene is often seen in elderly persons with severe blood circulation problems.

Moist or wet gangrene is accompanied by decay or putrefaction of the dead part, which is swollen and discolored. The bacterial infection that causes the decay may cause the dead tissues to have an extremely unpleasant odor. The line of demarcation between the dead and the healthy tissues is not as sharp as in dry gangrene. Moist gangrene may spread fairly quickly and pose a serious threat to life. In addition, bacteria may enter the bloodstream and cause generalized poisoning (*septicemia*) of the body.

Moist gangrene can sometimes be controlled with prompt medical treatment, including the prescription of antibiotics and other drugs. The physician attempts to keep the area dry in the hope that the gangrene will be restricted to a limited area. If this is not possible, the only choice is surgical removal of the affected part at a point above the gangrenous area where the blood circulation is unimpaired.

Gangrene usually affects the toes or feet, but it can also occur in other areas, including the intestines.
SEE ALSO *necrosis*

gastrectomy Surgical removal of all or part of the stomach. Partial gastrectomy is sometimes necessary in the treatment of a severe case of *peptic ulcer* or stomach cancer.

gastric Relating to the stomach.

gastric juice A clear and highly acidic fluid produced by various glands in the walls of the stomach. It plays a major role in the digestion of food. Its constituents include the enzymes pepsin, mucin, and rennin, and *hydrochloric acid.*

gastrin A *hormone* secreted by glands in the lower part of the stomach. Its major role is to stimulate the secretion of *hydrochloric acid* and other digestive juices in response to the presence of food in the stomach.

gastritis Inflammation of the stomach lining. It may flare up suddenly (acute gastritis) following the excessive consumption of alcohol, coffee, highly spiced or indigestible foods, or after eating food that is contaminated with harmful (pathogenic) bacteria. Gastritis can also occur after taking certain drugs, especially aspirin, in those who are particularly sensitive. Gastritis can also be an accompanying feature of an acute illness such as a viral infection.

Symptoms and signs of acute gastritis include a sensation of fullness, nausea, and vomiting. In children gastritis may be caused by swallowing harmful or corrosive chemicals. Part of the stomach lining may be worn away, resulting in the vomiting of small amounts of blood (which is often also the case in persons with gastritis caused by aspirin sensitivity. In severe cases the condition requires immediate medical attention.

If it is known that the cause of acute gastritis is the swallowing of a corrosive substance (alkalies or lye, strychnine, strong acids, cleaning fluid, or petroleum distillates such as kerosene, gasoline, coal oil, fuel oil, or paint thinner), it is essential not to induce vomiting, which may further damage the mouth or esophagus. Call a physician or hospital emergency room at once for advice.

Prolonged inflammation of the stomach lining (chronic gastritis) often has no troublesome signs or symptoms, although the patient may complain of mild nausea and discomfort after eating. The condition is frequently associated with indigestion or appears to be similar to such symptoms. The cause is often unknown but may be related to prolonged use of aspirin, *pernicious anemia,* or the flow of bile salts back into the stomach from the first part of the small intestine.

The effective treatment of many types of chronic gastritis is difficult or impossible. Modifications in diet may be helpful, as may the taking of an antacid. Some cases of chronic gastritis may require the administration of vitamin B_{12} to prevent pernicious anemia.

The diagnosis of chronic gastritis may require an analysis of the *gastric juices,* examination of the stomach lining *(gastroscopy),* and a *biopsy* of tissue from the stomach lining.

gastroenteritis Inflammation of the stomach and intestines.
SEE *colitis, enteritis, gastritis, ileitis*

gastroenterology The branch of medical science concerned with the diagnosis and treatment of diseases and disorders that affect the stomach, intestines, and associated structures. A specialist in this field is known as a gastroenterologist.

gastroenterostomy The surgical formation of a new passage between the stomach and the small intestine, usually the jejunum. It may be performed to bypass a seriously damaged or permanently obstructed part of the pylorus or duodenum, the structures that form the beginning of the small intestine.

gastrointestinal Relating to the *stomach* and *intestines.*

gastrointestinal series
SEE *GI series*

gastroscopy A diagnostic procedure in which the lining of the stomach is examined with a gastroscope, a slender flexible instrument equipped with its own light source. It is passed into the stomach by means of the mouth, throat, and esophagus, usually after the patient has been given a local anesthetic.

generic Relating to the chemical name (as opposed to the brand name) of a drug or pharmaceutical product. For example, acetaminophen is the generic (chemical) name of the over-the-counter *analgesic* and *antipyretic* available under such brand names as Datril and Tylenol. Ampicillin is the generic name of an antibiotic available only with a prescription; it too is available under several brand names, including Penbritin and Totacillin.

In most cases the cost of generic prescription and over-the-counter drugs is significantly less than that of brand-name products. However, not all brand-name prescription drugs are available under their chemical names, often because the manufacturer holds a current patent granting exclusive right to manufacture and sell a drug under a brand name for a given number of years. When the patent expires, any company can manufacture the drug under its generic name or under a new brand name, with the approval of the Food and Drug Administration.

genes Tiny particles, normally found in pairs, occupying a specific position on a *chromosome*, capable of self-reproduction. They transmit hereditary traits from one generation to the next.

genitourinary Relating to the reproductive and urinary systems or to their organs or parts.

genus A term used in the biological classification of plants and animals to distinguish groups of organisms that are more closely related than members of a family (the next most general classification) but are not as alike as those of a *species*, members of which are usually capable of interbreeding.

geriatrics The branch of medicine concerned with the study and treatment of diseases that affect the elderly and the special problems of medical care in old age. A specialist in this field is known as a geriatrician.
COMPARE *gerontology*

German measles
SEE *rubella*

gerontology The branch of medical science concerned with the study of the aging process and the social and health problems of the elderly.
COMPARE *geriatrics*

gigantism Abnormal enlargement or overgrowth of the entire body or a limb, caused by an overproduction of growth hormone by the *pituitary gland*. Gigantism is distinguished from *acromegaly* in that the overactivity of the pituitary gland begins before puberty, when the long bones of the body are not fully developed. In extreme cases the patient may grow to a height of over eight feet.

gingivitis Inflammation of the gingivae (gums), a common condition caused by dental *plaque*, the invisible film of bacteria that accumulates on the surface of uncleaned teeth after twenty-four hours. Chemical irritants produced by plaque enter the gums by way of the shallow crevices at the junction of the gums and teeth; food debris also accumulates, and eventually hard deposits of *calculus* (tartar) form on the teeth.

Gingivitis causes the gums to become red and swollen and appear smooth or glossy; they tend to bleed easily, especially when brushing or eating hard foods. The bleeding may discourage the patient from brushing effectively, and plaque and food debris accumulate to make the condition worse. An unpleasant taste and halitosis (bad breath) may be noticeable. Persistent gingivitis requires a dentist's advice and treatment. If untreated, it can result in teeth falling out.

GI series Short for gastrointestinal series; a two-part diagnostic technique or procedure in which x-rays are taken of the stomach and small intestines after the patient swallows a mixture of *barium sulfate,* a *radiopaque* substance that makes the digestive tract clearly visible on x-ray film or a *fluoroscope* screen, and x-rays are taken of the large intestine or colon after giving the patient a barium enema. Such studies may reveal the presence of tumors, intestinal obstruction, ulcers, or other abnormalities.

gland Any of the various secreting organs situated throughout the body. *Exocrine glands* have ducts that empty their secretions onto the body surface or into a cavity, as do sweat glands and sebaceous glands, while *endocrine glands* have no ducts and secrete *hormones* directly into the blood-stream.

glans The rounded end of the penis (glans penis) or the head of the clitoris (glans clitoridis). Both are extremely sensitive to touch or friction and play a key role in stimulating *orgasm*.

glaucoma A disease of the eye caused by abnormally high fluid pressure within the eyeball. It is not related to blood pressure.

The space between the cornea and the lens of the eye is filled with a watery fluid known as the aqueous humor. Under normal conditions this fluid is constantly produced and then drained off through channels that empty into the optic veins. If too much fluid is produced or if the drainage channels are blocked or excessively narrowed, the fluid tends

glioma

to collect inside the eyeball and exert high pressure on the retina and optic nerve. If untreated, the pressure can cause permanent damage to the eye and result in partial or total blindness.

In cases of suspected glaucoma or as a general screening procedure, an ophthalmologist measures the pressure exerted by this fluid by means of an instrument called a tonometer placed against the cornea. This is an absolutely painless procedure because anesthetic eyedrops are first placed in the eyes.

There are two general types of glaucoma, although physicians sometimes classify the disease into several distinct categories. In one form the pressure within the eyeball suddenly increases (acute or subacute glaucoma). The eye is red and quite painful and vision may become blurred or misty. Sometimes lights appear to have a halo around them. Severe cases of an acute attack may be accompanied by nausea, vomiting, and severe headache; in such cases a physician should be consulted immediately. In the chronic form of glaucoma, which is more common, the disease may develop over a period of several years before a marked change in vision is noted.

The danger is that permanent damage to the retina or optic nerve may occur before the condition is diagnosed. It is therefore important, especially in those over forty, to have regular eye examinations. Tests of the field of vision are also helpful to the physician in determining the extent of possible damage.

Treatment of glaucoma depends largely on the type and severity. The physician may prescribe eyedrops or recommend a simple operation to reduce the pressure within the eyeball. The early detection of glaucoma usually leads to successful treatment or the arrest of the condition before serious damage occurs.

glioma A tumor of the connective tissue (glia) of the brain or spinal cord. Unlike other cancers, gliomas do not spread.

globulin Any one of a group of proteins found in the blood. The best known is *gamma globulin*, important in the formation of antibodies.

glomerulonephritis Inflammation of the filtering units (glomeruli) of the *kidneys*. The disease may be acute or chronic.

Acute glomerulonephritis is most often associated with a previous bacterial infection, especially a streptococcal one involving the throat, sinuses, or tonsils. Most researchers believe that the bacteria themselves do not cause the kidney inflammation (bacteria are rarely found at the site), but that they somehow disturb the body's natural defense system (*immunological* disturbance).

In nearly every case, signs of the disease will include both blood and protein in the urine (hematuria and albuminuria). The output of urine is reduced and the patient may show signs of facial puffiness and swelling around the eyelids. Pain in the small of the back and nausea and vomiting are also quite common. In severe cases blood pressure may be extremely high and the patient may experience shortness of breath on exertion.

Treatment primarily involves bed rest and the elimination of any current streptococcal infection with penicillin or other appropriate antibiotics. The physician may also recommend a salt-free diet and a temporary reduction in water intake. Possible complications are treated individually, such as the prescription of diuretics to control the excessive accumulation of fluids in the tissues *(edema)* or drugs to reduce high blood pressure.

Most patients make a full recovery, although in a few cases the urine will continue to show traces of blood and contain other abnormal sediments. The outlook depends largely on the original severity of the disease and the prompt initiation of treatment.

glossitis Inflammation of the tongue. The tongue is typically very sore, inflamed, and may be smooth and swollen. Among the many possible causes are anemia (particularly affecting women of childbearing age), a fungal infection, or a deficiency of B vitamins. Treatment is aimed at the underlying cause.

glottis The part of the *larynx* concerned with sound production. It consists of the two vocal cords and the space between them.
COMPARE *epiglottis*

glucose A simple sugar produced in the body by the partial breakdown of starch. It is the body's principal source of energy. Liquid glucose is often mixed with water for intravenous feeding.

glucose tolerance test A test used in the diagnosis of *diabetes mellitus*. The patient is given instructions about the type and amount of food to eat for three days before the test; no food may be eaten the night before the test. On the day of the test, an initial blood sample is taken (usually from a vein in the arm) to determine the fasting sugar level. The patient is then asked to swallow a solution of sugar and water, following which further blood samples are taken at intervals of approximately thirty minutes for the next two hours. The amount of sugar in the blood at each stage of the test gives the physician a good indication of the severity of the condition.

glycogen A complex carbohydrate (starch) made in the body from chains of *glucose*. It is stored in the liver and (to a lesser extent) muscles, and it is converted back into glucose when energy or heat is needed.

glycosuria The presence of sugar in the urine. It is one sign of *diabetes mellitus*.

goiter An abnormal enlargement of the *thyroid gland*. It is generally

101

associated with overactivity of the thyroid gland in secreting an excessive amount of hormones (except for simple goiter, which results from a lack of dietary iodine). In advanced cases of *hyperthyroidism* the thyroid gland may swell to several times its normal size and be seen as a large growth (goiter) over the front of the throat. The size of the goiter does not bear a direct relationship to the severity of the disease. In some severe cases of hyperthyroidism (or thyrotoxicosis) the thyroid gland remains nearly its normal size although it may feel somewhat hard or lumpy on physical examination.

Treatment often involves surgical removal of most of the thyroid gland *(thyroidectomy)*.

SEE *Graves' disease*

gonad The sex glands of both the female and male: an *ovary* or a *testicle*.

gonadotropin Any of several hormones secreted by the *pituitary gland* (anterior pituitary gonadotropins) or the placenta (chorionic gonadotropins) that stimulate the *ovaries* or *testicles*.

gonorrhea An infectious disease contracted during sexual intercourse with an infected partner; a very common *venereal disease*. It is caused by the gonococcus bacteria, which do not survive long outside the body. For this reason, it is quite rare to contract the disease from contaminated linen, towels, or toilet seats. The incubation period varies from about two to ten days.

In men, symptoms include a burning sensation when urinating and slight soreness or irritation of the end of the penis. This is caused by infection and inflammation of the end of the urethra, the passage through which urine is conveyed from the bladder. If not treated, the infection continues to spread backward along the urethra. This inflammation (urethritis) causes a sense of frequency and urgency in having to urinate.

At first a thin liquid discharge is seen around the tip of the penis. After a few days this may become thicker and creamy; it represents the discharge of pus from the inflamed passage. If the infection spreads to the testicles it may result in sterility, the inability to produce healthy sperm cells.

In women, the first indications of gonorrhea are usually painful and frequent urination and a milky or creamy discharge from the vagina. However, many women have no early signs or symptoms. In severe and untreated cases the infection may spread to the uterus and Fallopian tubes.

In both sexes, an untreated case of gonorrhea occasionally results in complications such as painful inflammation of the joints (arthritis), inflammation of the membrane that lines the eyelids and covers the eyeball (conjunctivitis), and inflammation of the lining membrane of the heart and its valves (endocarditis).

Treatment with penicillin or

other antibiotics (and sometimes sulfonamides) is usually effective in curing the disease, especially if administered early enough. Since one attack of gonorrhea does not provide future protection *(immunity)*, it is essential to take precautions against reinfection. Any sexual partner should seek immediate medical treatment.

The use of a prophylactic sheath (condom) may minimize the risk of spreading the infection, but is by no means reliable protection against gonorrhea.

SEE ALSO *syphilis*

gout A metabolic disorder in which *uric acid*, a waste product, accumulates in body tissues. It is characterized by extremely painful inflammation of one or more joints, typically the large toe.

The signs and symptoms of gout (gouty arthritis) are caused by the presence of too much uric acid; it is normally flushed out of the body in urine. Crystals of uric acid are deposited in and around movable joints, causing excruciating pain and subsequent acute inflammation and possible deformity. In some cases of chronic gout these crystals enter the soft tissues of the body, forming a deposit called a *tophus*. One site where they often form is the fleshy rim of the ear; other likely sites are the knees and elbows.

An acute attack of gout comes on suddenly, often during sleep. It may affect any joint, but those most commonly involved are the large toe, heel, and knee. The joint is usually red, swollen, and shiny and is so painful that even a light covering may be unbearable. In many cases there may be related factors in an acute attack, such as a minor injury to the foot or overindulgence in food or alcohol.

At one time it was thought that the primary cause of gout was related to eating rich foods or drinking port wine. It is now known that dietary factors are relatively unimportant and that the disorder is caused either by an overproduction of uric acid or a failure of the *kidneys* to excrete uric acid in sufficient quantities.

If gout is undiagnosed and untreated, a potentially serious complication may occur—the formation of kidney stones. For the crystals of uric acid that are deposited in the joints can also be deposited in the kidneys. Should this occur, the ability of the kidneys to function normally can be seriously impaired.

Fortunately, most cases of gout are diagnosed relatively early (by examination of a blood sample, which reveals the presence of uric acid in high concentrations) and treatment is started to prevent the formation of uric acid crystals. This treatment is fairly straightforward and is a good example of the development of a specific pharmaceutical product, allopurinol, to control a specific disorder. Most cases of primary gout (gout not a result of another disorder) cannot be cured in the strict sense, but the

Graafian follicle

drugs that are available to control gout are dramatic and virtually immediate in their beneficial effects.

In the case of an acute attack, the pain can be relieved by taking certain potent antiinflammatory drugs, such as phenylbutazone. Further attacks can be prevented or minimized by taking drugs that hasten the excretion of uric acid through the kidneys (uricosuric drugs) or those such as allopurinol that interfere with the formation of uric acid. To prevent the recurrence of an acute attack and minimize the danger of uric acid stones forming in the kidneys, these drugs are usually taken for life.

SEE ALSO *hyperuricemia*

Graafian follicle A small sac or vesicle formed in the *ovary*, containing an ovum. Only one of these follicles matures each month during the menstrual cycle and releases an ovum, which then enters the Fallopian tube.

graft The transplantation of healthy tissue (such as skin or bone) from one part of the body to replace similar but diseased or otherwise defective tissue in another part of the body (autograft). When the transplantation tissue is taken from another human subject it is known as a homograft; if it comes from another species (more commonly performed in animal experiments) it is known as a heterograft.

SEE ALSO *skin grafts*

grand mal A major epileptic seizure.

COMPARE *petit mal*
SEE *epilepsy*

Graves' disease A disease characterized by enlargement of the *thyroid gland, goiter,* and bulging eyes *(exophthalmos)* caused by oversecretion of thyroid hormones. It is named after the Irish physician Robert J. Graves (1797-1853).

SEE *hyperthyroidism*

gynecology The branch of medical science concerned with the diagnosis and treatment of diseases that affect women. A specialist in this field is known as a gynecologist.

gynecomastia Abnormal enlargement of one or both male breasts. The condition may arise in normal boys at puberty and usually subsides spontaneously (without treatment) after about six to twelve months. Its occurrence in later life may be a sign of some disorder of the testicles or adrenal glands.

H

habituation A psychological dependence on a substance or drug. COMPARE *addiction*

hair follicle A depression or indentation of the surface of the skin from which a hair develops. Each follicle produces one hair. The base of the follicle is supplied with blood vessels and nerves, but the hair itself is made up of dead cells filled with a tough protein called keratin.

Hair follicles show intermittent activity; each hair grows to a maximum length, is retained for a time without further growth, and is eventually shed and replaced.

An adult probably has about five million hair follicles, of which about one million are on the head. No new follicles develop after birth, so damage to follicles as the result of skin disease or scars from accidents leads to a permanent loss of hair. As a person gets older, he or she loses some active hair follicles and the hairs they produce. Some people lose them before others, depending largely on hereditary factors.
SEE ALSO *alopecia, follicle*

Hashimoto's disease A disease of the *thyroid gland* characterized by a particular type of *goiter*. As the disease (also called autoimmune thyroiditis and chronic lymphocytic thyroiditis) progresses and involves more of the thyroid, the gland fails to secrete an adequate amount of hormone. The cause is thought to be related to a disorder of the body's natural system of *immunity*; it is an *autoimmune disease* in which the thyroid gland is treated like a foreign body. Middle-aged women are more prone to the disease than men and children.

This chronic form of inflammation affecting the thyroid gland (thyroiditis) is named after the Japanese surgeon Hakura Hashimoto (1881–1934). Treatment is aimed at replacing the thyroid hormone, which will usually shrink the

heart

goiter. In most cases treatment continues for the rest of the patient's life. Surgical treatment is rarely necessary.
SEE ALSO *hypothyroidism*

heart A hollow muscular organ, traditionally described as the size of a clenched fist, that contains four chambers. The two chambers on the right, the right atrium and right ventricle, receive oxygen-depleted blood from two large *veins* and pump it into the lungs. After picking up a fresh supply of oxygen the blood passes through the two chambers on the left side of the heart, the left atrium and left ventricle, where oxygen-rich blood is pumped out through the *aorta* (the largest *artery* in the body) and arterial system to every organ and tissue of the body.

The chambers on the right side of the heart are connected by means of a flap of tissue with three little cusps or points (tricuspid valve), which acts as a one-way valve to prevent a backflow of blood. The chambers on the left side are connected by a flap of tissue with two cusps (bicuspid or mitral valve). These valves ensure that blood always flows in the proper direction through the heart.

The inner walls of the heart and the heart valves are lined with a smooth membrane (endocardium). Between this and the outer walls is a thick muscular layer (myocardium). The entire heart is enclosed in a double-walled moist membrane (pericardium) that reduces friction of the beating heart.

One part of the heart muscle, the *pacemaker*, embedded in the wall of the right atrium, is specialized to coordinate the pumping action. An electrical impulse sent out from the pacemaker in a rising and falling wave causes the heart chambers to contract. This action forces blood out of the heart and into the lungs (on the right side) and out of the heart into the arteries (on the left side).

About seventy times a minute, blood is pumped from a healthy heart to all tissues of the body and back again. This is the main circulation. A second and smaller circulation (but just as important) takes blood to and from the lungs.
SEE ALSO *capillary, cardiac arrest, cardiac catheterization, cardiology, cardiomyopathy, coronary, coronary artery disease*

heart attack
SEE *coronary, coronary artery disease, coronary occlusion, coronary thrombosis, myocardial infarction*

heartburn A burning sensation in the chest (having nothing to do with the heart) caused by some of the stomach's acid contents flowing upward into the lower part of the esophagus. Technically known as pyrosis, it is one sign of indigestion, which can usually be relieved by taking an antacid.

heart failure A condition in which the heart fails to pump an adequate amount of blood through the arteries and veins. A serious defect or disease of the heart muscle (myocardium), the valves of the heart, or the major blood vessels may eventually result in a deficiency of blood being circulated to the organs and tissues of the body.

In heart failure one or more chambers of the heart may not completely empty of blood with each heartbeat (congestive heart failure). This residual blood tends to stretch the walls of the chambers and may lead to a gradual enlargement of the heart (cardiomegaly), often with a thickening of the walls. The heart may also begin to fail due to the increased workload of pumping against the pressure caused by narrowed and inelastic arteries *(arteriosclerosis* or *atherosclerosis)*, which most commonly occurs in the elderly. Abnormally high blood pressure (hypertension) may force the heart to increase its pumping action, which in turn maintains or increases the already high blood pressure.

The person with a failing heart may experience shortness of breath (dyspnea) on exertion, a little swelling at the ankles (edema), and occasionally a sensation of the heartbeat (palpitations). In more severe cases there may be a sudden sense of suffocation (especially at night), wheezing, sweating, and sometimes the coughing up of watery, bubbly sputum. To help relieve these obviously distressing symptoms, the physician may recommend a limit to physical activity and a restricted food intake if the patient is obese. If swelling of the tissues is a problem, a diuretic may be prescribed to rid the body of excess fluids. In many cases digoxin is prescribed to help improve the efficiency of the heart's pumping action.
COMPARE *cardiac arrest*

heart-lung machine A device used in open surgery on the heart that allows the blood to bypass the heart completely while still maintaining its oxygenation and circulation to all organs and tissues. This technique or procedure is used so the heart can be stopped during surgery.

Most of the delicate internal repairs on the heart that are common today would be impossible without the heart-lung machine. This device takes blood from the veins, supplies it with oxygen, rewarms it to body temperature, filters it, and pumps it back into the aorta and coronary arteries at the proper pressure.

heart massage Emergency treatment to restart the beating of the heart by massaging or compressing the exposed heart during chest surgery or by pressing firmly and regularly on the chest; a procedure that demands training to avoid injuring the patient.
SEE *cardiopulmonary resuscitation*

heart murmur Any abnormal sound heard (usually through a stethoscope) from the *heart*. This is often absolutely harmless, but on occasion it is the first sign of some physical defect in the heart or its valves.

A murmur is not one specific sound but any of various sounds that may be related to an abnormal contraction or relaxation of the heart, defective opening or closing of the heart valves, or the vibration of the blood as it enters and leaves the heart chambers. Thousands of people live full and active lives with some form of heart murmur without requiring medical or surgical treatment of any kind.

heatstroke
SEE *sunstroke*

Heimlich maneuver A potentially lifesaving technique or procedure for the emergency treatment of a person who shows signs of choking because the trachea is obstructed by food or some other foreign body. Often the victim will display the "choking sign" by grabbing at his or her throat. Since the trachea is obstructed, a choking victim (unlike a heart-attack victim) will not be able to speak. Any delay in applying the Heimlich maneuver may result in the death of the victim.

Although it is difficult to learn this technique from any book, it basically involves the following steps: wrap arms around the victim's waist, make a fist and place the thumb just above the navel and below the ribs, grasp the fist with the other hand and press into the victim's abdomen with a quick upward thrust. If the force of air thus expelled from the lungs does not dislodge the food particle or foreign object, repeat the procedure several times if necessary.

If the choking victim is sitting down, stand or kneel behind him or her and perform the steps exactly as outlined above. If the victim is lying down or has fallen, turn the victim's face upward and kneel astride the victim's hips, face to face. Place one hand on top of the other, with the heel of the bottom hand on the victim's abdomen just above the navel and below the ribs. Press into the victim's abdomen with a quick upward thrust. Repeat several times if necessary.

Many American restaurants now display details of the Heimlich maneuver with helpful illustrations. The procedure is named after the American physician Henry J. Heimlich, who first described it in 1974.
SEE ALSO *cardiopulmonary resuscitation*

hemangioma A benign (harmless) tumor of the blood vessels, especially the capillaries (capillary hemangioma). It typically forms a raised bright or dark red patch on the skin and represents a type of birthmark.
SEE *angioma*

hematocrit A diagnostic *blood test* used to determine the percentage of red blood cells (erythrocytes) after a sample of blood has been spun around at high speed in a centrifuge. It is used together with other blood tests in the diagnosis of conditions such as *anemia* (suggested by a low hematocrit) and *polycythemia* (suggested by a high hematocrit).

The values of the test results vary considerably. However, the normal range for men is between 42 and 54 percent; the normal range for women is between 38 and 46 percent.

hematology The branch of medical science concerned with the blood, blood-forming tissues (bone marrow), and diseases and disorders that affect the blood. A specialist in this field is known as a hematologist.

hematoma A swelling composed of dried or clotted blood. It can occur at the site of any injury in which blood vessels are broken. A common example is a bruise, which is a hematoma caused by the rupture of the tiny blood vessels (capillaries) just beneath the skin. A more serious site is between the outer covering membrane of the brain (dura) and the surface of the brain; this is called a subdural hematoma. If such blood clots do not resolve spontaneously, and if they cause problems because of the pressure they exert on the brain, they may have to be removed surgically.
Compare *ecchymosis, extravasation*

hematuria The presence of blood in the urine. Among the many possible causes, the likeliest is a disease or injury to the kidneys or bladder.

hemochromatosis A disorder that is caused by the accumulation of *iron* in body tissues. It can lead to *cirrhosis* from iron deposits in the liver, *diabetes* from iron overload in the pancreas, and various disturbances of heart function including *arrhythmia* and congestive *heart failure*. The skin typically takes on a bronze pigmentation.

The underlying cause is sometimes unknown (idiopathic hemochromatosis), although a *hereditary* basis is suspected. In other cases the cause is a disorder of the blood-forming tissues (erythropoietic hemochromatosis), a liver malfunction that promotes absorption of iron or impairs the body's normal use of iron (hepatic hemochromatosis), or (rarely) the excessive ingestion of dietary iron or iron supplements over prolonged periods.

Primary treatment is aimed at removing excess iron from the blood by means of *phlebotomy*, the opening of a vein to withdraw blood.
Compare *hemosiderosis*

hemodialysis A procedure used to purify the blood of patients with *kidney failure*. When the function of both *kidneys* becomes impaired so that the waste products of metabolism accumulate in the circulating blood instead of being filtered out and eliminated from the body in urine, life is directly threatened if the patient does not receive prompt treatment. This may involve either the surgical transplant of a donor kidney (kidney transplant) or the periodic use of an artificial kidney ("kidney machine"), known as a hemodialyzer.

The artificial kidney works on the principle of osmosis through a semipermeable membrane. The patient's blood passes on one side of a membrane while a solution of the dialyzing fluid flows in the opposite direction on the other side. Particles dissolved in the blood pass through the membrane, which is just porous enough for them to pass. This continues until the concentration of the waste products in the blood is the same as that of the dialyzing fluid (which is controlled). This provides the filtration of the blood normally performed by healthy kidneys. The procedure is sometimes referred to simply as *dialysis*.

There are different types of access for connecting the patient's bloodstream to the kidney machine. To maintain a good flow, blood is drawn out from an artery and returned to a vein. One way of doing this is to surgically insert two small external tubes into an artery and a neighboring vein and connect the outer ends. When the machine is not in use the tube is kept open with a continuous flow of blood. Or an artery and a neighboring vein inside a limb can be surgically joined, in which case access is achieved by the use of two needles inserted into the vessels and removed at the end of each hemodialysis.

The average patient has to undergo hemodialysis for twenty hours a week: ten hours twice a week or six-and-a-half hours three times a week. More efficient hemodialyzers can reduce the time required. Recently, some portable machines have become available.

Unfortunately, hemodialysis in the United States is an extremely expensive procedure and equipment may not always be readily available for the thousands of patients with kidney failure who need it. The process also involves a great deal of psychological stress for the patient.

There is no satisfactory substitute for healthy kidneys. Although a kidney transplant is the ideal means to solve the problem of kidney failure (only one healthy kidney is necessary), too few donor kidneys are available. Patients who are fortunate enough to have a successful kidney transplant can avoid many of the unpleasant problems associated with long-term hemodialysis.

SEE ALSO *peritoneal dialysis*

hemoglobin The iron-containing red pigment of the red blood cells *(erythrocytes)*. Its function is to take up oxygen from the lungs and deliver it to all the organs and tissues of the body. Hemoglobin forms a loose combination with large volumes of oxygen. As is does this it changes from the dull purplish tinge of reduced hemoglobin to the bright scarlet of oxyhemoglobin. This change accounts for the difference between the dark venous blood returning to the lungs from the tissues (where it has given up its oxygen) and the bright red of arterial blood leaving the lungs loaded with oxygen.

SEE ALSO *anemia, blood test, polycythermia*

hemolytic anemia
SEE *anemia*

hemophilia A rare inherited blood disease characterized by the failure of the blood to clot as quickly as normal following a cut or other injury. This can result in potentially fatal bleeding unless the patient receives immediate medical treatment.

Hemophilia is fully manifested only in males; females are usually symptomless *carriers* of the disease. A carrier has a 50–50 chance of passing the disease to her daughters, who will themselves become carriers, and an equal chance of passing it to her sons, who will be affected by the disease. A male hemophiliac cannot pass the disease to his sons but all his daughters will be carriers.

Hemophilia is characterized by a tendency to produce large and deep-seated bruises, which occur as a result of very minor injuries. Bleeding into joints may be recurrent and, unless promptly treated, leads to crippling deformities. External bleeding may also occur from cuts and abrasions or (particularly) as a result of surgery.

Treatment of each bleeding incident involves the injection or transfusion of the missing clotting factors and should be given by a physician as soon as the bleeding occurs. Very young children must be kept under close supervision to minimize the danger of injury and older children must take great care to avoid injuries.

hemoptysis The spitting or coughing up of blood. The cause is usually bleeding into the trachea, bronchi, or lungs. The condition demands prompt medical treatment.

hemorrhage An abnormal discharge of blood within the body (internal hemorrhage) or onto the body surface from a damaged vein, artery, or the capillaries. The severity of the bleeding depends on many factors, such as the type and size of blood vessel involved and its location.

SEE ALSO *cerebral hemorrhage, stroke*

hemorrhoids A condition in which the veins just inside the anus become swollen and form an itching and often painful mass; popularly known as piles, this condition is a special example of *varicose veins.* The development of hemorrhoids is associated with straining during bowel movements, obesity, pregnancy, persistent failure to evacuate all waste matter during defecation, or (rarely) the formation of an obstructing tumor within the rectum.

111

hemosiderosis

A common sign of hemorrhoids is slight or moderate bleeding from the rectum, particularly during bowel movements. It is very important to have a physician confirm that any rectal bleeding is caused by hemorrhoids and not due to some other, more serious condition.

Hemorrhoids are generally not serious, but they are unpleasant and can be extremely painful. Treatment includes ingesting mineral oil or some other substance to soften stools and using ointments or suppositories prescribed by a physician; in severe cases, the distended veins are surgically removed (hemorrhoidectomy).

hemosiderosis A condition in which the tissues become overloaded with deposits of *iron* without an associated damage to various organs.
COMPARE *hemochromatosis*

heparin A substance produced in the liver and certain other tissues that inhibits the clotting of blood. A preparation of heparin is used by physicians as an *anticoagulant* to prevent the formation of blood clots in certain disorders or to prevent a sample of blood from clotting before it can be tested.
SEE ALSO *embolism, embolus, thrombosis, thrombus*

hepatic Relating to the liver.

hepatitis Inflammation of the *liver*. This can occur in several ways. Toxic hepatitis is the result of poisoning of the liver by chemicals such as carbon tetrachloride or other industrial solvents, drugs, or (rarely) general anesthetics. The liver can also become inflamed as the result of infection with various microorganisms, including bacteria and protozoa. But the most common cause of hepatitis is a viral infection.

Acute viral hepatitis occurs in two forms, both of which present many similar clinical problems. The two forms were previously referred to as infectious hepatitis and serum hepatitis, based on what were thought to be the two distinct routes of infection. Infectious hepatitis was thought to be transmitted solely by the drinking of water or milk or the eating of shellfish or other food that had been contaminated with infected human feces, whereas serum hepatitis was thought to be transmitted solely as the result of using contaminated needles or syringes or inadvertently using contaminated blood during blood transfusions. It is now known, however, that both forms of viral hepatitis can be transmitted to people by either the parenteral (by injection) or oral route. Although these terms are still used, many experts in diagnosing and treating liver diseases (hepatologists) now refer to hepatitis A and hepatitis B.

Hepatitis A (infectious hepatitis or short-incubation hepatitis) is more common in children and young people. It is largely transmitted orally, with an incubation

hepatitis

period of approximately two to seven weeks. It is rarely fatal and typically runs it course within a few weeks or months.

Hepatitis B (serum hepatitis or long-incubation hepatitis) is a potentially more serious form of viral hepatitis. The incubation period ranges from approximately seven to twenty-six weeks. The infecting virus usually enters the body by means of contaminated blood during a blood transfusion or as the result of using contaminated needles or syringes (a special risk for drug addicts using unsterilized needles). In both forms of acute viral hepatitis the damage to the liver is similar. However, many cases (especially those of hepatitis A) are mild, and troublesome symptoms may never develop.

The first indications of the disease typically include a general feeling of being unwell (malaise), fever, and later *jaundice*, or a yellowish discoloration of the skin and whites of the eyes. The acute forms of viral hepatitis may not progress to jaundice, especially in those who have had a previous infection and thus have at least partial immunity to the disease. The patient usually has no desire for food and may become weak and drowsy. (The early symptoms often resemble those of influenza.) The urine may appear dark or reddish and the stools take on a grayish color.

In many cases the liver and spleen become enlarged. Jaundice, if present, becomes most prominent within the first two weeks after the onset of symptoms, after which it gradually disappears as the jaundice subsides, the stools regain their normal color. In the absence of complications, patients with hepatitis A usually recover within six to eight weeks. Those with hepatitis B may not fully recover for a year or more, during which time the consumption of alcohol is prohibited to avoid further irritation of the liver.

Treatment of both forms of acute viral hepatitis demands strict bed rest; in some cases, hospitalization is required. A few patients suffer from prolonged bouts of nausea and vomiting, during which essential body fluids are lost. In such cases it may be necessary to replace the lost fluids with an intravenous glucose solution. Patients who are treated in a hospital during the period when the symptoms of hepatitis are particularly severe include the elderly, diabetics, and pregnant women.

There is no specific drug therapy for patients with viral hepatitis. Nevertheless, the outlook is favorable in the vast majority of cases, although recurrences may occur. Even a severely damaged liver has a remarkable capacity for regeneration and recovery.

Chronic hepatitis is a form of liver disease of uncertain origin, although some cases are thought to follow viral hepatitis. The condition is also known as chronic active hepatitis and is seen most frequently

hepatomegaly

in young women. The disease is characterized by an enlarged and tender liver but without the development of jaundice. The condition may clear up after several years or progress to *cirrhosis*.

hepatomegaly Abnormal enlargement of the liver.

hereditary Relating to diseases, disorders, or symptoms that are inherited or caused by genetic factors.
SEE *genes*
COMPARE *congenital, familial*

hernia The protrusion or rupture of an internal organ through the muscle layers or other structures that normally enclose it. The hernia may be caused by a congenital weakness or developmental failure of muscles that hold an organ in place, weakness of the muscles following prolonged illness, injury, obesity, sudden strain from lifting heavy loads incorrectly, or even intense coughing.

The commonest form of rupture is called inguinal hernia, which can involve the scrotum and testicles; it usually requires surgical repair.

The treatment of a hernia depends on several factors, including its severity and site, the age of the patient, and whether or not it is reducible (capable of being depressed to the level of the surrounding skin by pressing gently on the bulge). In some cases the hernia does not cause much problem: the bulge can be compressed and the otherwise protruding organ can be held in position by a support (truss or abdominal belt) worn over the bulge. A support must fit properly and be approved and prescribed by a physician. In other cases the hernia is treated surgically.

Surgery is essential in cases when a herniated section of intestine becomes compressed into a loop and its blood supply is cut off. This is known as a strangulated hernia, an extremely serious condition demanding immediate surgical repair to avert disastrous consequences.

Many cases of hernia can be prevented by sensible attention to the correct method of lifting heavy objects—keeping the back straight while squatting and lifting with the muscles of the legs and arms without tensing the abdominal muscles. People who are overweight are more likely to develop hernias because of the weakening of the abdominal muscles and the heavy load these muscles must support.
SEE ALSO *hiatus hernia*

herpes simplex An infectious disease caused by the herpes simplex virus characterized by the formation of groups of small blisters at the corners of the mouth (cold sores or fever blisters), the eyes (ocular herpes), on the genitals (herpes genitalis), or occasionally on other parts of the body.

Infants born to women with herpes genitalis may become infected during passage through the birth canal (neonatal herpes). This can lead to a potentially life-threatening inflammation of the child's brain and its covering membranes (meningoencephalitis). If genital herpes is diagnosed as being active near the time a woman is scheduled to give birth, a cesarean section is usually performed to avoid infecting the baby.

Genital herpes is a sexually transmitted *(venereal)* disease affecting both men and women. It is becoming extremely common throughout the United States. Although several drugs are being tested, at present there is no effective cure for herpes.

Genital herpes sometimes tends to come and go in those persons who become infected. It is a good idea to keep the genital area clean and dry to prevent the additional complication of a bacterial infection and to consult an appropriate specialist (a gynecologist or urologist). The use of a prophylactic sheath (condom) during sexual intercourse may minimize the risk of spreading the infection.

The diagnosis of genital herpes can be difficult, especially for a physician who does not specialize in such disorders.

Herpes simplex infections are often referred to simply as "herpes." It should not be confused with a totally different disease, *herpes zoster.*

herpes zoster An acute infection of the central nervous system, commonly called shingles, caused by the same virus responsible for chickenpox. The virus typically attacks the roots of sensory nerves just outside the spinal cord and causes pain, which is followed a few days later by a red rash and then the eruption of blisters (vesicles) along the course of the affected nerve. Within a week or so the tiny clusters of blisters start to dry up and form scabs. Since the virus attacks one nerve or group of nerves, the rash and blisters typically appear only on one side of the body or one limb.

Complications following an attack of shingles are relatively rare and most patients recover completely within about two to five weeks. As with chickenpox, one attack normally provides lasting immunity against future attacks. The elderly are most likely to suffer from a severe infection than are younger people.

No known specific medical treatment for shingles exists. Analgesics or *corticosteroids* are often prescribed to relieve irritation and pain. If the eyes are involved, a physician will probably prescribe eyedrops.

As with most viral infections, shingles is a self-limiting infection in almost every case—that is, the virus runs its own course, and only symptomatic relief is possible. Antibiotics are basically ineffective against the virus but are sometimes used to control associated bacterial infections. COMPARE *herpes simplex*

hiatus hernia An abnormal condition in which a portion of the top part of the stomach protrudes up into the chest through a gap (hiatus) in the diaphragm. Hiatus hernia (or hiatal hernia) has nothing at all to do with an ordinary *hernia*.

The diaphragm forms a thin muscular dome separating the chest cavity from the abdomen. It has three natural openings; through two of these pass the largest artery and the largest vein, and through the third passes the esophagus.

In some persons the gap through which the esophagus passes may become abnormally enlarged because of muscular weakness in the diaphragm or a congenital deformity. Occasionally, prolonged violent coughing can weaken the muscles surrounding the opening. When this happens, the upper part of the stomach may be pushed up through the weakened opening or aperture. It is a fairly common condition in persons of middle or old age, especially in those who are severely overweight.

Hiatus hernia often presents no serious symptoms but they can include pain in the upper part of the abdomen (which is made worse by lying down), a feeling of abdominal swelling, and heartburn (pyrosis) caused by the stomach's acid contents flowing up into the esophagus and irritating its sensitive lining. Relief may often come from simple measures like raising the head of the bed, avoiding bending down, and not wearing tight undergarments that constrict the abdomen.

It is important to see a physician at the start of any troublesome symptoms. In most cases he or she may suggest a change in diet to blander foods, a reduction in the amount of food consumed at a single meal, the use of antacids to control excess stomach acidity, and weight loss.

high blood pressure
SEE *hypertension*

histamine A substance normally present in the cells of animals and plants. In humans it is concentrated largely in those tissues that have a direct or indirect contact with the air: skin, lining of the nose, lungs, and digestive tract.

Certain amounts of histamine are normally released into the tissues in response to an injury or infection. Histamine dilates (widens) the smaller blood vessels at the site of the injury, thus contributing to the inflammatory response, a natural feature of healing. It also results in the escape of some of the blood plasma through the walls of the tiny blood vessels into the surrounding tissues, which accounts for the swelling that accompanies many injuries and infections.

The sudden release of histamine is responsible for the signs and symptoms of *allergy* in many cases. In a sensitized individual, when an invading allergen comes in contact with a body cell to which an allergic *antibody* is attached, a dramatic reaction results. Histamine is released from such cells in greater amounts than would be normal in response to an infection or injury. Depending on the site of the allergic reaction, this can cause swelling, redness, and itching of the skin or the formation of welts; inflammation and swelling of the mucous membranes of the nose, and constriction or spasm of the small air passages of the lungs.

The symptoms and signs of allergic disorders in which histamine plays a role can usually be relieved by taking *antihistamines*, a class of drugs available either over-the-counter or prescribed by a physician to neutralize or inhibit the action of histamine.

histoplasmosis An infectious disease affecting the lungs and other organs, caused by the fungus *Histoplasma capsulatum*. The spores of this fungus are found in soil worldwide; in the United States the disease is especially prevalent in the Midwest. It is associated with the contaminated droppings of pigeons, chickens, starlings, grackles, and other birds, and bats. Human infection may result from breathing in the dust from a contaminated chicken house or working in soil beneath trees that serve as roosting places for various birds. The spores of the fungus can also be spread by the wind over large areas.

The primary site of infection is the respiratory tract, usually resulting in a mild and often symptom-free infection of the lungs. Some patients may experience coughing, fever, and a general sense of being unwell (malaise). A chronic form of the disease may produce early diagnostic evidence that closely resembles tuberculosis.

The severity of the disease appears to be closely related to the amount of contaminated dust inhaled. The acute primary form of the disease is usually benign (harmless). However, if the infection spreads through the bloodstream and remains undiagnosed and untreated, it can be fatal.

The diagnosis of histoplasmosis basically involves the examination of blood, urine, or tissue samples obtained for biopsy, in which the causative fungus can be demonstrated. Treatment of severe forms of the disease is the (usually intravenous) administration of the antifungal drug amphotericin B.

hives
SEE *urticaria*

Hodgkin's disease A rare *malignant* disease of unknown cause, characterized by progressive swelling of the *lymph glands* and *spleen*. It often appears initially as a widespread involvement of the entire lymphatic system, including the lymph glands in the neck, armpits, groin, abdomen, and chest. In addition to enlargement of the lymph glands and spleen, the symptoms include fever, loss of weight, poor appetite, fatigue, and itching of the skin. The diagnosis requires the surgical removal of one of the enlarged

117

holistic

lymph glands for examination under a microscope.

Treatment of Hodgkin's disease has been unsatisfactory in the past. Since the enlarged glands may arise simultaneously in many parts of the body, the surgical removal of all affected glands is impossible. However, in many cases the disease will be fairly well localized, which enhances the possibility of effective treatment. In some patients the disease will progress very slowly, while in others it becomes widespread within a relatively short time.

Within the past few years the treatment of Hodgkin's disease has greatly improved; most patients can be cured or at least have the disease arrested in its otherwise progressive severity. X-ray treatment (irradiation of the affected tissues) and *cytotoxic drugs* (which destroy cancer cells) alone or in combination can produce a remission of the disease in many patients.

More than 75 percent of patients with Hodgkin's disease can be cured if treatment is started early.

It is named after the British physician Thomas Hodgkin (1798–1866).

holistic Relating to the philosophy or principle of holism, which states that living organisms function as complete units that cannot be reduced to the sum of their parts. Holistic medicine attempts to treat the entire person, not a specific disease state, taking into account psychological, social, and environmental influences that have a direct or indirect bearing on health and well-being. Holistic health is a system of *preventive medicine* that emphasizes nutrition, exercise, and mental relaxation.

hormone A chemical substance secreted directly into the bloodstream by any of the *endocrine* (ductless) *glands*, including the *ovaries, testicles, pituitary, thyroid, parathyroid*, and *adrenal glands*, as well as special cells in the *pancreas*. Hormones are complex substances that act to stimulate an organ or part of the body into increased functional activity by supplying a chemical stimulus.

The endocrine glands produce and store hormones until they are called upon to release them into the blood. This release may be triggered by a nerve impulse or by a sudden change in the amount of certain "messenger substances" carried in the blood.

The body automatically turns on and shuts off the supply of hormones at a moment's notice. Although the control exerted by the endocrine system is brought into play less quickly than the nearly instantaneous control of the nervous system, once hormones have been released into the blood they act for a considerably longer time. When a specific hormone is released and reaches its target cells or organ in sufficient quantities, a message is automatically released by that part

of the body to reduce or shut off a further supply of hormones.
SEE ALSO *corticosteroid, estrogen, insulin, progesterone*

humerus The bone of the upper arm, extending from the shoulder to the elbow.

Huntington's chorea A relatively rare hereditary disease of the nervous system, characterized by involuntary muscular twitching and irregular jerky movements. It is not usually noticed until early adult life or middle age.

Huntington's chorea is an extremely serious condition that progresses until nearly all the muscles of the body are affected by involuntary movements. In the advanced stages the patient has difficulty swallowing, breathing, walking, and talking. The mind also becomes severely affected, from a reduction in the faculty of judgment and thought to utter confusion. Changes of mood and irrational behavior may also occur.

Because of the grim prospect of incurable mental deterioration, members of a family with a known history of the disease may decide not to have children, since there is a high probability that the abnormal genes will be transmitted to a new generation. No medical treatment exists that can halt the progress of the disease, but certain sedative drugs can minimize the symptoms.

The condition is named after the American physician George Huntington (1850–1916).

hydrocephalus An abnormal condition popularly known as "water on the brain" that occurs when *cerebrospinal fluid* accumulates within the hollow spaces (ventricles) of the brain. The most common cause is an obstruction within the cerebrum that prevents the fluid from circulating around the surface of the brain and spinal cord. The obstruction may be caused by a congenital malformation of part of the brain. In such cases the accumulating fluid pushes against the soft areas of the baby's skull (fontanels) and may cause bulging or an unusually rapid increase in the normal rate of head enlargement. In older children and adults the obstruction may be caused by the formation of fibrous tissue following the healing of brain tissue damaged by injury or infection, or (rarely) it may be related to the formation of a brain tumor.

Congenital hydrocephalus is usually apparent in the physical appearance of the skull and the abnormally enlarged veins in the scalp. If the condition develops later than infancy, the symptoms will typically include headache, visual disturbances (blurred vision or double vision), nausea, and vomiting. Although the condition occasionally resolves spontaneously, especially in the very young, in most cases the only treatment is surgical.

hydrochloric acid

A definitive diagnosis is made with an x-ray of the skull or a *CAT scan*, which will reveal distorted or enlarged ventricles caused by the increased pressure of cerebrospinal fluid. The surgeon may bypass the obstruction by inserting a narrow tube (catheter) into one of the cerebral ventricles and draining off the fluid through a vein into a body cavity (such as the right atrium of the heart). If the blockage is accessible it may be removed directly. Infantile hydrocephalus is occasionally associated with *spina bifida* and other anatomical malformations present at birth.

hydrochloric acid A constituent of the *gastric juices*, secreted by cells in the walls of the stomach; its chemical formula is HCl. It aids digestion and inhibits the multiplication of bacteria within the stomach. An abnormally large amount of hydrochloric acid in the stomach can cause a burning sensation and may contribute to the development of ulcers.
COMPARE *achlorhydria*

hydrocortisone A synthetic form of *cortisol*, a *corticosteroid* hormone secreted by the *adrenal glands*.

hydronephrosis Distension of the renal pelvis, a funnel-shaped structure in the *kidney* that tapers to form the beginning of the ureter, which conveys urine to the bladder. It is caused by an obstruction of the urinary tract. In severe cases of hydronephrosis the entire kidney may become affected: the pressure of the blocked urine impairs blood flow through the organ, which can become seriously damaged if not treated.

Treatment is aimed at removal of the obstruction and surgical drainage of the accumulated urine. Antibiotics may be prescribed to control any associated infection.

hydrophobia
SEE *rabies*

hymen A fold of mucous membrane popularly called the maidenhead that covers part of the entrance to the vagina in females who have not had sexual intercourse. The apparent absence of the hymen (or lack of bleeding during sexual intercourse) is not reliable evidence of previous sexual experience.

hyperacidity The presence of an abnormally large amount of *hydrochloric acid* in the stomach. It is a fairly common condition that, especially in the absence of food in the stomach, can cause a burning sensation. If the condition persists or is not relieved by antacids, a physician should be consulted. Prolonged hyperacidity of the stomach can play a part in the development of *peptic ulcers*.

hyperglycemia An abnormal increase in the amount of sugar in the blood. It is one sign of *diabetes mellitus*.
COMPARE *hypoglycemia*

hyperplasia Excessive multiplication and growth of normal cells, resulting in the gradual enlargement of an organ or part. It has nothing whatever to do with tumors or cancer. Generally the result of hormonal stimulation, it occurs, for example, during puberty when the female breasts begin to enlarge.
COMPARE *atrophy*, *hypertrophy*

hyperpyrexia An extremely high *fever*, one in excess of 106°F(41.1°C). Although children occasionally experience such high fevers during the course of various illnesses from which they usually recover following proper diagnosis and treatment, hyperpyrexia is potentially much more serious in adults. High fevers in children may be reduced by giving them a gentle sponging with cool water or placing them in a cool bath for about fifteen minutes. If aspirin, acetaminophen, or a similar antipyretic drug does not bring the fever down, a physician should be consulted at once. Prolonged temperatures in excess of 106°F are fatal.

hypersensitivity An exaggerated and abnormal sensitivity of the body to the effects of an external agent or foreign particle entering the body. Hypersensitivity to pollen results in hay fever (allergic rhinitis).
SEE ALSO *allergy*, *desensitization*

hypertension High blood pressure, a condition in which the blood pumped out of the heart exerts an abnormally high pressure on the walls of the *arteries*. Hypertension is known to be associated with several disorders, including *arteriosclerosis* (hardening of the arteries), *atherosclerosis* (the buildup of fatty deposits on the inner lining of the blood vessels), chronic kidney disease, disorders of the endocrine glands, diabetes mellitus, nutritional disorders, cigarette smoking, and various nervous or emotional disorders. In many cases, however, the cause is unknown or *idiopathic*.

Patients with high blood pressure often have no symptoms and the first evidence of the condition may be discovered during a general medical examination. Rarely, symptoms may include pounding headaches at the back of the head (especially in the morning), insomnia, tiredness, irritability, emotional outbursts, dizziness, and a feeling of fullness in the head. Occasionally an early sign of high blood pressure will include nosebleeds *(epistaxis)* and the rupture of tiny blood vessels in the retina of the eye (eyesight is generally not affected).

With prolonged hypertension there is usually a widespread narrowing of the smaller arteries, creating increased resistance to blood flow and making the heart pump much harder to maintain adequate circulation.

There is no exact point at which a person may be said to have high blood pressure. What is accepted as normal for a person of seventy would be considered abnormal for a

hyperthyroidism

person of thirty. Generally, hypertension is indicated if the *systolic* pressure is about 170 and the *diastolic* pressure 100. The diastolic reading is the more important in diagnosing hypertension.

Treatment of hypertension depends on the cause. It may be secondary to some other disorder, in which case it will be relieved only by treating the underlying condition. In essential hypertension, the physician may prescribe *diuretics* as well as drugs that dilate the blood vessels, thus lowering the resistance against which the heart must pump. A change in diet may be advised, including the restriction of salt.

Even among healthy people, blood pressure tends to rise in later life. With proper care and avoidance of emotional states that tend to increase blood pressure, persons with hypertension can live active and healthy lives. However, if blood pressure continues to rise and medical treatment is refused, serious consequences can occur, including *stroke*, heart disease, and *kidney failure*.

A single measurement of the blood pressure is rarely of diagnostic value. The pressure can rise, for example, because of the patient's anxiety in the physician's office. Usually, several measurements must be made on separate occasions, ideally involving the same person taking the measurement and using the same equipment under conditions in which the patient is relaxed. However, if the initial measurement is excessively high for the patient's age, the physician may recommend immediate treatment to lower the pressure.

Often blood pressure can be reduced without medical treatment: weight loss, restriction of salt, and stopping smoking.

Because the blood pressure tends to increase with age, an unusually high blood pressure is potentially more serious in a younger person than in an older one. Also, for unknown reasons, men tend to suffer more from the complications of hypertension than do women.

Most patients who are prescribed drugs to control their blood pressure must continue taking them for life. It can be dangerous to stop taking these drugs without a physician's approval.

SEE ALSO *angina pectoris, coronary artery disease, myocardial infarction*

COMPARE *hypotension*

hyperthyroidism A condition in which the *thyroid gland* is abnormally overactive and secretes an excessive amount of hormones. The early signs and symptoms include restlessness or nervousness, sweating, rapid heartbeat, and sensitivity to heat. As the disease progresses there may be breathlessness (dyspnea), a pronounced loss of weight (despite an increased appetite), muscular tremor, and staring eyes; the patient becomes increasingly nervous. In effect, the increased supply of thyroid hormones acts to speed up the metabolism of the body unnaturally. Some patients also complain of bouts of troublesome diarrhea, which are caused by increased activity of the digestive system. A tentative diagnostic sign is unusually warm and perspiring hands.

The disease can occur at any age, and it is about five times more common in women than in men. In advanced cases the eyes may appear to bulge outward *(exophthalmos)* or the thyroid gland may swell to several times its normal size and be seen as a large growth *(goiter)* over the area of the throat. The size of a goiter does not bear a direct relationship to the severity of the disease. In some cases of severe hyperthyroidism (thyrotoxicosis) the thyroid gland may remain nearly normal in size, although the physician may be able to feel lumps or hard areas on physical examination.

Treatment depends on the individual case and the degree of severity. Some patients improve with the administration of drugs that interfere with the production of thyroid hormones or with the use of radioactive iodine, which destroys part of the gland and thus reduces hormone output. In other cases the only successful means of treatment is to remove a large part of the thyroid gland, a surgical procedure known as partial thyroidectomy.
COMPARE *hypothyroidism*

hypertrophy An increase in the bulk of an organ or body part as the result of tissue enlargement or thickening, not cell multiplication. It does not involve the formation of a tumor. It is the characteristic response of muscles to work or exercise.
COMPARE *atrophy, hyperplasia*

hyperuricemia The presence of an abnormal amount of *uric acid* (a waste product of metabolism) in the blood. If untreated it can lead to *gout* or the formation of kidney stones.

hypnotic Relating to any drug that induces drowsiness or sleep, usually by acting directly on certain nerve centers in the brain. Hypnotic drugs, especially those that contain barbiturates, are known popularly as sleeping pills. An overdose, especially if taken with alcohol, can be fatal.

hypodermic Relating to or characterized by the introduction of medical remedies under the skin, as a hypodermic injection. A hypodermic needle is a hollow needle attached to a syringe and is used for injections.

hypoglycemia An abnormally low level of sugar (glucose) in the blood.

hypotension

It may be associated with overactivity of the cells in the pancreas that secrete insulin or in diabetic patients may follow the injection of too much insulin.

The symptoms of low blood sugar include nervousness, cold sweats, weakness, a feeling of acute fatigue, irritability, and (in severe cases) mental disturbances (confusion, hallucinations, or bizarre behavior), loss of consciousness (hypoglycemic coma), or even death.

Hypoglycemia is treated by reducing the amount of sugar in the diet and eating foods that are rich in proteins. Although one might assume that low blood sugar should be treated by taking more sugar, doing so causes the pancreas to secrete more insulin, which tends to further decrease the overall amount of sugar in the blood.

In rare cases, hypoglycemia may be caused by a tumor of the pancreas, which results in the overproduction of insulin. Surgical removal of the tumor is then necessary.

SEE ALSO *diabetes mellitus*
COMPARE *hyperglycemia*

hypotension Abnormally low blood pressure. Persistently low blood pressure is a condition that may be normal in some people, however; as a feature of disease it is extremely rare.

Blood pressure is considered to be abnormally low if the *systolic* pressure is below about 100. In cases of severe bleeding, especially from an artery, the blood pressure may reach dangerously low levels and require immediate medical attention to preserve life.

Transient cases of hypotension may follow a severe attack of influenza, prolonged bed rest, acute coronary thrombosis, or severe malnutrition. The brief feeling of faintness or dizziness sometimes experienced when getting up too quickly from a bed or chair is not an example of systemic or general hypotension, it is merely the result of a rapid change in posture in which the brain is deprived of sufficient blood for a few moments.

Low blood pressure is no longer generally regarded by physicians to be responsible for tiredness or weakness, although a person with hypotension may indeed feel weak from other or indirectly related causes. Some cases of low blood pressure seem to be related to being seriously underweight; the physician will recommend an appropriate change in the diet to improve general nutrition.

Other factors being equal, there is nothing to worry about if one's blood pressure is slightly below normal. In fact, some physicians consider that a mild state of hypotension is a sign of long life, based on the fact that the opposite condition, *hypertension*, is often associated with disease of the kidneys and heart.

hypothalamus A small and not very sharply defined area of the brain situated below the *thalamus*. Its functions include originating emotional urges, regulating body temperature (indirectly causing sweating and shivering), controlling food and water intake by adjusting appetite and thirst, and preserving the body's energy balance through the control of sugar and fat metabolism.

hypothermia A serious condition in which the body becomes abnormally cold. It is potentially fatal.

Those living alone are more at risk than those living with others. Elderly people have a tendency to become abnormally chilled in cold weather, especially because their bodies have a slightly lower temperature than that of younger people. In addition, the temperature-regulating mechanisms of their bodies are no longer able to adjust automatically and quickly to sudden changes of environmental temperature.

Accidental hypothermia is the name given to the condition in which a person's temperature sinks dramatically. From the norm of 98.6°F (37°C) it can descend to well below 86°F (30°C).

Many factors play a part in this. Poor nutrition and inadequate clothing and home heating can stem from financial difficulties. Poor blood supply as the result of narrowed arteries (arteriosclerosis or atherosclerosis) is common in the elderly, as is reduced activity of the thyroid gland, which helps to maintain body temperature. During sleep the elderly move less than the young and lack the muscle activity (including shivering) that helps to produce heat. Tranquilizers and sleeping pills have a side effect of lowering the body temperature.

Although hypothermia is more common in the elderly, anyone can be affected. Exposure to cold weather, immersion in icy water, and similar causes of lost body heat can result in hypothermia.

hypothyroidism A condition in which the *thyroid gland* is underactive and fails to secrete a sufficient amount of thyroid hormones. The symptoms of the disease depend largely on the age of the patient. If the disorder is present at birth because the thyroid gland has failed to develop normally during the prenatal period, the result may be *cretinism*.

In older children and adults, the development of hypothyroidism may first be manifest as unusual fatigue, weakness, loss of energy and drive, hoarseness, and increased sensitivity to cold. As the disease progresses the physical appearance changes. In a typical case of advanced hypothyroidism the patient develops *myxedema*, which is characterized by puffiness of the face and hands, enlarged tongue (which makes speech slow and difficult), abnormal weight gain, dry and dull skin and hair, slowed pulse rate, and general sluggishness of movement.

Hypothyroidism in adults is often the result of medical or surgical treatment to relieve an overactive thyroid gland *(hyperthyroidism)*. Other causes include inflammation of the thyroid gland (thyroiditis), a failure of the thyroid gland to trap or make use of dietary iodine, or an insufficient dietary intake of iodine.

In practically every case, hypothyroidism can be successfully treated by hormone-replacement therapy, which may have to be continued for life. An adequate dietary intake of iodine should also be maintained, which is possible with the regular use of iodized table salt.

hysterectomy Surgical removal of the *uterus*. The procedure may be performed for a variety of reasons. Uncontrolled bleeding from the uterus during a menstrual period (menorrhagia) or between menstrual periods (metrorrhagia) is one indication that the uterus may have to be removed. Sometimes benign uterine growths called *fibroids* enlarge and cause bleeding and severe pressure against the bladder and rectum, in which case the most appropriate treatment may be removal of the uterus. Less commonly, hysterectomy may be performed in cases of cancer of the uterus and *cervix* or to provide therapeutic termination of pregnancy (usually combined with *sterilization*).

The uterus may be removed through an incision into the abdomen (a procedure similar to cesarean section) or through the vagina.

There has been much criticism of the increasing number of hysterectomies performed in the United States. Some people feel that a significant percentage of these operations are being performed more for the economic benefit of the surgeon rather than for medically justifiable reasons. This unfortunate state is another valid reason to obtain a second opinion before agreeing to any elective (nonemergency) surgical procedure.

I

iatrogenic Relating to any abnormal or adverse physical or mental condition induced by a physician or surgeon. The term implies that the practitioner failed to give a patient adequate care and that the resulting condition was preventable. A disease or disorder caused by medical or surgical treatment that is inept, inadvisable, inadvertent, or otherwise shows a lack of professional concern, ability, or judgment is said to be iatrogenic.
SEE ALSO *malpractice*

ICU Abbreviation for *intensive care unit*.

idiopathic Relating to any disease or condition whose cause is not known.

ileitis Inflammation of the *ileum*, the lowest section of the small intestine.
SEE *enteritis*

ileostomy The surgical formation of a passage through the abdominal wall into the *ileum*, the lowest section of the small intestine, thus bypassing the large intestine and forming an artificial means for solid wastes to pass outside the body. It may be temporary (as part of the treatment of an intestinal obstruction) or permanent (as in removal of a cancerous section of the large intestine).
SEE *colostomy*

ileum The lowest section of the small intestine, the other two being the duodenum and the jejunum.

IM Abbreviation for *intramuscular*.

imaging The production of an image, shadow, or picture that represents an organ or part being investigated. In medical diagnosis this can be accomplished with x-rays or with such newer methods as CAT scans (computerized axial tomography), ultrasound, and infrared techniques.

immunity The condition of being resistant to a particular disease, microorganism, poison, or other foreign substance. Immunity is usually

immunization

established as the result of the formation of specific protective *antibodies* that circulate in the bloodstream. Immunity to one of the most serious infectious diseases, smallpox (which has now been virtually eradicated worldwide), was made possible by the English physician Edward Jenner, who introduced *vaccination* in the late eighteenth century.

In 1798 Jenner published a report of his successful experiments in inoculating patients against smallpox with material taken from persons with a similar but much less virulent infection, cowpox. In smallpox as in other infectious diseases the specific antibodies produced in response to the infecting microorganisms may remain in the body for years or even a lifetime, thus providing partial or total immunity to further attacks of the same disease.

SEE ALSO *allergy, autoimmune diseases, immunization, immunology, immunosuppressive, immunotherapy*

immunization The process or technique of bringing about or increasing a state of immunity in an individual, as by injecting a vaccine or other agent into the body or swallowing a substance that provides protection against a specific disease. SEE ALSO *vaccination*

immunology The branch of medical science concerned with the study of the body's natural mechanism of defense against disease *(immunity)*. A specialist in this field is known as an immunologist.

SEE ALSO *autoimmune disease, immunization, immunosuppressive, immunotherapy*

immunosuppressive Relating to a class of drugs that inhibits the body's natural system of *immunity*. Without the use of such drugs before the surgical transplant of a foreign organ (such as a kidney), the body would tend to attack and reject the transplanted organ or tissues in the same way that it would attack and destroy invading microorganisms.

immunotherapy A therapeutic method, still largely experimental, of controlling the growth of certain malignant tumors by stimulating the production of specific *antibodies* in the patient.

impacted Wedged, pressed, or jammed together or against something else. An impacted tooth is one that cannot erupt through the gums normally because it is emerging at an incorrect angle and is jammed against a neighboring tooth.

impetigo A contagious bacterial skin disease, most common in children. It is characterized by the formation of blisters that eventually break open and spread the infection to nearby areas of the skin. As the blisters dry they form yellow scabs. Early diagnosis and treatment with an appropriate antibiotic usually results in prompt recovery.

impotence The inability of a man to achieve erection of the penis. In some cases there is a physical cause such as a disease of the genitals or a hormone deficiency, but sexual anxiety is most often responsible.

Most men have one or more spontaneous erections during sleep; should this be noted, it is evidence that a physical disorder is not the cause of impotence.

A man who is impotent is not necessarily incapable of producing healthy sperm cells *(spermatozoa)*.
SEE ALSO *sterility*

incontinence The inability to control bowel or bladder emptying, usually as the result of a disorder involving the muscles or nerves that control the voluntary opening of the outlets of the bladder or rectum.

incubation period The interval between a person's exposure to an infectious disease and the appearance of the first signs and symptoms.

indication Any circumstance, condition, or sign that indicates a particular drug, pharmaceutical agent, or other means of treatment is appropriate for a patient.
COMPARE *contraindication*

indigestion
SEE *dyspepsia*

infarction The death and consequent formation of scar tissue in an organ that has been deprived of an adequate blood supply. When this occurs in the *heart* it is known as *myocardial infarction*.
COMPARE *necrosis*

infectious Relating to a disease that can be transmitted with or without direct contact with someone who has it; specifically, a disease caused by microorganisms.

Infection is the state or condition in which the body is invaded by bacteria, viruses, or other disease-causing microorganisms.
SEE ALSO *communicable*, *contagious*

infectious mononucleosis
SEE *mononucleosis*

infertility The inability or greatly reduced ability to conceive children. The condition may be present in either males or females and may be the result of immature or underdeveloped sex organs (testicles or ovaries), a hormonal disorder, a disorder or obstruction of the Fallopian tubes, or a congenital abnormality of the uterus.

It has been estimated that approximately 10 percent of married couples in the United States are affected by infertility. In about 40 percent of these cases, the cause is the male's inability to produce an adequate number of healthy sperm cells (spermatozoa). In 50 percent the problem is either a deficiency of female hormones or a disorder of the Fallopian tubes. The remaining 10 percent fail to produce children as the result of a hostile environment in the woman's genital tract (especially near the cervix), which renders en-

inflammation

trance of sperm cells impossible. This can be caused by various factors, including infections of the cervix, erosion of the cervix, or other local disorders.

Treatment is aimed at the underlying cause. To stimulate defective ovulation, clomiphene citrate or human menopausal gonadotropin, may be prescribed. Anatomical defects in the Fallopian tubes can often be corrected surgically. Male infertility may be associated with a physical problem that can be corrected surgically (such as a deformity of the penis that interferes with the passage of sperm cells), or a hormonal deficiency that can be treated by administering replacement hormones.

The failure of a couple to conceive children is often associated with psychological or emotional problems. (Frequently, a couple unable to conceive will adopt a child and within a short time the woman will become pregnant.

SEE ALSO *sterility*

inflammation The changes that occur in living tissues when they are injured, which are characterized by the following signs and symptoms in the affected area: pain, heat, redness, swelling, and an interruption of normal function. The process of inflammation is a natural function of the body's mechanism of self-repair following injury.

Pharmaceutical products that are prescribed to relieve these signs and symptoms are known as anti-inflammatory drugs. The suffix *-itis* denotes inflammation.

influenza An acute infectious and highly contagious disease, popularly known as flu, caused by a virus. The incubation period varies from about twenty-four to forty-eight hours and symptoms usually appear suddenly. They include severe headache, aches in muscles and joints (especially backache), chills, loss of appetite, sweating, and fatigue or prostration. The body temperature rises sharply to about 101–103°F (38–39.5°C). During the next two or three days the fever and pain gradually diminish, although in severe cases the temperature may briefly reach 104–106°F (40–41°C) and remain above normal for five or six days. A physician should be seen immediately if the fever lasts longer; the cause may be a secondary bacterial infection of the lungs that could lead to pneumonia, an extremely serious complication in the elderly and those with chronic diseases.

Drugs have no direct effect on the influenza virus; once a person has influenza the best that can be done is to treat the symptoms. It is important to rest during the period of fever and to drink plenty of liquids and eat sensibly (many people lose their appetite completely for two or three days). Aspirin or acetaminophen can be taken to reduce fever and relieve headache.

Vaccines are available that protect against specific strains of the influenza virus; these are especially important for the elderly or those with a chronic disease. A physician will advise about the desirability of vaccination.

During the worldwide influenza pandemic of 1918–1919, nearly 20 million people died. Although such a virulent strain of influenza virus is rare, any outbreak can be potentially serious.

informed consent The explanation to a patient by a physician or surgeon of the nature of a disease, its likely prognosis, and the possible risk involved in a particular course of therapy or surgical procedure including the availability of alternative methods of treatment.

This principle is often used by a medical or surgical practitioner to avoid litigation in cases of alleged *malpractice* or claims that a patient did not understand the implications of therapy and the resulting side effects or complications.

Many state courts have disagreed on the extent and nature of the information that an individual patient should be given. If a patient has been informed of all relevant aspects of a proposed method or course of treatment, and willingly submits to it, the patient's consent is considered to have been obtained. The patient is usually asked to read and sign an informed consent form.

injection The introduction of drugs or other substances under pressure into the tissues (skin or muscles) or into the blood vessels. An *intravenous* injection is into a vein, a *subcutaneous* or *hypodermic* injection is under the skin, an *intraarterial* injection is into an artery, and an *intramuscular* injection is into a muscle.
SEE ALSO *inoculation, syringe, vaccination*

inoculation The deliberate introduction into the body of microorganisms, serums, or toxic substances to stimulate *immunity* to a specific disease through the subsequent development of protective *antibodies*.
SEE ALSO *vaccination*

in situ In position; remaining in the original area of formation or development. A carcinoma that has not spread beyond its original site of formation is referred to as a carcinoma in situ.

insomnia An abnormal difficulty in falling asleep or in staying asleep; periodic wakefulness when trying to *sleep.*
COMPARE *narcolepsy*

insulin A hormone produced in the *pancreas* by so-called beta cells in an area known as the islets of Langerhans. It is essential in regulating the utilization and blood levels of glucose (sugar) and in the normal metabolism of carbohydrates and fats.

The isolation of insulin as an active hormone of the pancreas was made in 1922 by two Canadian physicians, Frederick Banting and Charles Best, who were also the first to use it in the treatment of *diabetes mellitus.*

intensive care unit (ICU) A room or area within a hospital in which sophisticated electronic monitoring devices (such as electrocardiographs) and trained personnel are concentrated for the continuous observation and care of patients with life-threatening diseases or disorders.

The intensive care unit began many years ago as a recovery room for patients who had just undergone major surgery. Gradually, it evolved as an area in which to monitor the progress of patients with a known or suspected heart attack (myocardial infarction), serious disturbances of the heart's rhythms (arrhythmias), heart failure, acute kidney failure, severe lung disease, and other urgent problems that demand immediate and continuous medical and nursing attention.

interferon A class of small soluble proteins produced in the body, especially by the white blood cells *(leukocytes)*, in response to a viral infection. Interferons act to inhibit ("interfere" with) the multiplication of the invading viruses and thus offer a degree of protection for those cells that have not yet been infected. Some researchers believe that interferon may be a previously unrecognized hormone, based on the way in which it appears to interact with cells. The substance was first identified in the late 1970s, although exactly how and why it works is still largely a mystery.

Preparations of interferon have been used experimentally since about 1980 in the treatment of various types of cancer, particularly breast cancer. The possible long-term benefits of such treatment are as yet unclear.

intestines
SEE *colon, duodenum, ileum, jejunum, large intestine, small intestine, rectum*

intraarterial Within an artery or arteries.
COMPARE *intradermal, intramuscular, intravenous, subcutaneous*

intradermal Within the substance of the skin (dermis).
COMPARE *intraarterial, intramuscular, intravenous, subcutaneous*

intramuscular (IM) Within a muscle. It is a common route for the injection of some drugs or pharmacologic agents.
COMPARE *intraarterial, intradermal, intravenous, subcutaneous*

intrauterine device (IUD) A small flexible object, typically in the shape of a loop or coil made of plastic or copper, placed within the *uterus* as a means of contraception.

It is possible for an intrauterine device to be expelled by the natural action of the uterus, so women should examine themselves regularly to see if the device is in place. All IUDs have thin threads attached to them, which can be easily found when they are to be removed or checked.

It has not been definitely established how IUDs prevent pregnancy, but it is believed that they make the lining of the uterus hostile to the implantation of a fertilized ovum. The IUD is not as effective a method of contraception as oral contraceptives but it has a much higher success rate than other mechanical devices. However, unlike those other methods, IUDs have undesired complications and side effects. Many women experience heavy and painful periods for the first two or three menstrual cycles after the IUD has been inserted, though this generally subsides.

In the main, IUDs used to be recommended for women who have had a child, but now special devices have been developed for childless women. If a woman wishes to become pregnant, the loop or coil can be removed very easily by a physician.

intravenous (IV) Within a *vein* or veins. This term is used primarily to describe the method of injecting a drug, nutrient, or x-ray contrast medium directly into a vein.

COMPARE *intraarterial, intradermal, intramuscular, subcutaneous*
SEE ALSO *injection, intravenous feeding, intravenous pyelography, radiopaque*

intravenous feeding The supply of liquid nutrients (such as glucose) through a tube inserted into a vein in the arm.

intravenous pyelography (IVP) An x-ray technique or procedure for examining the kidneys, ureters, and bladder; also called excretory urography. Just before a series of x-rays is taken of these structures, a contrast medium or *radiopaque* dye is injected into a vein in the arm. The dye enters the blood circulation and soon reaches the *kidneys*, where it is excreted and enters the hollow urine-collecting area (renal pelvis) of each kidney. The dye then passes through the ureter, the slender tube that conveys urine from each kidney to the bladder.

As the patient reclines on a table, the radiologist takes a series of x-rays as the dye quickly passes through the urinary system. Because the dye is not easily penetrated by x-rays, it permits a clear outline on the x-ray film of the structures it passes through. The radiologist can then get a fairly good idea of the size and shape of the kidneys and detect various abnormalities. For example, the dye will take longer to appear and fill the hollow structures of the urinary system in the presence of

intubation

a tumor, cyst, or certain other disorders.

Dyes to provide contrast on x-rays contain iodine. If the patient is hypersensitive to this substance, it can cause a potentially serious allergic reaction shortly after injection. More commonly, however, patients may experience a sudden and spreading sensation of warmth as the dye passes through the blood vessels.

Intravenous pyelography is one of the most important diagnostic procedures available to study the structure and function of the urinary system.

intubation The insertion of a tube into a body cavity, canal, or passage. A tube may be inserted through the nose and down the esophagus into the stomach (nasogastric intubation) for diagnostic or therapeutic purposes, or down the throat and into the trachea (endotracheal intubation), for the maintenance of an airway, removal of thick secretions, or administration of anesthesia.
COMPARE *catheterizaton*

intussusception The abnormal infolding or "telescoping" of one segment of the intestine within another segment; invagination. It occurs mainly in children and is usually an emergency that requires immediate surgical correction.

invasive Relating to any diagnostic technique or procedure that involves the introduction of foreign material into the body (such as the injection of x-ray contrast material into a vein prior to the taking of x-rays), the puncture or incision of the skin, or the insertion of an instrument into the body. It also is used for a malignant growth or tumor that spreads to ("invades") surrounding areas of previously healthy tissues.

inversion The turning inside out of a hollow organ; this occasionally happens to the *uterus* following childbirth (uterine inversion). In mild cases of uterine inversion the symptoms are minimal and spontaneous correction sometimes occurs. In other cases the woman may experience pain and bleeding, either soon after childbirth or up to several weeks or months later. Treatment depends largely on the severity of the symptoms and the lapse of time before the condition is diagnosed. In severe cases surgical correction may be required.

in vitro Within glass or occurring in a test tube. The term refers to a chemical or biological reaction or response that occurs outside the living body.
COMPARE *in vivo*
SEE ALSO *in vitro fertilization*

in vitro fertilization A technique or procedure used to fertilize an ovum outside the uterus. When it is used to fertilize a human ovum successfully, the result is known popularly (but incorrectly) as a "test-tube baby."

The process involves the surgical removal of a ripe ovum from the prospective mother by means of an instrument known as a laparoscope, which is passed through the abdominal wall to the ovary. The ovum is then placed in a shallow dish containing nutrient fluids and sperm cells from the prospective father. Approximately thirty-six hours following fertilization, or after the ovum has divided into about sixteen cells (forming a hollow ball of cells known as a blastocyst), it is removed and implanted in the woman's uterus.

The resulting baby continues embryonic and fetal development within the uterus of the natural mother. The only artificial aspect is that for any of several reasons (such as blocked Fallopian tubes that cannot be corrected surgically) the ovum is prevented from meeting the sperm within the Fallopian tubes, where natural fertilization takes place.

The technique was first performed successfully in England in 1977. Since then, many other healthy children have been born following in vitro fertilization. The technique requires specially trained medical experts and is extremely difficult. The success rate thus far has been disappointing, although the procedure offers hope for women who have otherwise been unable to conceive.

SEE ALSO *in vitro*

in vivo Occurring in living cells within an organism; taking place in the body. The term is used to describe a chemical or biological process or response.

COMPARE *in vitro*

involution The return to normal size of a temporarily enlarged organ, such as the uterus following childbirth. It also refers to the rolling or turning inward of the edges of a structure or part.

iodine A nonmetallic element that, in extremely small quantities, is essential for the normal functioning of the *thyroid gland*.

ipecac syrup A natural chemical compound, available over the counter in syrup form, used as emergency treatment to induce *vomiting* (emesis) in persons who have taken a potentially lethal (fatal) dose of drugs or poisons. Products or compounds used to induce vomiting are known as *emetics*.

Ipecac syrup should be administered to adults or children exactly as the label directs. If vomiting does not occur within twenty minutes, a second dose may be given. However, if vomiting does not occur within a maximum of thirty minutes, a physician should be consulted immediatly. Emetics (such as ipecac syrup) should not be used if the victim has swallowed a corrosive substance, such as alkalies (lye), strychnine, strong acids, cleaning fluid, or petroleum distillates such as kerosene, gasoline, coal oil, fuel oil, or paint thinner.

It is a good idea before administering ipecac syrup (or any emetic) to a possible victim of poisoning or drug overdosage to first seek professional advice by calling a physician, hospital emergency room, or a poison control center. Time is critical in providing emergency treatment.

No emetic (including ipecac syrup) should ever by given to an unconscious person.

iris The ring of colored tissue between the cornea and the lens of the eye. It expands or contracts to control the amount of light entering the eye and reaching the retina.

iritis Inflammation of the iris.

iron A metallic element essential in the diet for the formation of the oxygen-carrying blood pigment *hemoglobin*. It is prescribed in compound form for the treatment of iron-deficiency *anemia*.

irradiation The use of x-rays, ultraviolet light, or other forms of radiation in the treatment of disease; exposure to electromagnetic waves of any kind.

irritable bowel syndrome A disorder of the *small intestine* and *large intestine* (colon) characterized by abdominal pain and alternating episodes of constipation and diarrhea. The most common disease of the gastrointestinal tract, it is also known as spastic colon, irritable colon, and mucous *colitis*. The cause is unknown but in most cases is associated with anxiety, emotional stress, or other psychological factors; no *organic disease* is present. The severity of symptoms varies considerably from patient to patient, as does duration. The onset of the problem typically occurs in early adult life with intermittent or recurring symptoms; each episode may last from a few days to several weeks.

Treatment of irritable bowel syndrome is aimed primarily at encouraging the patient to reduce stressful factors in daily life. Bulk-producing laxatives such as psyllium hydrophilic mucilloid may be useful, and antispasmodic drugs may also be prescribed to reduce the incidence and severity of painful intestinal spasm.

ischemia An inadequate supply of blood to a structure or part, such as that caused by a local obstruction of the blood vessels that supply it.

islets of Langerhans Clusters of specialized cells in the *pancreas* that produce the hormone *insulin*.

They are named after the German pathologist Paul Langerhans (1847–1888).

itching Irritation of the skin that provokes a desire to scratch; medically, *pruritis*. If itching is persistent it may be a sign of allergy, heat-rash (prickly heat), or an occasional feature of some other problem (such as a fungal skin infection) that requires medical attention.

IUD Abbreviation for *intrauterine device*.

IV Abbreviation for *intravenous*.

IVP Abbreviation for *intravenous pyelogram*.

J

jaundice A yellowish discoloration of the skin and the whites of the eyes, caused by the abnormal presence in the blood of excessive quantities of bile pigment *(bilirubin)*.

Jaundice (once known as icterus) is not in itself a disease but a sign of some underlying disorder of the *liver* or *gallbladder*. The discoloration is caused by the deposition in the affected tissues of bilirubin, which is mostly derived from the breakdown of hemoglobin in dead red blood cells *(erythrocytes)*. The pigment finds its way into body tissues for one of three basic reasons: failure to excrete bilirubin because of liver diseases such as infective *hepatitis*, drug damage, or *cirrhosis* (hepatic jaundice); obstruction to the normal flow of bile due to blockage of the common bile duct, as by gallstones (obstructive jaundice); and excessive destruction of red blood cells, as in hemolytic *anemia*.

The treatment of jaundice depends on successful treatment of the underlying condition. One of the most common causes of jaundice is the formation of gallstones *(cholelithiasis)* that block the outflow of bile from the gallbladder to the duodenum, the first part of the small intestine. Dramatic improvement is usually seen following surgical removal of the obstructing gallstones.

Jaundice is always a sign that requires immediate medical attention, for the risk exists of permanent damage to the liver. Although jaundice does not represent a true medical emergency—as does, for example, appendicitis—failure to obtain a prompt medical diagnosis and permit the start of treatment can have serious consequences.

jejunum The part of the small intestine between the *duodenum* and the *ileum*.

jugular veins Any of the four veins (one pair on each side of the neck, the internal and external jugular veins) that return blood to the heart from the brain, face, and neck.

juvenile rheumatoid arthritis
SEE *Still's disease*

K

keloid The formation or presence of an excessive amount of raised scar tissue at the site of a healed wound, burn, or surgical incision. Keloids are more common in persons of dark complexion or black skin and tend to recur if they are surgically removed. They are harmless though unattractive.

keloidosis The formation of *keloids* on the skin.

keratin The tough protein substance present in the nails, hair, and other horny tissues; it is insoluble in water, weak acids, or alkalis.

kidney Either of two purplish brown organs at the back of the abdominal cavity, one on each side of the vertebral column, responsible for filtering out waste products such as urea from the blood, maintaining the body's delicate balance of salts and water, and forming and excreting *urine*.

The kidneys are the most important structures of the urinary system and (without medical intervention) at least one healthy kidney is necessary to maintain life. In the adult, each kidney is about 4 inches (10 cm) long, 2 inches (5 cm) wide, and 1 inch (2.5 cm) thick, forming a structure somewhat resembling a tiny, curved boxing glove.

Each kidney is surrounded by a tough fibrous membrane and the entire organ is embedded in a mass of protective fatty tissue. Seated on top of each kidney is an *adrenal gland*. Nerves and blood vessels enter and leave the kidney through a fissure (hilum) on its concave (inner) side. It is also through this fissure that the *ureter* emerges, conveying urine collected from the kidney to the bladder.

The kidney is a highly complex organ consisting of a relatively thin outer layer (renal cortex) and a much larger inner portion (renal medulla). The functional and structural unit of the kidney is the *nephron*, over a million of which lie in the cortex of each kidney. The nephrons are the kidney's filtering units: they remove waste products and permit the reabsorption into the tissues of useful material, including

kidney failure

about 95 percent of the water that was originally filtered out.

Blood enters the kidney by means of the renal artery under relatively high pressure, since it is directly linked with the aorta, the largest artery of the body. The renal artery branches out into smaller vessels, which in turn branch into a coiled mass of microscopic blood vessels that form the first part of the nephron and are known collectively as a glomerulus. It is within this coil of capillaries that the incoming blood is filtered under pressure; almost all of the dissolved constituents of the blood are removed with the exception of proteins, because protein molecules are too large to be forced through the capillary walls. The filtered fluid is collected in the space known as Bowman's capsule that surrounds the glomerulus.

Fluid is drained off from Bowman's capsule through a coiled tube with three distinct sections. By the time the fluid reaches the final portion of this tube, it can properly be called urine. As the newly formed urine reaches this point it enters a larger channel known as a collecting tubule. Eventually the urine flows into a funnel-shaped area of the kidney known as the renal pelvis, which tapers to form the beginning of the ureter.

Only a very small amount of the blood entering the kidneys through the renal arteries is used as a source of nourishment; the rest is filtered through the glomeruli. However, it takes several passes through the kidneys (about forty-five minutes) for all the blood to be filtered, and during any one pass through the kidneys not all the blood will be fully filtered.

SEE ALSO *diuretic, glomerulonephritis, hydronephrosis, intravenous pyelogram, kidney failure, nephrolithiasis, pyelitis, pyelonephritis*

kidney failure A failure of the *kidney* to perform its essential functions; also called renal failure. Acute kidney failure is characterized by the sudden accumulation in the blood and other body fluids of urea and other waste products that are normally excreted in the urine, and by severe disturbances in the body's normal balance of water and essential salts, acids, and minerals. The amount of urine is usually abnormally low over a given twenty-four hour period; in rare cases the excretion may be suppressed altogether.

Acute kidney failure can be caused by any disease that directly or indirectly interferes with urine production or excretion, a crushing injury to the kidneys, obstruction to the flow of urine, poisoning of the kidneys (as with mercury, carbon tetrachloride, or ethylene glycol), severe burns, blood poisoning, sudden interruption or diminution of the normal blood supply to the kidneys, and mismatched blood during transfusions.

The parts of the kidneys commonly involved in acute kidney fail-

kidney machine

ure are known as the lower renal tubules. They convey urine from the coiled mass of microscopic blood vessels called a glomerulus. These tubules typically become necrotic—that is, small portions of them die. Since the filtering portion of the kidneys (the cortex) is not usually affected in acute tubular necrosis, the patient may pass a very dilute urine. If the cortex is affected, the condition is potentially more serious and may not be reversible with medical treatment.

Many forms of kidney failure can be successfully treated, but all represent extremely serious conditions that require prompt medical attention.

SEE ALSO *hemodialysis peritoneal dialysis*

kidney machine
SEE *hemodialysis*

kidney stones
SEE *nephrolithiasis*

Koch's law A postulate that establishes the following four conditions as necessary to prove conclusively that a specific microorganism is the sole cause of a particular disease: it must be present in the affected tissues in every case of the disease; it must be capable of being cultured in a pure form (containing only the one species); it must produce the same disease when the cultured microorganisms are inoculated in susceptible animals; it must be recovered from the inoculated animals and grown again in a pure culture.

The law is named after the German bacteriologist Robert Koch (1843–1910).

Koplik's spots A diagnostic sign of measles that is sometimes noted by a physician just before the typical rash appears. It consists of tiny white spots on a red base on the inner surface of the cheeks. These spots often disappear as the rash develops.

The term is named after the American pediatrician Henry Koplik (1858–1927).

kwashiorkor A *tropical disease* caused by severe protein malnutrition. It is primarily a problem affecting babies and children under the age of two who have been weaned from breast milk and given a substitute low in protein. The disease is characterized by a distended abdomen, enlarged liver, inactivity, apathy, and subnormal growth and development.

In many parts of the world, particularly the developing countries of Africa, breast milk is the main source of protein for infants. When a child is abruptly deprived of this essential food he or she may be given dilute cereal gruels or other high-carbohydrate foods. The child's energy requirements may be met, but he or she may develop severe emotional and physical problems.

Children with kwashiorkor are typically underweight, although high-carbohydrate diets may give them a deceptively chubby appearance. Common signs of the disease include watery diarrhea, swelling of the tissues (edema), and, in dark-skinned children, a patchy loss of skin pigment. The prolonged lack of a well-balanced diet predisposes children to a wide variety of health problems and makes them far less able to cope with the infectious diseases common during childhood.

Immediate treatment involves the administration of potassium, iron, and vitamins (especially vitamins A and C) together with a diet based on milk or milk substitutes. Except for severely ill children, in whom the death rate may be as high as 40 percent, the correction of vitamin, mineral, and protein deficiencies results in the regaining of lost strength and vitality. The long-term effects of prolonged malnutrition during infancy are unclear.

L

lactation The production of breast milk during the last stage of pregnancy. At first, the engorged breasts may be painful; this can be relieved by analgesics, a nursing bra, support halter, or ice packs applied to the breasts. If the mother does not choose to breast feed, lactation can be suppressed in several ways, including by an intramuscular injection of testosterone enanthate and estradiol valerate just after delivery.

laminectomy A surgical procedure involving the removal of the posterior arch (part of the rear portion) of a vertebra, especially to relieve pressure on the spinal cord as in cases of a severe *slipped disk*.

lanugo The fine, downy hairs on the body of a fetus or newborn baby that form from about the fifth month of life; also, the similarly short, delicate hairs that occur on body surfaces with the general exception of the soles of the feet and the palms of the hands.

laparotomy A surgical incision through the abdominal wall, especially an operation performed to investigate the cause of an acute illness for which the diagnosis or affected abdominal site is not yet known (experimental laparotomy).

large intestine The lower part of the digestive tract; also known as the colon or large bowel. It is about 5 feet (1.5 meters) long and extends from the ileum, the lowest section of the *small intestine*, to the *anus*, forming a single loop that passes upward, across, and then downward in the abdominal cavity. Its main function is to absorb water from indigestible food residues passed along from the small intestine and prepare them for expulsion from the body as *feces* (stools).

When indigestible food residue reaches the last section of the large intestine, the *rectum*, it is temporarily held by the muscular ring (anal sphincter) at the anal opening.

laryngectomy Surgical removal of the *larynx*. Various types of growths are occasionally found on the larynx, particularly on the vocal cords. The most common of them, *polyps*, are smooth, glistening, blisterlike swellings. These and other relatively simple growths can usually be removed by a simple operation.

However, potentially serious tumors that are not simple and that tend to spread can affect the mucous membrane lining of any part of the larynx. Those that interfere with the action of the vocal cords are the first to be diagnosed because of the obvious voice alteration. In such cases x-ray treatment is generally used to destroy the malignant cells. If this fails, surgical removal of the entire larynx is almost always necessary to prevent the cancer from spreading. On rare occasions a partial removal of the larynx may be effective.

Once the larynx has been removed, voice production can be relearned; the individual forces air into the top of the esophagus and brings it back again under pressure. The vibratory noise produced is then modified in the throat and mouth to create recognizable sounds. This esophageal voice can become quite distinct, although lacking in range.

Numerous types of artificial larynxes have been constructed in the past and in recent years as alternatives to esophageal speech. There are models that can be kept inside the mouth or inserted into the mouth while in use, and also those that can be placed against the throat to provide the audible vibrations necessary for speech (this electrolarynx is fairly common today). Other devices require further surgical intervention and enable air expelled from the lungs to produce an artificial voice.

laryngitis Inflammation of the *larynx*. It may occur suddenly as a result of overuse of the voice (commonly experienced by singers, actors, and public speakers) or it may develop as an extension of a viral infection of the upper air passages. It may also occur as a complication of a wide variety of other infectious diseases, including bronchitis, tonsillitis, pharyngitis, sinusitis, whooping cough, or measles. Alcohol, tobacco smoke, and the common cold can also provoke laryngitis.

The symptoms of laryngitis vary according to the severity of the infection and include hoarseness, a tickling sensation or pain in the throat, difficulty in swallowing and, if the larynx is swollen, shortness of breath during physical exertion or other difficulties in breathing (dyspnea).

Chronic laryngitis results from the inadequate treatment of repeated acute attacks or from the resumption of activities that put a strain on the voice before the larynx has fully recovered. The swollen laryngeal tissues may become thickened with scar tissue, causing

laryngoscopy

permanent damage to the voice. Irritants like tobacco smoke can lead to the thickening of vocal cords and cartilages as the result of cellular changes.

Treatment of laryngitis demands careful investigation of the nasal passages by a physician to detect the possible presence of microorganisms that may be responsible for the infection, prevention of irritation by dust, and in some cases an examination of the larynx *(laryngoscopy)*. Antibiotics are prescribed to treat bacterial infections, and steam inhalation, bed rest, and total disuse of the voice (whispering as well as talking) are required until the condition clears.

laryngoscopy Examination of the interior of the *larynx*. The procedure may be either direct or indirect.

Direct laryngoscopy involves the use of an illuminated instrument called a laryngoscope or fiberoptic endoscope that is passed through the mouth and throat to the larynx. The specialist can then detect any damage, swollen tissue, the location of an obstructing foreign body (which can be removed by means of an attachment on the laryngoscope), and help confirm the possibility of laryngeal cancer.

Indirect laryngoscopy, a far less complex procedure, involves the examination of the larynx by means of an instrument with a mirror on the end. It is held near the back of the throat and reflects light down to the larynx, the surface structure of which is examined in the laryngeal mirror by the physician.

larynx A structure in the throat consisting of the enlarged upper end of the trachea that contains the vocal cords; it is known popularly as the "voicebox."

The larynx consists of a series of cartilages situated between the trachea and the base of the tongue, where the *epiglottis*, a leaf-shaped piece of cartilage, acts as a valve; it blocks off the larynx during swallowing and opens to allow breathing or talking. The epiglottis is attached to the largest cartilage in the body, the thyroid cartilage (Adam's apple), which is particularly prominent in men. Below this is the cricoid cartilage, which is frequently fractured in cases of strangulation.

The vocal cords are two tense elastic bands covered with mucous membrane that stretch across the larynx from front to back. Below them is a small space called the subglottic space, the narrowest part of the larynx; choking occurs if a foreign particle such as a piece of food or a tiny bone becomes trapped there. Normally the larynx is closed off by the epiglottis when swallowing or vomiting takes place, but the cough reflex may temporarily interfere with this natural blockage. Should this occur, especially in an unconscious patient, there is a danger that some food or vomit may be inhaled into the lungs.

When the laryngeal muscles pull together they close the gap that is normally open between the vocal cords. When air from the lungs is forced through the closed vocal cords it causes them to vibrate and produce a sound. The pitch of the sound depends on the length and tension of the cords: the higher the tension, the higher the sound. Loudness is directly related to the force and volume of the air forced through the vocal cords. The formation of intelligible speech requires this sound to be modified by the combined action of the teeth, tongue, and lips.

SEE ALSO *Heimlich maneuver, laryngitis, laryngoscopy*

laxative Any substance or chemical agent that acts to loosen the bowels and relieve constipation; also called purgative or cathartic. Many *over-the-counter* laxatives are considered too harsh for use in small children; most pediatricians recommend the use of mineral oil to soften stools, thus reducing straining during bowel movements. The usual dosage is one tablespoonful (15 ml) in the morning and one at night (an additional tablespoonful may be given during the afternoon) until loose bowel movements occur four or five times a day. If significant improvement is not noted within one or two weeks, it is important to consult a physician.

A laxative should never be taken in the presence of abdominal pain, high fever, or nausea and vomiting. The overuse of laxatives can aggravate constipation or even create it.

lead poisoning Poisoning from the ingestion of lead, characterized in the chronic form by nausea, vomiting, severe abdominal pain, impairment of the nervous system, and a wasting of the muscles. It can be caused by prolonged industrial exposure to lead dust, eating or drinking from lead vessels, or by chewing on lead toys or lead-based paints.

Diagnosis is made by means of blood tests to determine the presence of lead; a urine test is also sometimes used in the diagnosis of lead poisoning in children (coproporphyrin test). X-rays may also reveal typical "lead lines" in the wrists and knees.

Treatment involves taking chelating agents, compounds that engulf molecules of lead in the body and aid in its eventual elimination in the urine.

Legionnaires' disease A form of pneumonia caused by bacterial infection. It is so named because in July 1976, 149 American Legion conventioneers developed a disease characterized by fits of coughing, fever, and pneumonia. An additional 72 people who had been in or near the hotel were also affected,

lens

and 34 died of pneumonia or directly related complications.

The species of bacteria found to be responsible for the infection was named *Legionella pneumophila*. Among the sites where the bacteria have been found to thrive are air-conditioning cooling towers. It is thought that the bacteria are distributed in the fine mist of water vapor that emanates from such sources.

Several outbreaks of Legionnaires' disease have been reported in the United States. In 1980, two outbreaks occurred in Burlington, Vermont; eighty-eight cases were confirmed and seventeen patients died.

Symptoms of the disease usually develop from two to ten days after exposure to the bacteria and include muscular aches, mild headache, coughing, and a rising fever (up to 105°F/41°C). Patients may experience pain in the chest and abdomen, and breathing typically becomes difficult. Diarrhea is fairly common, and some patients may appear confused or sluggish, perhaps as a result of involvement of the central nervous system.

Death from pneumonia or circulatory collapse (shock) has been reported in approximately 20 percent of untreated patients. Erythromycin, the antibiotic first found effective in treating Legionnaires' disease, is still used.

SEE ALSO *Pontiac fever*

lens A biconvex colorless transparent structure in the *eye* that automatically changes shape slightly to permit the sharp focus on the *retina* of both near and far objects.

leprosy A chronic and mildly *contagious* disease that occurs in nearly all tropical and subtropical climates and in certain other areas; for example, it is *endemic* to some warmer parts of the United States. The disease is caused by infection with the microorganism *Mycobacterium leprae*, which primarily affects the skin and nerves. It has been estimated that between 11 and 15 million people throughout the world suffer from the disease.

The incubation period of leprosy is unusually long, ranging from about one year to as many as twenty-five or thirty years in exceptional cases. Two major forms of the disease exist: lepromatous (the more contagious) and tuberculoid. The infection occurs most often in communities with inadequate hygiene. Children are particularly susceptible, although because of the disease's slow progress the signs and symptoms may not be recognized for several years following the initial infection.

In the lepromatous (or nodular) form of the disease, early signs of infection include intermittent attacks of fever and painful red swellings or nodules on the skin. In time the skin becomes thick and irregular, especially over bony prominences such as those above the eyes; the lines of the face may become distorted into a lionlike expression.

This form of the disease is progressive and in the absence of medical treatment fatal complications may eventually occur.

The tuberculoid form of leprosy primarily affects the nerves of the skin. The areas of skin supplied by the affected nerves lose their sense of touch and can often be felt as hard, thick cords. The patient may complain early in the course of the disease of a sense of tingling, numbness, and loss of the sense of pain and temperature in the limbs. The tuberculoid form is not contagious and usually runs a self-limiting course.

Treatment of leprosy involves the administration of antibiotic drugs such as dapsone or sulfoxone. With proper treatment, the prognosis is good.

lesion Any abnormal alteration in the tissues of an organ, structure, or part. Lesions include the pathological changes brought about by infectious diseases, wounds, metabolic or hormonal disorders, and tumors.

leukemia A malignant (cancerous) disease of the white blood cells *(leukocytes)*, characterized by a vast increase in their numbers in the bloodstream.

As with other forms of *cancer*, the cells cease to multiply in an orderly manner; leukemia involves the rapid and excessive production of immature white blood cells that lack normal effectiveness. This leads to the progressive infiltration of white cells into body tissues, particularly the *bone marrow*. As a result, bone marrow is destroyed and loses its ability to produce normal red blood cells *(erythrocytes)*, white blood cells, and *platelets*.

The failure of red cell production leads to anemia; the lack of normal white cells lowers the body's resistance to infection; and the failure of platelet production leads to the danger of severe bleeding. Thus, the main symptoms of leukemia are anemia, infection, and hemorrhage.

There are four main types of leukemia, two chronic and two acute. Chronic myeloid leukemia is a disease of adults and affects the neutrophils (one type of white blood cell); chronic lymphatic leukemia affects the elderly and involves the *lymphocyte* series of white cells. Both chronic leukemias are responsive to treatment, although as yet they are not curable. Patients with these disorders may live for many years even without medical treatment.

Acute lymphatic leukemia is almost entirely a disease of childhood. Its onset is usually rapid and, if untreated, it leads to death within a few weeks or months. Fortunately, there has been rapid progress in its treatment by *chemotherapy*, with the result that about 50 percent of children with the disease can be cured, although the course of treatment required is as long as two years or more.

Acute myeloid leukemia is largely a disease of adults and it runs a similar course to the childhood disease. It is not nearly as responsive to treatment and can rarely be cured. Nevertheless, with early and adequate treatment some patients can survive for up to three years, compared to three months for untreated cases.

leukocyte White blood cell. Although they are much less numerous than red blood cells, a drop of blood contains about half a million white cells. Some are manufactured in the bone marrow while others are made in the lymph glands and spleen. The lifespan of many of them is a day or two, so many new ones must be produced to maintain a steady number.

White cells exist in several types. The neutrophils are the most numerous and act as a direct defense against bacterial infection. They actively approach bacteria and engulf, kill, and digest them. They are very active cells, capable of moving through body tissues to concentrate in areas of bacterial invasion. The monocytes, less numerous than the neutrophils, have a similar function. They combine the ability to attack bacteria with scavenging activities that assist in the removal of dead or damaged tissue, bacteria, or foreign material.

The main function of the *lymphocytes* is the production of *antibodies*. Lymphocytes react to the presence of foreign material or organisms by producing complex proteins (antibodies) that can attack and neutralize the invader. *Immunity* to many diseases is established by the production of specific antibodies following the first attack.

Two minor classes of white cells, the eosinophils and basophils, have important but less well understood roles in allergic disorders.

Many of the neutrophils are destroyed in the process of destroying invading bacteria; their bodies are part of the pus that forms. Lymphocytes, however, have a relatively long lifespan and continue to produce essential antibodies for months or years.

SEE ALSO *leukocytosis, leukopenia*

leukocytosis An increase in the number of white cells *(leukocytes)* in the blood, most commonly caused by the presence of a bacterial infection. This increase is the normal reaction of the body's defense system to foreign invaders, especially to pathogenic bacteria.

leukopenia An abnormally low number of white blood cells *(leukocytes)* in the circulating blood. It is most commonly the result of decreased production of new white cells because of infection, drug reaction, or irradiation.

leukoplakia The formation of irregular white patches or spots on the surface of the tongue and the mucous membrane of the cheek. The condition requires immediate medical attention because it may be a sign of cancer.

leukorrhea A white or yellowish discharge from the vagina. It may precede or follow menstruation and be normal, but it may also be caused by an infection of the vagina or the lining of the cervix. Unless the discharge is copious, undergoes a change in color or consistency, or develops an unpleasant odor, medical attention may not be necessary.

lichen planus Any of a variety of inflammatory skin diseases characterized by itchy rough or scaly patches, especially on the legs, wrists, forearms, and inside the cheeks. The cause is unclear but an emotional basis has been postulated. There is no specific treatment, although an ointment to relieve the itching can be used. The problem is self-limiting but may last for some time.

ligament A tough band of fibrous tissues that supports various bodily organs and structures and connects the bones that form joints.

ligature A fine wire or thread of various materials (such as catgut, silk, nylon, dacron, or cotton) used to tie or constrict a blood vessel or other structure.

lipemia An abnormally large amount of fat or fatty substances in the circulating blood.

lipid Any of various true fats and fatlike substances such as *cholesterol*.

lipoma A benign (harmless) tumor or growth composed of fatty tissues.

lipomatosis An accumulation or deposition of several benign tumors composed of fatty tissues *(lipomas)*.

lithotomy The surgical removal of a *calculus* (stone) from a kidney or other affected organ.

liver The largest organ of the human body, situated on the right side of the abdominal cavity just beneath the diaphragm. It is responsible for the production of bile, the storage of glycogen, and a wide variety of essential metabolic activities. This gigantic chemical factory, which is essential for life, also acts to detoxify various poisonous substances that may be absorbed into the blood from the intestines.

The major functions of the liver depend largely on its distinct system of blood vessels, known as the portal circulation. In most organs the oxygen-depleted blood that enters the veins is conveyed directly to the heart, where it is pumped into the lungs to pick up a fresh supply of oxygen and returned through the heart to the arteries. The veins from the stomach and intestines, however, first pass through the liver, where they branch out and form a new network of capillaries. On the other side of this capillary network the blood again enters the veins and is conveyed to the heart.

Blood that enters the liver's capillary network carries with it all the nutrients and waste products absorbed from the digestive tract. One of the major functions of the liver is to remove glucose (sugar) from this blood; the glucose is converted to glycogen and stored. Glycogen is the energy-reserve carbohydrate of the body; on demand by the muscles, it is converted back into glucose to supply energy or heat.

The liver is also able to build proteins from the *amino acids* present as a result of protein digestion.

The liver contains cells known as Kupffer's cells that surround and destroy cellular debris, bacteria, and other unwelcome particles that enter the portal circulation. Various chemicals that are not needed by the body, or that may be potentially dangerous if left in the circulation, are rendered harmless by the liver and then removed from the body in the urine.

Fibrinogen and prothrombin, constituents of the blood that are essential for clotting, as well as the anticoagulant *heparin*, are manufactured in the liver. Other functions of the liver include the storage of the fat-soluble vitamins (A, D, E, and K) and vitamin B^{12}, the formation of cholesterol, the secretion of bile, and the production of a large proportion of normal body heat.

It has been estimated that the liver is responsible for performing nearly 500 separate functions in its essential role as the body's chemical factory.

SEE ALSO *cirrhosis, gallbladder, hepatitis, jaundice*

loading dose   An especially high dose of an antibiotic or other drug prescribed for a patient the first time the product is taken. This 'loads" the drug in the bloodstream and accelerates the attainment of a therapeutic blood level of the drug. Thereafter, the drug is taken exactly as prescribed. Continuing to take higher doses than recommended can result in potentially serious side effects.

lobar pneumonia   Inflammation of one or more lobes of the lungs. SEE *pneumonia*

lochia   The normal discharge from the uterus and vagina that begins shortly following childbirth and persists for about two weeks. It is at first largely composed of blood but becomes yellowish, pale, or whitish during the second week.

lockjaw   SEE *tetanus*

low blood pressure   SEE *hypotension*

lumbago   A general term for any dull, aching pain in the lower part of the back.

lumbar puncture   The insertion of a hollow needle between two of the lumbar vertebrae at the lower part of the spinal column to extract a sample of *cerebrospinal fluid*. A lumbar puncture, also known as a spinal tap, is usually performed under a local anesthetic, with the patient lying on one side and the knees drawn up.

The fluid is examined with the naked eye (it is normally clear) and subjected to various laboratory tests. The procedure is relatively common and quite safe; the only discomfort to the patient is a headache, which may persist for a few days.

lumpectomy The surgical removal of a malignant (cancerous) lump of tissue, especially one in the breast, that is confined to a relatively small area. Under appropriate circumstances it is used as a less disfiguring alternative to removal of the entire breast *(mastectomy)*.

lung One of a pair of light spongy organs situated in the *thorax* (chest) that provides a vast surface area of specialized tissues for the absorption of oxygen by the blood and the release of the waste product carbon dioxide during breathing. Each lung is shaped somewhat like a cone, with the narrow part pointing upward. At birth the lungs are grayish pink, but with age they gradually turn a bluish black from the inhalation of various pollutants in the air.

Air reaches the lungs through the *trachea*, a tube about 4 inches (10 cm) long and 1 inch (2.5 cm) wide that begins at the base of the larynx and ends behind the sternum (breastbone). It divides into the two main air passages, the bronchi.

The lungs occupy most of the chest cavity, extending up beneath the collarbones and down to the diaphragm, or the dome-shaped muscular wall that separates the thorax from the abdomen.

The right lung consists of three separate segments or lobes and the left lung of two lobes. Each lung is covered with a membrane (pleural membrane), which also lines the chest wall and diaphragm. There is an airless cavity between the lungs and the chest wall lying within the pleural membrane. A thin film of fluid separates these membranes, allowing the lungs and chest wall to expand smoothly during breathing without rubbing together.

The basic functional unit of the lung consists of a bronchiole (the smallest subdivision of the air passages) with its cluster of alveoli (air sacs) at the end. Together they form a primary lobule. On a larger scale, each lung consists of ten major branches or segments of the bronchi, each of which forms self-contained units. (Some types of lung disease may be localized for a time in one of these segments and be treated without involving an entire lung or major lobe.)

All the living cells of the body need oxygen to survive, and all produce carbon dioxide as a waste product. When a person inhales, air is drawn into the lungs through the nose, trachea, bronchi, and bronchioles. This is called inspiration and is brought about by the action of the muscles between the ribs, which expand the chest upward, outward, and sideways, and the diaphragm, which moves down. The internal volume of the chest and the chest wall (pleural cavity) becomes larger, creating a suction effect on the lungs that causes them to expand.

Because the volume of the lungs increases, a partial vacuum is created and air rushes in through the nose and air passages to fill the enlarged space. Exhaling (expiration) is a passive action; it is the result of the natural escape of air held momentarily in the lungs at slightly more pressure than that outside the lungs.

At rest, a normal person inhales and exhales about sixteen times a minute, during which a gas exchange takes place in the lungs. Oxygen passes from the air in the lungs through the thin walls of the alveoli and capillaries into the blood. At the same time, carbon dioxide passes in the opposite direction into the lungs and is then breathed out. The oxygen-rich blood passes to the left side of the heart and is pumped out to all organs and tissues of the body through the arteries.

SEE ALSO *asthma, bronchiectasis, bronchitis, pleurisy, pneumonia, pneumothorax*

lung cancer Cancer that occurs in various structures of the lungs and major air passages; also called bronchogenic *carcinoma*. It is responsible for nearly 40 percent of all male deaths from *malignant* disease; it is seen most often between the ages of 50 and 75, and has been known to be five times more common in men than women, although that is changing. There is no doubt that most cases of lung cancer are caused by cigarette smoking; the more cigarettes smoked per day, the greater the risk. For every nonsmoker who contracts lung cancer, thirty heavy smokers will die from the disease.

Lung cancer typically begins with nonspecific signs and symptoms such as a persistent cough and a secondary infection that may produce bloodstained sputum. Partial obstruction of the bronchus by the tumor can cause *emphysema*, and total obstruction can collapse the lung. Another frequent symptom is pain beneath the ribs, which increases during inhalation. Late symptoms include weight loss and weakness.

The *prognosis* for most patients with lung cancer is negative, although in a few cases early treatment can prolong life considerably. Chest x-rays are an important aid in diagnosis; however, by the time x-ray evidence is clear the disease may have progressed to the point where surgery or other treatment is ineffective.

SEE *asbestosis, chemotherapy, metastasis*

lupus erythematosus A chronic and disfiguring systemic (affecting large portions of the body) and cutaneous (affecting the skin) disease of unknown origin. It is characterized by the formation of red, scaly patches and, in the so-called disseminated form, by inflammation of the body's connective tissues, whose chief constituent is the protein collagen. Lupus erythematosus is one of the collagen diseases, and it takes two distinct and unrelated forms: disseminated (systemic) lupus erythematosus and discoid lupus erythematosus. Both conditions are thought to represent examples of an *autoimmune disease*, in which an impairment in the body's natural defense system results in the abnormal production of *antibodies* against some of its own tissues.

Discoid lupus erythematosus is more commonly seen in women than men and usually occurs in middle age. The first sign is a red patch on the face, especially the bridge of the nose or other skin exposed to sunlight (which seems to induce the skin eruptions). Often this rash spreads over the nose and cheeks to form the shape of a butterfly ("butterfly rash"). The application of a cream or ointment containing *steroids* and the administration of antimalarial drugs such as hydroxychloroquine are often effective treatment.

Disseminated lupus erythematosus is often characterized by the same type of butterfly rash. In addition, the patient may experience fever, painful joints (arthritis), and various malfunctions of the lungs, kidneys, and heart. Disseminated lupus erythematosus is a progressive and potentially serious disease. The treatment depends on the severity of the disease and the organs involved. Mild forms of the disease are usually treated with drugs to relieve pain and inflammation and the administration of antimalarial drugs such as hydroxychloroquine. Severe forms of systemic lupus erythematosus require the administration of *corticosteroids* such as prednisone.

Patients with both forms of this disease should avoid excessive exposure to strong sunlight.

lymph The clear, yellowish, and slightly alkaline fluid drained off from the body tissues and conveyed to the bloodstream by the *lymphatic vessels*. It is similar in composition to the fluid portion of the blood, although in some parts of the body its composition varies; for example, the milky white lymph derived from vessels that drain the intestinal tract is rich in absorbed fats.

lymphatic vessels The vessels that form a vast network in the body for the transport of *lymph*, the clear fluid that bathes all tissues of the body. In addition to lymph, these vessels carry *lymphocytes* (a type of white blood cell) and other substances essential for the body's natural defense (immune) system.

lymph glands Bean-shaped swellings or protuberances composed of small masses of lymphatic tissue occurring at intervals along the network of *lymphatic vessels*. Also

lymphocyte

called lymph nodes, they act as filters through which the lymph passes. They may become infected and greatly enlarged during the course of various diseases, a condition popularly known as "swollen glands."

lymphocyte A type of white blood cell *(leukocyte)* that plays an important role in the body's natural defense (immune) system.

lymphoma A general term applied to any of various malignant diseases that involve lymphoid tissue, the tissue that comprises the lymph glands. Hodgkin's disease is an example.

M

malaise A general feeling of being unwell or of general bodily discomfort. It is an extremely common symptom of a wide variety of diseases and disorders.

malaria An acute and sometimes chronic infectious disease caused by any one of four distinct species of parasitic *protozoa* of the genus *Plasmodium: P. falciparum, P. vivax, P. malariae,* and *P. ovale.* The ovale form of malaria is relatively rare and primarily seen in West Africa; the other three forms are fairly widespread in tropical and subtropical climates. The most serious form of malaria is caused by *Plasmodium falciparum;* it is this form that will be discussed.

Malaria is the gravest parasitic disease in the world; nearly 100 million new cases are reported each year in Africa, Asia, and Central and South America. In Africa alone, malaria kills about 1 million people annually—an average of more than 2,700 people every day!

Malarial parasites are transmitted to humans by the bite of an infected female mosquito of the genus *Anopheles;* less commonly the disease can be transmitted by the transfusion of infected blood. The parasites need two hosts to complete their life cycles: the *Anopheles* mosquito, in which the sexual phases of reproduction and development occur, and a human. The only way a mosquito can acquire the parasites is by biting a person already infected with malarial parasites.

In the early stages of an acute malarial infection the symptoms may be confused with those of influenza. They include headache, pain in the muscles and joints, chills, and a slight rise in body temperature, all of which may last for up to a week before the disease takes hold. The typical attack occurs in three stages. The first is the so-called cold stage, characterized by a sensation of extreme chilliness even though the body temperature may be higher than normal. This is followed by the hot stage, in which the patient feels an increasing sensa-

malignant

tion of warmth or has periodic hot flashes. Eventually the body temperature may go as high as 106°F (41.1°C) and remain there for several hours. As the fever begins to subside after the hot stage has reached its maximum, the symptoms are gradually relieved and the patient begins to sweat profusely.

The falciparum form of malaria (also known as malignant tertian malaria) is distinct from the other forms in several respects, in addition to being the most deadly. Attacks rarely occur in a predictable manner; the onset may be gradual and the fever irregular, intermittent, or continuous. This is because the cycle of reproduction and release of parasites within the red blood cells is not as well synchronized as in other forms of the disease.

The incubation period for malaria is generally from about ten to thirty-five days, although in some forms (certain strains of vivax) it may be several months. Falciparum malaria can be fatal: among the major complications are severe *anemia* (as a result of the destruction of vast numbers of red blood cells by the parasites), acute *kidney failure*, blockage of blood vessels in the lungs and brain by clumps of parasites, and *coma*. In most cases of untreated malaria the *spleen* and *liver* eventually become enlarged.

The definitive diagnosis of malaria of any form involves the microscopic identification of the parasites in a blood sample. Partially successful attempts to control malaria have been made by draining swamps and other areas where the mosquitoes breed and by using insecticides; unfortunately, mosquitoes have a tendency to become resistant.

Research is under way to develop a *vaccine* that will render people *immune* to malarial parasites. Currently, however, the most successful means of controlling and treating malaria is by administering drugs such as chloroquine; combinations of drugs are used when the parasites have become resistant to chloroquine.

Before traveling to a malarial region it is important to consult a physician well before departure; he or she can prescribe small doses of an antimalarial drug to be taken regularly before arrival in the malarial region and continuing until the return home.

malignant Resisting treatment; growing worse; life-threatening. The term is used especially to describe *cancer*.
COMPARE *benign*

malpractice The faulty, incorrect, negligent, or injurious treatment of a patient by a physician, surgeon, nurse, or other member of the health-care profession. It can lead to legal action against the practitioner by the patient. As a result, most physicians and surgeons are covered against such litigation by malpractice insurance. They also tend to cover themselves against malpractice accusations by ordering many types of *diagnostic* tests and procedures when treating an individual patient, many of which would not be necessary were it not for the threat of misdiagnosis and the subsequent lawsuit. Malpractice insurance and questionable tests add to the medical expenses that the patient must pay.

SEE ALSO *iatrogenic*

mammography X-ray or other radiographic examination of the breast, used especially in the diagnosis of *breast cancer*. The resulting x-ray film is known as a mammogram. Because of the possibility of injury to a fetus during such a procedure, the American Cancer Society and the American College of Radiologists urge that this test not be performed on pregnant women, despite the relatively low radiation levels involved.

It is generally agreed that mammography should not be used as the only evidence of breast cancer. Although the procedure can accurately detect breast cancer in over 90 percent of cases, it also provides a false positive result in about 75 percent of cases: that is, it offers false evidence that a woman has breast cancer when she does not.

SEE ALSO *thermography, ultrasonography*

mastectomy Surgical removal of a breast, usually as treatment for *breast cancer*. Nearly 106,000 American women each year are diagnosed as having breast cancer, and despite the best efforts to treat this disease in its earliest stages, mortality from breast cancer has remained basically unchanged for the past three or four decades.

A total mastectomy involves surgical removal of the affected breast as well as the lymph nodes in the armpit (axillary nodes). A radical mastectomy goes one step further and removes the underlying chest muscles as well.

There is growing evidence that a radical mastectomy, the most extensive surgical procedure, is not more effective than a total mastectomy followed by radiation therapy. Many physicians now believe that radical mastectomy has been accepted by many surgeons without convincing evidence of its superiority. On the contrary, there is abundant evidence supporting the proposal that more conservative procedures provide at least equal benefits with substantially less disfigurement.

SEE ALSO *lumpectomy, mammography, thermography, ultrasonography*

masturbation The stroking, rubbing, or other manipulation of the penis or clitoris to produce an *orgasm*. Absolutely no physical harm can come from this practice.

measles A highly contagious childhood disease caused by a virus infection and spread by airborne droplets. The incubation period is from about ten to fourteen days. The first signs are fever, runny nose, red and watery eyes, sneezing, and a hacking cough. The temperature generally continues to rise slightly every day for about three or four days and may go as high as 104°F (40°C). At about this time the typical rash can be seen, beginning behind the ears and spreading to the face and back. Within the next two days it spreads to the body and limbs, becomes blotchy in places, increases in size, and changes to a slightly darker red. Just before the rash appears it is often possible to see tiny white spots on a red base on the inner surface of the cheeks (Koplik's spots).

The child's eyes will be especially sensitive to light for a few days; it is not necessary to put the child in a darkened room, but strong light should be avoided.

A child can be infectious from the moment the symptoms appear until about three to five days after the rash has disappeared. It is important to keep the child isolated during this period so that others are not exposed to the disease. Although most cases of measles present no serious problems or complications, a physician may want to make sure that there is no associated infection of the eyes, ears, or lungs. If a child has not yet had measles, a physician may suggest *vaccination* against it, which is usually possible from about the age of one year.
COMPARE *rubella*

medulla The central or innermost part of an organ, as distinguished from its *cortex*. The term is also used to refer to the *medulla oblongata*.

medulla oblongata The lower part of the *brain stem*, consisting of the enlarged portion of the spinal cord as it enters the skull. It contains several important nerve centers including those responsible for the regulation of breathing, swallowing, and heart action. The vomiting center of the brain is also located in the medulla oblongata; when nerves in this part of the medulla are stimulated, as by the action of some drugs, vomiting occurs.

melanin A black or dark brown pigment that occurs especially in the hair, skin, part of the structure of the eye (the choroid), and a specific mass of nerve cells deep within the brain, the substantia nigra. Exposure to sunlight stimulates the production of melanin. It is also present in some malignant growths.
SEE *melanoma*

melanoma A skin tumor containing the dark pigment *melanin;* also, a rare and extremely malignant (cancerous) tumor that starts in a black mole and rapidly spreads (metastasizes).

melena Stools (feces) that appear black and tarlike because of the presence of blood that has been altered by the action of intestinal juices, as from a bleeding ulcer of the stomach or duodenum.

membrane A thin layer of tissue, especially one that surrounds an organ or part, separates adjacent cavities, or connects related structures.
SEE ALSO *mucous membrane*

menarche The beginning of *menstruation*, occurring at puberty.

meningitis Inflammation of the three delicate membranes (meninges) that cover the brain and spinal cord. The condition is especially common in children. The infection may be bacterial or viral, and can spread to these membranes as a result of a local infection of the ears, sinuses, or tonsils, or it may be carried by the bloodstream.

The first symptoms of meningitis are common to many other infections, and include high fever, chills, severe headaches, and vomiting. These symptoms are frequently followed by stiffness of the neck and back, and in severe cases the head bends back and cannot be bent forward. As the disease progresses there may be convulsions or loss of consciousness. In such cases a physician should be consulted immediately, since many cases of bacterial meningitis respond well to antibiotics. The doctor may also arrange a *lumbar puncture* to obtain a sample of the fluid in the spinal canal *(cerebrospinal fluid)* to confirm the diagnosis.

menopause The end of *menstruation* and female reproductive ability. The ovary gradually stops producing ova (eggs) and secreting the hormones estrogen and progesterone, which create and control the monthly cycle. These changes usually take place between the ages of forty and fifty-five, most commonly between forty-seven and fifty.

The way in which the periods cease varies greatly. In about 75 percent of women, the interval between each period lengthens and menstrual bleeding is lighter and shorter. About 25 percent of women experience irregular and sometimes very heavy bleeding. However, it must never be taken for granted that such out-of-pattern bleeding is due to menopause, and a medical examination should be made to exclude other possible causes. For a small percentage of women the periods may cease quite suddenly.

Many women have no symptoms other than the end of menstruation. Some women experience "hot flashes," feelings of warmth at the head and neck and over the rest of the body. Sweating may also occur. These sensations are momentary and appear unpredictably and irregularly. They may be caused by deficiency of the hormone *estrogen*. Other physical changes at the time of the menopause include a tendency to gain weight. Sexual desire and the ability to reach orgasm are not affected.

Medical treatment to relieve menopausal symptoms is seldom required, although hormone replacements may be prescribed.

menorrhagia An abnormally prolonged menstrual period or one during which the blood flow is excessive. It may be associated with some disorder of the uterus, such as *fibroids*, and if persistent requires a medical examination.
SEE ALSO *metrorrhagia*

menstruation The monthly discharge of blood-containing fluid from the lining of the uterus through the vagina in sexually mature women who are not pregnant. The onset of menstruation *(menarche)* usually begins between the ages of eleven and thirteen, and the menstrual cycle continues until *menopause*.

From puberty onward many ova (eggs) begin to ripen in the ovaries each month, but only one becomes fully mature. This ovum ripens during the first half of the menstrual cycle, when the uterine lining (endometrium) thickens under the influence of the hormone estrogen. As the ovum moves from the ovary to the uterus via the Fallopian tube, the ovary produces another hormone, progesterone, which makes the endometrium thicker and moist with many blood vessels in preparation for a fertilized ovum.

If the ovum is not fertilized by a sperm cell during its passage to the uterus, it breaks up and dies and is not implanted in the uterine lining. As a result of this, the lining begins to break down. Cells die, the uterus contracts and expels the top layers of the endometrium into the cervix, where they are passed outside the body through the vagina.

The menstrual flow consists mainly of reddish-brown blood; the volume and duration vary from woman to woman over three to five days. During menstruation, normal exercise should be continued and sexual intercourse is perfectly harmless to both partners. Menstrual flow can be absorbed by cotton pads or tampons; a menstrual tampon will not damage the hymen (maidenhead), which has an opening to release the flow of blood.

Many women experience pain and discomfort during their menstrual periods *(dysmenorrhea)*. Should these symptoms become severe, a physician should be consulted.

Women who take oral contraceptives continue to have menstrual periods even though they do not ovulate.
SEE ALSO *menorrhagia, metrorrhagia, toxic-shock syndrome*

mesentery A large fold of tissue formed by the *peritoneum* that helps support the small intestine, to which it is attached.

metabolism The sum of all the chemical processes within a living organism that are responsible for its growth, maintenance and repair (anabolism) and the conversion of complex substances into simpler ones (catabolism) mainly for the release of energy. The rate at which these processes or changes occur in the cells and tissues is under the control of hormones, particularly those secreted directly into the bloodstream by the *thyroid gland.*

metastasis The spread of *cancer* cells from their original site in a malignant tumor or growth to other parts of the body through the bloodstream or lymphatic system.
SEE ALSO *in situ*

metrorrhagia Bleeding from the uterus, especially at times other than during the menstrual period. It may be caused by a disease or disorder of the cervix (neck) of the uterus or a disorder of the hormonal control system that regulates ovulation and prepares the lining of the uterus for reception of the fertilized ovum. In some cases the cause may be cancer of the cervix or other part of the genital tract. Prompt medical attention is essential to discover and treat the underlying cause.
SEE ALSO *menorrhagia, menstruation*

mg
SEE *milligram*

microorganism Any living organism too small to be seen with the naked eye, such as *protozoa, bacteria, fungi, rickettsiae,* and *viruses.* Only a very few species of microorganisms are pathogenic (capable of causing disease).
SEE ALSO *Koch's law*

microsurgery Any surgical procedure performed with the direct use of a microscope and usually involving a micromanipulator, a device that permits the surgeon to manipulate extremely small instruments within the field of view.

micturition Urination.

migraine A severe headache that typically occurs in sudden attacks and may be preceded or accompanied by symptoms such as visual disturbances, acute sensitivity of the eyes to light (photophobia), and frequently nausea and vomiting. Very often the headache eases with the onset of vomiting.

Some migraine sufferers have advance warnings of an impending attack; these include the impression of bright streaks or flashes of light, blurred or temporarily lost vision, depression, or (rarely) the partial loss of feeling in an arm or leg. These sensations may last for ten or twenty minutes and disappear with the onset of the headache, persist throughout, or first occur during the migraine attack itself.

The headache is often throbbing and characteristically begins in or is limited to one side of the head, although in a few patients it gradually becomes more diffuse and appears to affect the entire head. The attacks vary greatly in severity. They may last from a few minutes to several hours, and in particularly troublesome and untreated cases they may last for three or four days.

Different patients are affected in different ways. In many patients there is no advance warning of the attacks; the pain may affect the entire head from the beginning, with no visual or gastrointestinal symptoms (nausea and vomiting).

The exact cause of migraine is not known. Among the implicating factors are a family history of migraine (which suggests a genetic predisposition), some disturbance of blood circulation in the brain, or emotional disturbances. Attacks occur in a few people following exposure to rapidly flashing lights or certain foods. Many cases are undoubtedly related to stress.

Treatment of migraine depends largely on the severity of the attacks and the interval between them. Some patients find relief by lying down in a darkened room or by taking prescribed doses of aspirin, codeine, or another analgesic, or a tranquilizer. In more severe cases the physician may prescribe a drug to prevent, delay, or reduce the severity of the attacks. Some of these drugs are prescribed to be taken at the first warning symptoms; the earlier it is taken, the greater the chance that it will be effective. These drugs include barbiturates, codeine, and ergotamine tartrate.

milligram One-thousandth of a gram, the measurement commonly used to identify the strength of a tablet or capsule of a prescription or over-the-counter drug. Abbreviation: mg
SEE *dose*

miscarriage
SEE *abortion*

mole A congenital discolored spot raised above the surface of the skin, sometimes containing hairs. Moles should never be irritated or interfered with in any way; only a physician should attempt to remove one. Most moles are benign (harmless), but if they start to bleed or undergo a change in color or size a physician should be consulted, since this may be an early indication of *cancer*.

mongolism An abnormal genetic condition in which a child is born with a small and slightly flattened head, eyes that are narrow and slanted, and a large tongue that protrudes from the mouth, and mental deficiency.
SEE *Down's syndrome*

moniliasis
SEE *candidiasis*

mononucleosis An acute infectious disease caused by a virus. It tends to affect children and young adults and is rare in persons over the age of forty. Outbreaks of the disease (also called glandular fever) occur most frequently where large groups of young people live or work together, as in schools. It is popularly thought that the infection can be transmitted by kissing, which is highly probable.

The incubation period varies from about four to ten weeks. The onset is gradual and the symptoms are often mild. They include sore throat, swollen lymph glands (especially in the neck, armpits, and groin), fatigue, and fever. In a few cases a rash develops (similar to that of German measles) and, rarely, the patient becomes jaundiced. In severe cases the symptoms are more pronounced and may last for several weeks. Depression and general debility may continue for months following a particularly severe attack.

The diagnosis is possible only with the examination of a blood sample. People with the disease have an increased number of certain types of white blood cells (lymphocytes and monocytes) in their circulating blood. Many of these cells also have a characteristic abnormal appearance when examined under a microscope. The other major diagnostic test (Paul-Bunnell-Davidsohn test) is based on the fact that the blood serum of someone with infectious mononucleosis contains a factor capable of making the red blood cells of sheep agglutinate (stick together).

It is now virtually certain that infectious mononucleosis is caused by one of the many herpes viruses—specifically, the Epstein-Barr virus. As with most viral diseases, there is no specific treatment. Therapy is aimed at making the patient feel better during the course of the disease, including bed rest during the acute phase. In most cases the patient will fully recover within one to four weeks, although in stubborn cases recovery make take up to three months.

morphine A potent *narcotic* analgesic obtained from opium and used to relieve severe pain. The medical use of morphine is under strict governmental control because of its abuse potential and the fact that prolonged use can result in *addiction*.

mucous colitis
SEE *irritable bowel syndrome*

mucous membrane The moist tissue that lines the various bodily organs and passages that are directly or indirectly exposed to air. These include the digestive tract (a hollow tube from the mouth to the anus), the air passages (from the nose to the lungs), and the urinary and genital organs. Cells within these membranes secrete *mucus* to prevent them from drying out.

mucoviscidosis
SEE *cystic fibrosis*

mucus The viscid fluid secreted as a protective coating by the *mucous membranes*.

multiple sclerosis A chronic disease of the central nervous system (brain and spinal cord). The disease, also known as disseminated sclerosis, is characterized by a scattered or patchy degeneration of the myelin sheath, the fatty insulation around nerve fibers in the brain and spinal cord. The symptoms of multiple sclerosis are extremely variable and depend on the original functions of the damaged nerves. The condition may therefore mimic a wide variety of other neurological disorders.

The cause is not yet known, despite evidence reported in 1976 that a virus might be responsible for some forms of the disease. Other investigators have implicated a disturbance in the body's normal defense mechanism *(autoimmune disease)*, metabolic disorders, and metal poisoning.

The onset of multiple sclerosis is not dramatic and can occur at any age. The first symptoms may include minor visual disturbances, dizziness, weakness or stiffness of the arms and legs, and partial loss of sensation in a specific area of the body. A characteristic and diagnostic feature of the disease is that the symptoms often tend to disappear or diminish for a time before flaring up again; some patients are perfectly normal for intervals of several months or years. In severe cases, however, the symptoms persist and become progressively more incapacitating.

There is no known medical cure, although in acute attacks some of the symptoms can occasionally be relieved by adrenocorticotropic hormone (ACTH) or prednisone. Most physicians advise against excessively strenuous activity, but with proper supportive care many patients can maintain a fairly normal and active life. No test can conclusively demonstrate the presence of multiple sclerosis; its diagnosis depends largely on the evaluation of signs and symptoms by a physician.

mumps An acute contagious viral disease common in childhood, characterized by inflammation of the salivary glands, especially the largest, the parotid gland, situated just below the ear; for this reason the infection is also known as epidemic parotitis (inflammation of the parotid glands). The disease is spread by airborn viruses from an infected person. The incubation period is between two and three weeks. Children between the ages of five and fifteen are most often affected, although it is possible to catch mumps at any age. The first attack generally provides *immunity* (protection against future attacks) for life.

The first signs of mumps are stiffness and a slight pain in the neck, followed by a swelling of the parotid gland, which enlarges the entire side of the neck. Often both sides of the neck are swollen. The patient may have difficulty opening his or her mouth wide, the mouth may become very dry, and there is a fever. In severe cases there may be vomiting and the temperature may go as high as 104°F (40°C). Most cases are mild, however, and the swelling usually goes down within five to ten days.

There is no specific treatment for mumps other than keeping the child in bed comfortable. If the symptoms persist or become worse, a physician should be consulted immediately.

Complications are rare in children, but in adolescents or adults the possibility exists of complications such as an infection of the pancreas, thyroid, testicles, or ovaries. This can cause serious problems and it is important to keep all older persons who have not had mumps away from an infectious child until all signs of illness have disappeared.

In rare cases the complications of mumps may involve inflammation of the brain and the membranes that surround it (encephalitis and *meningitis*). The outlook is favorable in most of such cases, although some children may suffer deafness in one ear or partial paralysis of the face muscles as the result of nerve damage.

A live mumps virus *vaccine* is available; a single vaccination provides protection against the disease. It is not yet known if vaccination against mumps provides lifelong immunity.

murmur
SEE *heart murmur*

muscular dystrophy A relatively rare hereditary disease characterized by progressive weakness and wasting of the muscles. In at least half the cases of this disease one member of the direct family is affected. The age at onset is usually during early or late childhood, with boys being more often affected than girls. The onset of the symptoms is insidious. The muscles of the chest, abdomen, and buttocks are affected first, and the disease progresses steadily to affect other parts of the body. In some instances, muscular weakness is experienced after prolonged physical activity. As a general rule, disability develops much faster in patients in whom the disease appears in early life.

Some muscles, particularly those of the calves and buttocks, may enlarge but remain weak. Later the muscles may waste and contract, which can lead to deformity. The absence or diminution of the tendon-jerk reflexes is a characteristic finding. There is no pain with the condition unless the contraction of the muscles is advanced, but progressively the muscles refuse to operate in response to nervous stimulus or voluntary control.

Muscular dystrophy is thought to be associated with an inherited enzyme deficiency and consequent defect in the muscles' ability to use certain amino acid in the manufacture of protein. There is no cure and no specific treatment for muscular dystrophy. Particular attention is given by the physician to the risk of respiratory infections—without a forcible cough reflex, there is a constant danger of pneumonia. Physiotherapy can reduce the risk of muscle contraction, and antibiotics are prescribed to minimize the consequences of infection.

Most children with muscular dystrophy are confined to a wheelchair by the age of ten or twelve, especially in the most common form of the disease, Duchene or pseudohypertrophic muscular dystrophy, which typically affects boys between the ages of three and seven.

myalgia Tenderness or pain in the muscles.

myasthenia gravis A rare chronic disease characterized by progressive loss of function of various groups of muscles. It can occur at any age, but is most common in women between the ages of eighteen and twenty-five and in men over forty. In the early stages muscular fatigue can be relieved by a period of rest. Attacks of generalized muscular weakness in the body after prolonged activity may occur, but the disease is also characterized by periods of remission that may last for months or years.

In the early stages the symptoms of myasthenia gravis include drooping eyelids, double vision, some difficulties in speech, and facial weakness or sagging of the jaw after talking for a few minutes. In the advanced stage there may be difficulty swallowing, breathing (due to involvement of the chest muscles), and lifting the head (due to weakness of the neck muscles).

Myasthenia gravis, which is thought by some researchers to be an *autoimmune disease*, is caused by the failure of the signal from the nerve endings to produce a response in the muscle fibers. Although no cure for this condition has yet been found, the use of neostigmine and related drugs is effective for varying periods of time. Some patients respond favorably to the surgical removal of the *thymus gland*.

mycosis Any disease caused by a *fungus;* a fungal infection.

mydriasis An abnormal dilation (widening) of the pupil of the eye. Among the many possible causes are the effects of various drugs, coma, general anesthesia, fright, and sudden emotion. Any drug used by a physician (especially an ophthalmologist) to dilate the pupils during examination or treatment is known as a mydriatic.

myelin A fatlike substance that forms a protective insulating sheath around certain nerve fibers; these nerves are said to be myelinated.

myelitis Inflammation of the spinal cord or (less commonly) the bone marrow. It represents a potentially serious condition that demands prompt diagnosis and treatment. The symptoms include back pain (which may radiate to the limbs), loss of appetite, moderate fever (101°F/38.5°C), various types of partial loss of sensation (such as numbness, burning, or tingling of the skin), and constipation. The nature of the symptoms depends on the site of the inflammation. If certain spinal nerves are affected, the patient may suffer partial or total paralysis. Diagnosis may necessitate a *lumbar puncture* to obtain a sample of *cerebrospinal fluid*. Treatment depends on the underlying cause. In some cases a patient is given an intravenous injection of *corticosteroids* to decrease the inflammation.

myelography A technique or procedure for examining the spinal cord after the injection of an x-ray contrast *(radiopaque)* medium into the space between the spinal cord and the innermost membrane that surrounds it (subarachnoid space). The procedure usually combines the use of both fluoroscopy and x-ray films.

The patient lies prone on a fluoroscopic table, which can be tilted up or down. This tilting causes the contrast fluid to flow up or down the outside of the spinal cord, an outline of which can be seen on the fluoroscope screen. A series of x-rays is usually taken simultaneously to provide a record of the findings. These may include the identification of a tumor of the spinal cord or some blockage to the normal flow of cerebrospinal fluid, such as a slipped disk.

The x-ray film made during this procedure is known as a myelogram.

myeloma A tumor of the bone marrow, originating in the tissues concerned with the production of blood cells. The term multiple myeloma (also known as plasma cell myeloma or myelomatosis) refers to a rare cancerous disease of the bone marrow that is gradually progressive and life-threatening. The prognosis depends largely on how early in the course of the disease it is recognized and treated, as well as the patient's response to chemotherapy.

myocardial infarction One of the medical terms used to describe what is popularly known as a heart attack; the others are *coronary thrombosis* and *coronary occlusion*. Each emphasizes a slightly different event, although in each case part of the heart muscle is suddenly deprived of blood. This may be caused by spasm or narrowing of the coronary arteries, which nourish the heart muscle, or it may be caused by the formation of a blood clot *(thrombus)* in a branch of these arteries that blocks the blood flow to the heart muscle. In certain cases the part of the heart muscle that is deprived of blood dies and is gradually replaced by a fibrous scar *(infarction)*.

During a heart attack the coronary arteries are suddenly blocked. This usually causes intense chest pain, similar to *angina pectoris*. One distinction is that pain from a heart attack is not relieved by resting. The victim often turns pale and begins to sweat.

In most cases the victim of a nonfatal heart attack is able to resume mild activity after a period of bed rest, often in as little as three weeks. During this time the heart muscle is given a chance to repair damage,

myocarditis

although full healing may take several months. The physician may advise some form of mild physical exercise, such as short walks, after the initial recovery period. It is important for the patient to avoid overexertion, strenuous work, or emotional stress.

The physician's advice should be rigidly followed regarding physical activity, diet, and the continued danger of smoking cigarettes. The conscientious victim of a heart attack should be able to return to a normally active life.

SEE ALSO *coronary artery disease, coronary bypass*

myocarditis Inflammation of the myocardium, the muscular tissue of the heart.

myocardium The *heart* muscle.

myoma Any tumor composed of muscular tissue.
SEE *fibroid*

myomectomy Surgical removal of a portion of muscle, muscular tissue, or a tumor formed of or in muscular tissue. An example is the surgical removal of uterine fibroids.

myopathy Any disease of the muscles.
SEE *muscular dystrophy, myasthenia gravis, myotonia*

myopia The condition of being nearsighted, occurring when the eyeball is slightly too long from front to back. The light entering the *eye* is focused by the *lens* at a point in front of the *retina*, resulting in a blurred image as the light rays redisperse before reaching the retina. This happens when viewing objects at a distance; objects close to the eye are usually in focus.

Myopia is rarely present at birth. It may be observed in school-age children who hold a book or other object very close to the eyes to obtain the proper focus. Various degrees of myopia exist, depending on how far the focal point of the light rays is from the retina.

Myopia usually develops slowly and may not be recognized until distant objects become noticeably more difficult to see clearly. When the defective vision is corrected with eyeglasses or contact lenses, the myopic person is often amazed at how much clarity of vision has been missing over the years.

myosarcoma A malignant (cancerous) tumor of the muscles.

myositis Inflammation of a muscle.
COMPARE *fibrositis*

myotonia Muscular spasm or temporary rigidity of a muscle group following contraction. Myotonia is an inherited disease characterized by a failure of the muscle to relax after contraction has been induced voluntarily. Myotonia congenita is the name given to the disease when it first appears in childhood. It is rare but dominant in its genetic pattern so that there is always a history of its presence in one parent.

Myotonia congenita is generally

not serious; it does not progress, nor does it affect life expectancy. It is probably caused by a congenital defect in one of the enzymes associated with the chemistry of nerve control of muscle fibers. The condition is aggravated by cold and emotional excitement but diminishes with age. The muscles are well developed and function normally but remain contracted.

When myotonia appears for the first time in adulthood it may, very rarely, be associated with eye defects (due to cataract) and with degeneration of the testicles or ovaries. Atrophy (wasting) of the muscles can also occur.

Electromyography, the recording of the electrical activity of selected muscle groups at rest and during voluntary contraction with the use of a needle electrode inserted into a muscle, is used to define or diagnose the true congenital form of myotonia and distinguish it from the temporary effects of excessive muscular activity.

The muscle stiffness and cramping associated with myotonia congenita may be relieved by the administration of drugs such as phenytoin, quinine sulfate, or procainamide.

myringitis Inflammation of the *tympanum* (eardrum); also called tympanitis. It can occur as the result of physical injury or infection. Sudden and dramatic changes in air pressure (as in diving or very rapid ascent or descent in an aircraft) may stretch the eardrum and cause it to become inflamed. Infection of the eardrum is often a consequence of a disease of the respiratory tract or a complication of influenza. Most such infections seem to be viral in origin. Bleeding blisters occasionally form on the eardrum and nearby areas of the external ear passage; in severe cases these blisters break and partial or total deafness can temporarily occur in the affected ear.

Specific treatment of myringitis is usually not required, unless the inflammation is caused by bacterial infection, in which case antibiotics or other drugs are prescribed. In the presence of bleeding blisters on the eardrum, however, the physician may apply antibiotic eardrops or a warm solution of an antiseptic agent. Earache can usually be effectively relieved with the proper dose of aspirin or another analgesic.

myxedema A condition caused by prolonged underactivity of the *thyroid gland (hypothyroidism)* characterized by dry skin, swelling of the tissues of the face and limbs, and an increased sensitivity to cold.

N

narcolepsy An abnormal, sudden, and uncontrollable desire to *sleep*. It is a rare chronic condition often first experienced during adolescence as periodic bouts of unexpected drowsiness; if untreated, these gradually become more intense throughout the person's life. The subject tends to fall asleep during the day in spite of a full night's sleep, even in the most inappropriate situations, such as driving a car.

Since scientists understand very little about why people need sleep, trying to understand why a person has an abnormal desire to sleep presents even greater difficulty. The causes of both normal sleep patterns and the abnormal sleep patterns of narcolepsy are unknown, although several interesting theories have been put forward.

Most narcoleptics can be easily aroused from their abnormal slumber, after which they usually feel refreshed. The dream state occurs almost immediately; by contrast, in normal sleep dreaming generally occurs only after the first ninety minutes. The significance of this phenomenon is unknown, but the finding is so consistent that some experts have suggested that immediate dreaming be used as part of the definition of narcolepsy.

The treatment of narcolepsy is simply to keep the subject alert during the appropriate periods of each day. In a few cases this can be accomplished merely by having the subject drink coffee or tea, both of which contain the stimulant caffeine. More commonly, a physician will prescribe a stimulant, particularly amphetamine.

narcosis The state of unconsciousness brought about by the use of *narcotic* drugs.

narcotic Producing sleep or inducing stupor; said of various potent drugs, especially such opium derivatives as *morphine, codeine,* and heroin, with the ability to relieve severe pain. They also have a profound effect on behavior and mood, and prolonged use can cause *addiction*.

nasopharynx The part of the *pharynx* behind and above the soft palate. It is directly continuous with the nasal passages.

naturopathy A therapeutic system that abandons the use of drugs and surgery. It is based on the belief that natural remedies such as light, heat, cold, water, fruits and other natural foods are sufficient to prevent and cure any disease.

nausea The sensation that usually precedes *vomiting*, characterized by a peculiar feeling in the region of the stomach and an aversion to food. It is a common early symptom (especially in association with vomiting) of many diseases.

necropsy Medical examination of the body after death.
SEE *autopsy*

necrosis The death, as by deprivation of an adequate blood supply or by infection, of a small area of tissue or bone. Necrosis implies involvement of a much smaller area of destruction than does *gangrene*; often, necrosis is noticeable only under a microscope. The dead area is surrounded by healthy cells.

needle biopsy
SEE *biopsy*

neonatal Relating to a newborn baby or to the first four to six weeks after its birth.

neoplasm Any abnormal formation of new tissue, especially a tumor or growth. It can be benign (harmless) or malignant (life-threatening).
SEE *cancer*

nephrectomy Surgical removal of a *kidney*.

nephritis Inflammation of the *kidney*.
SEE *glomerulonephritis*

nephrolithiasis Stones *(calculi)* in the *kidney*. Kidney stones can be found at any point in the urinary tract from the kidneys to the urethra, but they are formed only in the kidney and urinary bladder (although all such stones are commonly referred to as kidney stones). The stones vary in size from tiny particles the size of a grain of sand to huge concretions (staghorn calculi) that can fill up a large portion of the renal pelvis.

About 90 percent of all kidney stones contain calcium and 2–5 percent contain *uric acid;* some stones have a mixed content of calcium, uric acid, and other minerals, such as xanthine, cystine, and magnesium. In cases of obstruction of the urinary tract the urine accumulates in the bladder and renal pelvis and provides an excellent breeding ground for bacteria. It is well known that stone formation is frequently associated with urinary infections.

Stones formed and retained in the kidney itself may present no problems unless they interfere with the drainage of urine into the ureter. However, if even a small stone

171

nephrology

enters the ureter and becomes temporarily or permanently trapped at one of its three particularly narrow points, it can cause severe pain (renal colic). Even if the stone does not become lodged it may cause severe pain during its passage through the ureter; this is typically experienced as a radiating sensation from the kidney over the abdomen and into the groin.

Many kidney stones are eventually passed out in the urine. In some cases it is necessary to remove the stones surgically, either by cutting them out *(lithotomy)* or by inserting a surgical instrument through the urethra and into the bladder or ureter.

SEE ALSO *cystoscope*

nephrology The branch of medical science concerned with the structure and function of the kidneys and the diagnosis and treatment of kidney disease. A specialist in this field is known as a nephrologist.

nephron The structural and functional unit of the *kidney*. Each kidney contains approximately one million nephrons.

SEE *glomerulonephritis*

neuralgia A sharp often burning pain along the course of a nerve. Among the possible causes of neuralgia are inflammation of the nerve (neuritis), pressure on nerve trunks, toxins (poisons), and faulty nerve nutrition.

neural-tube defect Any of various defects in the brain or spinal cord formed during embryonic development.

SEE *anencephaly, spina bifida*

neuritis Inflammation of one or more nerves, usually associated with degenerative changes resulting in various degrees of loss of sensation, movement, or function. Neuritis is not a disease but a symptom; in spite of the suffix *-itis*, it is only rarely associated with significant signs of inflammation.

Some degree of pain along the course of the affected nerve is fairly common. There may also be at times a tingling, burning, or "pins and needles" sensation or, conversely, numbness. Mononeuritis is the name given to the condition when only one nerve is involved; it is often caused by an injury such as the tearing or crushing of the nerve fiber following a bruise, direct blow, or the fracture or dislocation of a bone. Another mechanical factor is prolonged pressure against a nerve, especially one that lies over a bone; this may occur as the result of prolonged squatting, the use of improperly padded crutches, or (more rarely) the formation of a tumor.

Polyneuritis is used to describe any condition in which many nerves are simultaneously affected by neuritis. The cause may be associated with infectious diseases, metal poisoning, vitamin deficiencies, pernicious anemia, diabetes, or other primary disorders that can affect the health of the nerves. In one form, acute idiopathic polyneuritis, the cause is unknown. The condition is characterized by progressive muscular weakness and tenderness similar to the symptoms of poliomyelitis and acute inflammation of the muscles, diminished reflex actions, and often involvement of some of the cranial nerves.

Treatment of polyneuritis is aimed at eliminating the underlying cause. Most forms of the disorder respond favorably to prompt medical treatment. If isolated areas of the body are affected, they should not be exposed to possible injury and should be rested (but not rigidly immobilized). A physician may prescribe physical exercises and suggest the application of heat to relieve pain.

neurology The branch of medical science concerned with the nervous system and the diagnosis and treatment of various diseases and disorders that affect it. A specialist in this field is known as a neurologist.
SEE ALSO *neurosurgery*

neurosis A functional disorder, also known as psychoneurosis, characterized by various degrees of mental conflict and disruption of normal thought processes without serious impairment of the sense of reality. Psychiatrists generally agree, however, that no truly satisfactory definition of neurosis exists (as compared with *psychosis*). In the mildest form, neurosis is difficult to distinguish from familiar and everyday human reactions to disturbing situations or prolonged mental conflicts.

The general personality of a neurotic person is essentially preserved, in that the subject does not appear to those around him or her as completely irrational or outside the context of fundamental human contact. Neurotics typically possess insight regarding their emotional disturbances.

neurosurgery Surgery involving any part of the nervous system, especially the brain and spinal cord (central nervous system). Operations on the living human brain are among the most delicate and exacting in the entire field of surgery.

There is evidence of prehistoric neurosurgery; sections of the skull were removed and some patients survived for several years after such operations (called trephining) despite the lack of antiseptics. They were performed to release evil spirits believed to take hold of the victim and cause unbearable headaches, convulsions, or other serious symptoms.

Modern brain surgery did not develop until a great deal had been learned about the brain's localization of function, particularly in the cerebral cortex. This knowledge was provided largely by tests in which a mild electric current was applied to areas of the brain surface. A specific part of the body would respond, and eventually a detailed map of cortical function was compiled. Without such knowledge a neurosurgeon could not be sure that in removing a deep-seated tumor he would not also be removing brain tissue essential for voluntary movements, speech, or intellectual function.

Most of the knowledge of cerebral function has come from the work of neurosurgeons such as Wilder Graves Penfield (1891–1976), who founded the Montreal Neurological Institute and provided the surgical treatment of certain forms of epilepsy (removal of brain tumors responsible for periodic convulsions).

COMPARE *neurology*

nevus A birthmark resulting from either a localized depositon of pigment or dilation of a mass of tiny blood vessels just under the skin.

nicotinic acid A vitamin of the B complex also known as niacin, present in lean meat, liver, fish, yeast, beans, and the germ of cereals. A deficiency of this essential vitamin can result in gastrointestinal disturbances and pellagra.

nitrogen A gas that occurs in a free state in the atmosphere and forms approximately 80 percent of the air people breathe. In the form of various compounds, especially proteins, it is essential for the buildup of tissues in both plants and animals.

nitroglycerin A chemical used medically for its ability to relieve the pain of *angina pectoris*. It acts by dilating (widening) the blood vessels.
SEE *coronary artery disease*

nuclear medicine The branch of medicine concerned with the diagnostic and therapeutic use of minute amounts of radioactive substances (radionuclides or *radioisotopes*). When used in medicine or medical research, these substances are also known as radiopharmaceuticals. They are injected into a blood vessel, swallowed, or placed in a body cavity and emit high-energy radiation that can be detected outside the body. The radiation emitted is generally detected by devices called scintillation detectors or scintillation cameras.
SEE ALSO *brain scan*

nystagmus A constant involuntary movement of the eyeball. Both eyes are usually affected. The eyes often move in a somewhat circular direction, although the movements are jerky in some cases and may be both horizontal and vertical in turn. The disorder is most commonly present at birth, related to poor vision resulting from a congenital abnormality of the eyes. Nystagmus seen in later life may be associated with a disease of the nervous system or a disorder of the inner ear. It is sometimes called miner's disease because it used to be a common affliction of miners who worked long years in dim light; improvements in the illumination of coal faces has made such cases relatively rare today. Nystagmus may also be caused by excessive eyestrain, fatigue of the muscles that control eye movements, or failure of light rays to focus properly on the retina.

Treatment of nystagmus depends on the cause. In many cases the disorder can be corrected by suitable eyeglasses. If the disorder is of nervous origin, prompt diagnosis and treatment of the underlying cause are essential. Occasionally the uncontrollable movements of the eyeball will last only a relatively short time. It is important to tell a physician of such an occurrence at once since it may be an important diagnostic sign.

In most cases nystagmus is not serious and vision is not adversely affected, even though correction of the rapid eye movements may not be possible.

O

occipital Relating to the back part of the head, skull, or brain.

occipital lobe A major division of each cerebral hemisphere of the brain. Roughly triangular in shape, it is situated at the back of the skull and concerned mainly with the interpretation of visual impulses transmitted to it by the optic nerve, which conveys nerve impulses from the light-sensitive retina.

occult blood The presence of minute traces of blood (as in feces) that can be detected only by means of chemical tests or other laboratory procedures.

occupational disease Any disease acquired primarily as the result of adverse or unhealthy working conditions. In certain jobs the continued inhalation of dusts and other harmful particles can cause changes in the tissues of the lungs that lead to respiratory diseases. Toxic gases and fumes such as ammonia, chlorine, sulfur dioxide, and toluene, which are encountered in the chemical, plastic, and rubber industries, can also cause lung disease. Dust particles in the lungs cause irritation that, if prolonged, may result in *fibrosis* of the tissues.

In most types of occupational lung disease a long period of exposure to the dust is necessary before these changes can be detected. It can take even longer before symptoms appear, sometimes up to twenty or thirty years as in *asbestosis*.

The first symptom of lung disease is usually shortness of breath on exertion (dyspnea) that progressively worsens and may eventually become severe and incapacitating. The diseases do not always follow this progressive course; many miners, for example, suffer few if any symptoms. However, complications may occur at any time; tuberculosis is a common complication of *silicosis*, and lung cancer may cause early death in asbestosis.

Taking such precautions as wearing respirators (face masks) to prevent the inhalation of dust particles and installing effective ventilation systems are now required by law in

certain industries in many countries, and do much to lessen the risk of certain lung diseases.
SEE ALSO *pneumoconiosis*

olfactory Relating to the sense of smell, as olfactory nerves.

oliguria A reduction or diminution in the amount of urine passed during a given period. This may or may not be of specific diagnostic importance to a physician. Prolonged oliguria, however, is usually evidence of some disorder of the kidneys or abnormal enlargement (hypertrophy) of the prostate gland. Oliguria may also be associated with drug poisoning, brain disease, or coma.

oncology The branch of medical science concerned with the study and treatment of malignant and benign tumors. A specialist in this field is known as an oncologist.

oophorectomy Surgical removal of an ovary; also known as an ovariectomy.
SEE ALSO *hysterectomy*

ophthalmology The branch of medical science concerned with the eye and its diseases and disorders. A physician who specializes in this field is known as an ophthalmologist.
COMPARE *optician, optometrist*

ophthalmoscope An instrument fitted with lenses and its own light source used to examine the inside of the eye, especially the *retina*. By shining the light directly into the eye through the central opening (pupil), the physician can look through the ophthalmoscope and see the retinal blood vessels at the back of the eye, as well as the spot (optic disk) where the optic nerve leaves the eyeball and enters the brain.

The retina may reveal signs of several bodily disorders in addition to those that primarily involve the eyes. High blood pressure (hypertension), for example, can often be recognized by the general condition of the retinal blood vessels. The abnormally increased pressure of the blood circulating through the tiny retinal vessels may cause some of them to break and release a small amount of blood within the retina. Diabetes can also cause characteristic changes in the appearance of the retina and its blood vessels *(diabetic retinopathy)*, as well as of the central portion of the eye (vitreous humor). All of these changes can be seen by a physician with the aid of the ophthalmoscope, which permits early diagnosis and treatment of the underlying condition.
SEE ALSO *ophthalmology, retinopathy*

optic Relating to the eyes or the sense of sight.

optician A person, not generally a physician, skilled in the grinding and fitting of lenses and the preparation of optical instruments.
COMPARE *ophthalmology, optometrist*

optometrist A person who measures visual ability and prescribes corrective lenses and exercises, but not drugs, which can only be prescribed by a physician (*ophthalmologist*).
COMPARE *optician*

oral contraceptive Any of various pills designed to prevent conception; popularly known as "the pill" or birth-control pills. It is the most reliable method of *contraception*: if taken according to instructions, it is virtually 100 percent effective in preventing pregnancy. The pill is simple to use and no special action need be taken at the time of sexual intercourse.

The contraceptive pill acts in three ways. During pregnancy the body secretes increased amounts of the hormones *progesterone* and *estrogen*, which prevent the ovaries from releasing the regular monthly ovum. The pill contains synthetic hormones similar to those produced during pregnancy and thus inhibits *ovulation*. It also reduces the receptivity of the uterine lining to a fertilized ovum and makes the plug of mucus in the cervix hostile to sperm cells.

Most oral contraceptives are taken for twenty-one days and then stopped for seven, when bleeding occurs as in a normal menstrual period. Many women experience side effects when they first start taking the pill, including weight gain, nausea, or headaches; these usually disappear after the first few months. If side effects persist, a physician may recommend a change to another oral contraceptive.

Research has shown that women who take oral contraceptives have a statistically increased risk of developing clotting disorders, gallstones, depression, nausea, skin disorders, and weight increase. On the other hand, women who take oral contraceptives are statistically less likely to develop cancer, ovarian cysts, and nonmalignant diseases of the breasts.

orchidectomy Surgical removal of a testicle.

orchitis Inflammation of a *testicle*.

organic disease Any disease or disorder in which there are detectable or observable structural changes in the tissues or organs of the body.
COMPARE *functional disease*

orgasm The climax of sexual intercourse or masturbation. In men it is usually accompanied by the ejaculation of semen.

orthopedics The branch of medical science concerned with the prevention and correction of deformities of the bones and joints. A specialist in this field is known as an orthopedist or orthopedic surgeon.
COMPARE *rheumatology*

osteitis Inflammation of a bone.
SEE ALSO *osteomyelitis*

osteitis deformans SEE *Paget's disease*

osteoarthritis A chronic degenerative disease of the joints, especially those that bear part of the body weight. It is a fairly common disorder, particularly in those over the age of fifty who are also overweight. It is not considered to be a serious problem; more often it is a consequence of changes in bones with aging, although injury to a bone is often associated with the first manifestation of symptoms. These include pain and sometimes muscle spasm, particularly after exercise. The weight-bearing joints (spinal column, hips, and knees) are commonly involved.

The edge of the affected joint loses its smooth covering of cartilage (hyaline cartilage) and there is often a slight overgrowth of bone around the edges of the joint called osteophytes. These interfere with movement and cause pain when the joint is active and stiffness during periods of rest. The stiffness usually disappears when the joint is exercised again.

Osteoarthritis is not the best name for this disorder, since it implies inflammation; degenerative joint disease or osteoarthrosis describes the condition more accurately, since inflammation is rarely a problem. Only in cases of severe involvement of the hip joint is movement seriously affected; in many persons the damaged joint can be surgically replaced with a metal ball-and-socket joint.

The cause of osteoarthritis is unknown, although the predisposing factors of aging, injury, and obesity seem to play a part. Surgery may be required in cases where new bone growth is pressing on a nerve and causing pain or other difficulty. Otherwise treatment usually consists of symptomatic relief of pain with the use of appropriate doses of aspirin or a more potent prescription analgesic.

SEE ALSO *rheumatoid arthritis*

osteomalacia A disease characterized by an increasing softness of the bones from lack of vitamin D. This vitamin plays an important role in the formation of bone and in the body's ability to absorb calcium from the intestinal tract. The body's exposure to the sun's ultraviolet rays causes a chemical change that results in the manufacture of this vitamin under the skin. It is also available from the diet, particularly in fish and dairy products such as milk and cheese. A gross deficiency of vitamin D during childhood, when the bones are developing, results in rickets; if the deficiency occurs in adults, the disorder is known as osteomalacia.

Osteomalacia may affect any adult with a severely inadequate intake of vitamin D. It is seen in some women who have had several pregnancies one after the other. Early symptoms of osteomalacia osteomyelitis

(which are not specific to this disorder) include stiffness, skeletal pain, muscular weakness, and fatigue. In some cases the body weight on the weakened bones may cause painful fractures. In uncomplicated cases the treatment of osteomalacia is the same as for rickets: adequate amounts of calcium and phosphorus in the diet plus therapeutic dietary supplements of vitamin D (approximately 1,600 units daily) for about a month. The dose of vitamin D can then be gradually reduced to the normal daily requirement (400 units).

osteomyelitis A bacterial infection of the bone and its underlying marrow. The disease is much more common in children under the age of twelve than in adults, although before the advent of antibiotics a chronic form often persisted for many years. The infection may be the result of the spread of bacteria in the bloodstream from an abscess, penetrating wound, or infected tooth, or it may follow a local injury to the involved bone.

The long bones of the arms and legs are most commonly involved. Once the infection reaches the bone marrow it may spread along the shaft of the bone and cause extensive damage. Untreated cases may lead to necrosis (death) of a portion of the affected bone, which then becomes detached from the surrounding living bone and forms a mass called a sequestrum.

Because the symptoms of osteomyelitis are not specific for this disease, the diagnosis may pose a challenge for the physician. They include chills, fever, muscular weakness, and intensive pain and swelling (resembling a huge abscess) over the site of the infection.

The bacteria usually responsible for the infection, *Staphylococcus aureus*, are easily controlled with antibiotics if the condition is diagnosed early enough. If the infection goes untreated, dead areas of bone must be surgically removed. Medical treatment has made this condition relatively rare compared to only a few decades ago.

osteoporosis A disorder of the bones in which they lose calcium and other minerals and become much less dense than normal. It is fairly common in the elderly and affects women more often than men. With the progressive loss of bone mass the possibility of fractures increases, especially of the weight-bearing vertebrae (spinal column).

Some bone loss is a normal consequence of aging. Minute amounts of the skeletal bones begin to dissolve shortly after the skeleton has reached full development at the age of about twenty-five. This is a very slow process; if the bone loss is not related to an underlying disease, it will take about forty years before any symptoms or signs of bone loss are noted.

Calcium deficiencies in the bones could be due to an unsatisfactory diet or to diseases that result in insufficient calcium being absorbed into the body. It may also be associated with some upset in the hormones; it is sometimes seen in women after menopause as a result of an estrogen deficiency. Other causes include the prolonged administration of corticosteroids and prolonged bed rest. In the latter case, treatment includes keeping the patient as active as possible with mild exercise or physiotherapy. The physician may also advise a diet rich in proteins and calcium to minimize further loss.

There are many degrees of bone loss in osteoporosis and no dividing line exists between normal and abnormal bone density. However, by the time symptoms or signs are evident the bone loss is usually considerable. Common symptoms include pains in the back, trunk, or limbs. A limb bone may fracture fairly easily. Under spinal stress or jarring, a severely weakened vertebra may collapse suddenly and cause great pain, but there is rarely any damage to the spinal cord. In uncomplicated cases in which the patient receives proper supportive treatment, relief of any pain associated with osteoporosis is obtained within a few weeks.

OTC Abbreviation for *over-the-counter*.

otitis Inflammation of the ear. Otitis externa is an inflammation of the outer ear; an inflammation of the middle ear is known as otitis media; and inflammation of the inner ear is referred to as otitis interna.

otolaryngology The branch of medical science (also called otorhinolaryngology) concerned with the ears, nose, and throat (ENT), including the larynx, and the diagnosis and treatment of diseases or disorders that affect these structures. A specialist in this field is known as an otolaryngologist (otorhinolaryngologist).

otosclerosis A condition characterized by abnormal thickness and hardness of the structures of the middle ear, usually resulting in various degrees of hearing loss. The problem is caused by an overgrowth of bone around the part of the middle ear attached to the stapes, the third of the three tiny bones (ossicles) that transmit sound vibrations from the eardrum to the inner ear. As the condition becomes progressively worse it results in total deafness in the affected ear.

Otosclerosis is an extremely common cause of hearing loss in adults and is usually the result of an inherited condition (a family history of the disease is noted in about half of the cases). The symptoms of impaired hearing typically start in early adult life and the condition slowly progresses until loss of hearing is complete in the affected ear or ears. In most instances both ears are involved. Women tend to be affected more than men and the condition can be made worse during pregnancy.

This condition is known as a conductive type of deafness, which implies that in many cases surgical correction of the bony overgrowth will result in restoration of some degree of hearing. In appropriate cases, the surgical procedure is stapedectomy, the removal of the anchored stapes. This is replaced with an artificial device. The operation is relatively successful in about 80 percent of cases, and patients achieve a marked degree of restoration of hearing. Without the operation, some patients can improve their hearing with the use of a hearing aid.

otoscope An instrument for examining the ear canal and the eardrum. It basically consists of a small funnel-shaped cup with an attached light source. When the cup is gently inserted into the ear canal, the physician can see if the eardrum is inflamed and detect boils or other infections.

The eardrum (tympanic membrane) is normally pearly gray and reflects light from the otoscope. A healthy eardrum appears to be somewhat metallic in the reflected light; if it appears red, dull, or does not reflect light, the physician knows that something is wrong and immediate diagnosis and treatment is required.
SEE *otitis*

ovarian cyst An abnormal fluid-filled sac that occasionally develops within an ovary. It is a fairly common condition in women between the ages of thirty and sixty. If the cyst enlarges to the extent that it presses against other organs within the abdominal cavity, it can cause pain or a feeling of distension and a frequent urge to urinate. The definitive treatment for this and other troublesome cases is surgical removal of the cyst (cystectomy). In severe cases the entire affected ovary may have to be removed.

ovariectomy Surgical removal of an ovary; also known as *oophorectomy*.

ovary Either of two small oval organs, one on each side of the uterus, responsible for secreting the female sex hormones and producing ova (eggs). The two ovaries perform an essential role in reproduction and are the female counterparts of the *testicles*. The ovary releases a mature ovum (female sex cell) each month and manufactures and secretes the hormones *estrogen* and *progesterone*.

At birth a female child has within her ovaries all the potential ova she will ever have. Since only one mature ovum is normally released each month during ovulation, the maximum number of ova that can be released from the beginning of the menstrual cycle to menopause is in the range of four hundred. By contrast, at each ejaculation a man releases millions of sperm cells.

Every month in fertile women (unless an oral contraceptive is

taken), an ovum matures in the surface of one of the ovaries and is expelled into the *Fallopian tube;* this process is called *ovulation.*
SEE ALSO *Graafian follicle, oophorectomy, oral contraceptive, ovarian cyst*

over-the-counter drug Any drug or pharmaceutical product that can be purchased freely without a physician's *prescription.* In general, over-the-counter (OTC) drugs can be used with relative safety without medical supervision by the average person in general good health if dosage instructions on the label are carefully followed. It has been estimated that approximately 300,000 OTC products are available by brand name and generic name in the United States. In these products, however, only about 500 active ingredients are represented.

Most OTC products are useful only for the relief of symptoms in relatively minor ailments, although there are exceptions—such as the apparent ability of *aspirin* in appropriate doses to reduce the likelihood of future heart attacks in patients who have already experienced a myocardial infarction.

oviduct The *Fallopian tube.*

ovulation The release of a mature *ovum* (egg) by the *ovary* each month during the menstrual cycle of sexually mature females. It occurs approximately fourteen days before the onset of the next menstrual period. The exact time of ovulation can sometimes be determined by carefully taking body temperature daily during two successive menstrual periods; just before ovulation it falls slightly, and during ovulation it rises slightly. It then remains more or less constant before falling again at the onset of the next menstrual period.

ovum The female sex cell.
COMPARE *spermatozoa*
SEE *fertilization, ovary, ovulation*

oxygen A colorless, odorless gas that forms approximately 20 percent of the air people breathe. It is essential to life (except for anaerobic bacteria) and to support combustion.
SEE *hemoglobin*

oxyhemoglobin The combined form of *hemoglobin* and oxygen found in oxygen-rich arterial blood.

oxytocic Any chemical agent that stimulates the muscular contractions of the uterus during childbirth.
SEE *oxytocin*

oxytocin A hormone secreted directly into the bloodstream by the pituitary gland. It stimulates the muscular contractions of the uterus during childbirth and influences the secretion of breast milk (lactation). Pitocin is a trade name for a preparation of oxytocin, often used to induce labor, help expel the placenta, and aid lactation.

oxyuriasis Infestation of the body with pinworms (threadworms). This condition, also known as enterobiasis, is the most common parasitic infestation of children who live in temperate climates. In most cases there are no signs and symptoms and treatment is usually not necessary. Some children will experience intense itching in the anal area, which can usually be relieved with the application of antipruritic creams or ointments.

Although pinworm infestations are rarely harmful and tend to disappear spontaneously without treatment, a single dose of pyrvinium pamoate eradicates pinworms in approximately 90 percent of cases.

P

pacemaker A nerve center in the wall of the right atrium (the upper chamber of the right side of the *heart*), specialized to coordinate the heart's pumping action. An electrical impulse sent out from the pacemaker in a rising and falling wave causes the heart chambers to contract. This action forces blood out of the heart into the lungs (on the right side) and out of the heart into the arteries (on the left side).

An artificial pacemaker, a small battery-powered electronic apparatus that provides the same function, can be surgically introduced into the body to control disordered heart actions.

Paget's disease A chronic and slowly progressive bone disorder also known as osteitis deformans that most commonly affects adults over the age of forty. It is characterized by an increased breakdown and reforming of bone, leading to abnormal thickening and softening of the bones, especially of the spinal column, legs, and skull.

The first full description of osteitis deformans was made in 1877 by the English surgeon Sir James Paget (1814-1899); he also published a paper on a precancerous condition of the nipples, which eventually also came to be known as Paget's disease. To avoid confusion physicians often refer to Paget's disease of bone or osteitis deformans.

In a person with Paget's disease the new formation of bone (recalcification) does not occur in an orderly fashion. Not only is more new bone deposited than is normal, but the structure of the calcium deposits does not follow a normal pattern.

The symptoms of the disease depend largely on the extent of the involvement and which bones are affected. Many patients have no symptoms at all. In more extensive involvement, in which the long bones of the legs are affected, there may be pain and a disturbance in walking (often related to an increase in the length of the bones of the leg).

pain

When about a third of the skeletal bones are involved the disease may become more active. One potential problem is that the new bone mass requires new blood vessels for nourishment and the greatly increased number of vessels may put a severe strain on the heart to pump out more blood. In rare cases this may lead to a form of heart disease known as high-output heart failure.

After twenty or thirty years of slowly progressive bone changes, the accompanying deformities may lead to severe problems in movement and result in invalidism.

Pain may be relieved by prescribing estrogens, analgesics, and x-ray therapy.

pain A sensation of discomfort usually elicited as the result of an injury or disorder or exposure of the tissues to a stimulus of appropriate intensity.

Although obviously unpleasant, pain is a warning by the body that something is wrong, indicating the need for a careful examination and investigation to find the underlying cause. Pain is experienced as a wide variety of sensations—dull, aching, sharp, burning, throbbing—and the different types of pain and their location are important diagnostic clues for the physician.

Despite extensive research into the nature of pain, it is still not clear which nerve endings or receptors in the skin and internal organs and tissues are responsible for conveying to the brain the impulses that are interpreted as pain. Some researchers believe that the sufficient stimulation (above a certain threshold) of a wide variety of nerve endings will initiate impulses that are then interpreted as pain. If more lightly stimulated, some of these nerve endings appear to be responsible for the sense of mild irritation, tingling, and itching. Experiments have shown that these milder sensations can be transformed into painful ones if the intensity of the stimulus (such as heat applied to the skin) is increased.

Inflammation is invariably accompanied by pain, although the site of the pain may not indicate the location of injury, infection, or inflammation. The pain impulse may be projected along a specific nerve fiber to a distant point (for example, an injury to a spinal nerve may be experienced as pain in an arm or leg); this is known as projected pain. In other cases, the pain impulse may become linked with totally distinct nerve fibers, which also results in the sense of pain being experienced at a site other than that actually affected; this is known as referred pain.

palate The roof of the mouth. It consists of bone in the front (the hard palate) and a fleshy structure at the back (the soft palate).

palliative Serving to soothe or relieve the symptoms of a disease or disorder; said of a drug or agent that relieves symptoms but does not cure a disease disorder.

palpation A diagnostic technique or procedure in which the surface of the skin is prodded and otherwise explored by the hands and fingers. It is used to detect disease or abnormality in various organs; for example, an abnormally enlarged liver or spleen. The results of such findings usually demand additional and more sophisticated diagnostic tests to determine the cause of the abnormality.

palpitation Any heart action of which the patient is aware. The sensation is often associated with an unusually rapid heart rate *(tachycardia)* and is felt as a throbbing, fluttering, or pulsation in the chest. It can be experienced as a symptom of disease, stress, or as a side effect of various drugs.

palsy A temporary or permanent loss or impairment of muscular movement; *paralysis*.

pancreas An elongated gland situated behind the stomach, with its larger end resting in the curve formed by the duodenum, the first part of the small intestine. It secretes digestive juices into the duodenum through a duct and the hormone *insulin* directly into the bloodstream.

The pancreas is a soft, lumpy, elongated organ with a large head and a tapering body stretching across the back part of the abdominal cavity from the duodenum to the spleen. Most of the gland produces the enzyme-rich pancreatic juice, which aids in the digestion of fat. Only about 1 percent of the organ has an endocrine function, localized in the beta cells of an area called the islets of Langerhans, which manufacture and secrete *insulin*. The presence of insulin in the blood permits the liver and muscles to store and make use of glucose, the energy-giving sugar formed during digestion. If the islets of Langerhans fail to secrete an adequate amount of insulin, the result is a reduced rate of removal of glucose from the blood or an increased rate of release into the blood of glucose stored in the liver. This causes excessive accumulation of sugar in the blood (hyperglycemia), a feature of *diabetes mellitus*.
SEE *pancreatitis*

pancreatitis Inflammation of the *pancreas*. An attack can be very mild or extremely severe. In acute forms of the disease, the underlying cause may be related to an obstruction of the pancreatic duct, entrance of bile into the secretory channels of the pancreas, infection, alcoholism, metabolic and nutritional deficiencies, injury, or an adverse reaction to certain drugs. The exact mechanisms that cause an attack of pancreatitis are not clear. However, if the digestive enzymes secreted by the pancreas are blocked from flowing to the small intestine, they may start to digest the tissues of the pancreas.

The signs and symptoms of acute pancreatitis include severe and steady abdominal pain that occasionally radiates to the chest and back (often relieved by sitting upright), nausea, vomiting, fever, and sometimes total collapse. This is an extremely serious condition and requires immediate medical attention. Transfusions may be necessary to restore an adequate blood volume. In some cases surgery may be required to unblock and drain the pancreatic or bile duct and to drain any abscesses. Antibiotics are prescribed to control infection.

Chronic pancreatitis is frequently associated with alcoholism or gallstones and is marked by recurring attacks of varying severity. A physician will provide instructions on necessary dietary changes and perhaps prescribe drugs to relieve the condition. If the insulin-secreting portions of the pancreas are severely damaged, it may be necessary to treat the patient for a mild form of diabetes mellitus.

pandemic Relating to or being a disease that affects people over an entire land area or worldwide.
COMPARE *endemic, epidemic*

papilledema Swelling and inflammation of and around the optic nerve at the point where it enters the back of the eyeball. Also called choked disk, it may be a sign of increased pressure within the brain (increased intracranial pressure) caused by factors such as a tumor or abscess of the brain, meningitis, cerebral trauma or bleeding, severe disease of the kidneys, or hypertension.
SEE ALSO *ophthalmoscope*

papilloma A benign (harmless) growth such as a polyp or wart that affects the skin or mucous membranes.

Pap test A routine diagnostic test for cancer of the *cervix* (neck) of the uterus. Cervical cancer is one of the easiest types of cancer to detect and treat in its earlier stages.

The test is named after the American scientist George Papanicolaou (1883–1962).
SEE *cervical smear*

papule A small, firm spot raised above the surface of the skin. Papules may form as the result of a variety of diseases, including measles, syphilis, and eczema. In each case the papules present a fairly characteristic appearance and the underlying cause requires expert medical diagnosis.

paracentesis Surgical puncture of a bodily cavity for the removal of fluid, usually with a syringe.
COMPARE *amniocentesis*

paralysis Temporary or permanent loss of voluntary muscular movement in a part of the body. The control of the movement of a muscle, either voluntarily or by reflex action, depends on its nerve supply.

parathyroid glands

If the nerves are damaged in any way, the muscle will no longer act under any form of control and is said to be paralyzed. All forms of muscular paralysis are therefore expressions of a nerve disorder, and the most common ones are caused by injury.

Nerve injury can be present at birth due to brain damage or damage of a particular nerve. Tumors of the spinal cord can interfere with the nervous control of muscles and lead to the paralysis of groups of muscles. In poliomyelitis the virus can affect the nerve cells of the spinal cord and cause paralysis below the affected area.

Facial paralysis, often one-sided and causing drooping of the mouth, occurs after certain virus infections that are related to the common cold. Damage to the spine can be caused by severe accidents that fracture the vertebrae (spinal column), resulting in paralysis of the body from the waist downward (paraplegia). Secondary deposits of cancerous tissue (metastasis) can cause collapse of individual vertebrae, and this may result in paralysis. Strokes, which cause brain damage due to disruption of the blood supply to the brain, lead to one-sided paralysis (hemiplegia). The elderly are particularly subject to this, following either a blockage (thrombosis) or hemorrhage of the blood vessels in the brain.

A paralyzed muscle becomes flaccid, shrinks due to lack of use, and without care may contract to produce a deformity of the limb. Function may be regained if the nerve disorder is only temporary; surgery may be necessary to overcome movement difficulties.

paraplegia Paralysis of the lower part of the trunk and the legs, usually from injury to the spinal cord.

parathyroid glands Four small endocrine glands, one pair situated on each side of the thyroid gland, which regulate the amount of calcium and phosphorus in the circulating blood. They can vary somewhat in size and exact location within the neck.

If the parathyroid glands fail to secrete an adequate amount of parathyroid hormone or if they are accidently removed during surgical treatment of the thyroid gland, the amount of calcium in the blood will fall and the amount of phorphorus will rise. This can result in *tetany*, a condition in which the patient becomes very restless and the nerves are overly excitable, causing the limbs to twitch or go into spasm. It can be controlled by injecting parathyroid hormones or taking supplemental amounts of vitamin D, which corrects the deficiency by increasing the calcium level in the blood.

When the parathyroid glands secrete too much hormone the amount of calcium in the blood is increased. Some calcium is drawn directly from the bones. If parathyroid overactivity persists, the bones gradually weaken due to their loss of calcium. They become thin and brittle and tend to break easily. Long-standing excess of calcium in the blood can cause fatigue and muscle weakness, as well as the forming of kidney stones. Treatment of an overactive parathyroid gland depends on the cause, which is often a tumor; in such cases surgical removal of the tumor is the definitive treatment.

paratyphoid fever A disease caused by an infection of salmonella bacteria; it is similar to but less severe than *typhoid fever*. Paratyphoid fever is transmitted by contaminated food, milk, or water. In addition to human carriers, the feces of infected animals may spread the disease. The incubation period is from one to about ten days.

As with most infectious diseases, the first symptoms of paratyphoid fever usually include headache and fever. The temperature begins to rise daily for a few days, often reaching a high of 105°F (40.6°C). Other fairly common symptoms are chills, sweating, development of rose-colored spots on the chest and abdomen, aching in the limbs, and tiredness. Treatment consists of an appropriate antibiotic and bed rest until all signs of fever have disappeared.

parenteral Relating to or denoting any route of administration of a drug that does not involve direct absorption through the digestive tract. The parenteral route involves its *injection* into a vein, artery, or muscle group.

parkinsonism
SEE *Parkinson's disease*

Parkinson's disease A slowly progressive disease associated with damage to or disruption of the basal ganglia, nerve centers deep within the brain. The basal ganglia have complex connections with the *thalamus*, brain stem, and areas of the cerebral cortex that control voluntary movements. In a few cases the cause of Parkinson's disease and other diseases that have the same symptoms is known. These include viral inflammation of the brain (viral encephalitis), carbon-monoxide poisoning, and chronic manganese poisoning. Another cause is the taking of certain strong tranquilizers that interfere with the brain's use of dopamine, a chemical that occurs naturally in the basal ganglia and is thought to play a vital role in the transmission of the impulses that control muscular activity. In the vast majority of cases, however, no cause of Parkinson's disease can be found.

Parkinson's disease (paralysis agitans, shaking palsy) is characterized by the gradual development of a typical group of signs and symptoms: an expressionless, masklike face with the eyes rarely blinking; muscular tremor affecting the head, arms and legs (worsening during periods of excitement or stress); a "pill-rolling" movement of the thumb against the first two fingers of the hand; and rigidity or stiffness of some muscle groups, associated with delay and slowness in making voluntary movements. Curiously, the tremors often cease or become less noticeable during voluntary movement. Walking is usually slow, and consists of short shuffling steps, with the head and trunk held slightly forward and the arms at the sides.

The patient with Parkinson's disease may suddenly break into a brisk short-stepping run while walking, as if trying to catch up with the body's center of gravity. In a few patients the ability to write normally is affected—the letters are unusually small and cramped together (micrographia). Often these symptoms are experienced only to a minor degree. It is estimated that Parkinson's disease affects about one person in every thousand, making it one of the more common neurological disorders.

Until about 1970 the treatment of Parkinson's disease was less than satisfactory. Surgical disruption of part of the thalamus had been attempted successfully in some carefully selected types of the illness; this relieved the severe muscular tremors and rigidity that are the hallmarks of this disease. An important development took place in 1967 with the discovery of the clinical benefits of a drug known as levodopa (L-dopa). However, surgical treatment is still used on certain patients.

Taken in tablet or capsule form, levodopa is converted into dopamine in the digestive tract. Levodopa replaces the characteristically reduced amounts of dopamine and can bring about a marked improvement in many patients.

When levodopa was first introduced it sometimes caused serious side effects, including nausea, vomiting, dizziness, faintness, and occasionally nightmares. To obtain the maximum benefit from the drug each patient had to discover how much could be taken before the side effects became too serious; in some cases the process of discovering the correct dosage took up to six months.

More recently these problems have been considerably lessened by the introduction of new drugs combining levodopa with an additive that greatly increases its efficiency. Thus the patient now needs less of the drug and, it usually takes only one or two weeks to establish the correct dosage for maximum benefit. The condition of many patients is now significantly improved.

The disease is named after the English physician James Parkinson (1755–1824).

parotid gland Either of a pair of large salivary glands, one situated just below each ear.
SEE *mumps*

parotitis Inflammation of the parotid gland; epidemic parotitis is the medical term for *mumps*.

paroxysm A sudden attack or recurrence of the symptoms of a disease; also, a spasm, seizure, or convulsion.

patch test A method of identifying the cause of a suspected allergic reaction of the skin (contact dermatitis). A small amount of the suspected substance or substances is placed on the skin, and the area is later examined for evidence of an inflammatory response.

patent ductus arteriosus A congenital heart disorder in which the channel or duct between the pulmonary artery and the aorta fails to close at birth. Until the condition is corrected surgically, this permits oxygen-poor blood to mix with oxygen-rich blood.

pathogen Any substance or microorganism capable of causing a disease.

pathogenic Producing or causing a disease.

pathology The branch of medical science concerned with the study of the causes, processes, and effects of disease as reflected in the changes brought about in organs and tissues. A specialist in this field is known as a pathologist.

pediatrics The branch of medical science concerned with the diagnosis and treatment of diseases and disorders that affect children and adolescents. A specialist in this field is known as a pediatrician.

pediculosis Infestation of the body with lice. The first signs of pediculosis are usually intense itching, irritation, and inflammation of the skin. The disease is spread by close contact with an infected person or by using contaminated clothing or objects.

Lice are generally found on hair—on the head, around the genital organs, on the chest and under the arms—and on clothing, especially underclothing. The eggs they lay take about two weeks to hatch, during which time they are stuck to the hair with a kind of cement and cannot be brushed off. By careful examination they may sometimes be seen on the scalp at the back of the head. A physician can determine the most effective way to get rid of the lice and their eggs. Scratching must be avoided to prevent bacterial infection.
COMPARE *scabies*

pellagra A disease caused by a deficiency of *nicotinic acid*, a B vitamin. In severe cases it is characterized by inflammation of the mouth and tongue, skin eruptions, diarrhea, anemia, and impairment of mental abilities. Treatment is directed at establishing a diet rich in B vitamins in addition to the use of vitamin supplements until all evidence of the deficiency has disappeared.

penicillin A group of widely prescribed *antibiotics* produced by certain species of bacteria, molds, or other microorganisms, or manufactured (synthesized) in the laboratory. Penicillin can be injected or taken orally.

Penicillin was first discovered by Alexander Fleming in 1928, although it was not until the 1940s that it was widely used to treat bacterial infections. The original form, known as penicillin G, must be injected or taken on an empty stomach (one hour before or two to three hours after a meal) to make sure that its antibacterial effects are not destroyed by stomach acids. Penicillin V (or VK) is available only in oral forms. It has the same antibiotic effectiveness as penicillin G and is not easily destroyed by stomach acids; it can be taken without regard to meals.

All forms of penicillin can cause potentially serious allergic reactions in patients who are sensitive to its effects, including an *anaphylactic reaction*, which can be fatal. Less severe allergic responses to penicillin include skin rashes, painful joints, and drug-induced fever. Although allergic reactions can occur with any dosage form, they are most common when the drug is injected.

peptic ulcer An open sore that develops on the mucous membrane that lines the stomach (gastric ulcer) or the duodenum, the first part of the small intestine (duodenal ulcer). The most common symptom is a gnawing pain that usually occurs after a meal, either directly afterward or up to three hours later; it is relieved by eating more food or by taking nonprescription antacids. The pain becomes worse if alcohol or spicy foods are ingested and may sometimes by aggravated by lack of rest, emotional tension, or smoking.

In severe cases the ulcer may bleed. The chemical changes that occur as the blood passes down the intestinal tract cause the stools to have a black or tarry appearance (melena). Vomiting may bring up partially digested food mixed with blood, somewhat resembling coffee grounds. In such cases, medical attention is required at once to avert more serious complications. An x-ray examination may help confirm the diagnosis of peptic ulcer.

In most cases the amount of hydrochloric acid in the stomach is abnormally high. Treatment includes bed rest until severe symptoms have abated. The physician may recommend that the stomach not be permitted to empty. Small amounts of food at frequent intervals and the avoidance of stress can contribute a great deal toward recovery. With proper care and dietary attention, most ulcers heal completely.

Some physicians prescribe the drug cimetidine (Tagamet) in the short-term treatment of peptic ulcers. It acts to inhibit the secretion of stomach acid. First available to American physicians in 1977, cimetidine is now one of the most

perforation

commonly prescribed drugs in the United States. It should not be taken at the same time as other drugs (especially anticoagulants) without a physician's approval.

perforation An abnormal opening or hole through a bodily structure or part caused by injury or ulceration.

pericarditis Inflammation of the pericardium, the membranous sac that surrounds or encloses the heart. The condition is often accompanied by shortness of breath (dyspnea) and chest pains that may worsen during coughing or deep breathing. In some cases fluid collects between the walls of the pericardium and may interfere with the heart's pumping action. In severe cases, in addition to treating the condition with antibiotics, the fluid may have to be drained off by means of suction.
COMPARE *endocarditis, myocarditis*

perinatology The subspeciality of medical science concerned with the development and health of the fetus and infant during the perinatal period, the interval approximately six weeks before and six weeks following birth. A specialist in this field is known as a perinatologist.

peristalsis The forward wavelike movement of the walls of the esophagus and the intestines that propels food and waste products along the course of the digestive tract.

peritoneal dialysis An indirect method for removing waste products and certain toxic (poisonous) substances from the blood by filtering them through the peritoneum, the moist membrane that lines the abdominal cavity and covers its internal organs. This is in contrast to the direct filtering of waste products from the blood in the procedure known as *hemodialysis*. The technique is most often used in the treatment of selected patients with *kidney failure*.

Peritoneal dialysis involves the insertion (usually under local anesthesia) of a temporarily implanted catheter or a permanently implanted (Tenckhoff) catheter, which is passed through an incision in the abdominal wall until it reaches the appropriate site in the peritoneal cavity. A sterile solution (dialysate solution) is passed into the catheter under gravity and flows into the peritoneal cavity. This fluid helps stimulate the passage of waste products in the blood through the semipermeable membrane of the peritoneum into the abdominal cavity. After a predetermined period which varies from patient to patient, the end of the catheter is again opened to permit the outflow under gravity of the previously sterile dialysate fluid, which now contains various waste products and (in certain cases) toxic substances that have filtered into the fluid.

A typical dialysate solution includes the following substances: glucose, sodium (salt), chloride, potassium, acetate, calcium, and magnesium.

Peritoneal dialysis can be an

alternative to hemodialysis. Although the procedure is still performed in many hospitals, some patients have been trained to undergo peritoneal dialysis at home, using automated delivery systems in which the dialysate solution is delivered to the proper site from a bag attached to the patient's upper abdomen, after which the waste products flow into a similar bag.
SEE ALSO *dialysis, kidney*

peritoneum The moist membrane that lines the abdominal cavity and covers its internal organs.
SEE *peritonitis*

peritonitis Inflammation of the *peritoneum*. The cause may be associated with an infection in which microorganisms (especially bacteria) gain access to the membrane as a result of a rupture or perforation of an abdominal organ or part (as when an inflamed appendix bursts). The infection can also spread from the female genital tract, an injury of the abdominal wall (such as a piercing wound,) or surgical incisions into the abdomen (especially where strict aseptic techniques are not followed); bacteria can also reach the peritoneum through the bloodstream or lymphatic vessels.

Peritonitis is an extremely serious condition that demands prompt treatment with an appropriate antibiotic. Typical symptoms include chill, fever (up to about 103°F/39.4°C), rapid pulse, abdominal pain, extreme tenderness over the abdomen that sometimes is so intense that bodily movements are inhibited, and persistent vomiting. These symptoms are mainly seen when a relatively large area of the peritoneum is involved (acute diffuse peritonitis).

pernicious anemia A potentially severe blood disease characterized by a progressive decrease in the number of red blood cells (erythrocytes), muscular weakness, and marked disturbances of the gastrointestinal system and the nervous system. If not diagnosed and treated, it can be fatal.

Treatment of pernicious anemia involves the administration of appropriate amounts of vitamin B_{12}, in addition to dietary supplements of iron and correction of general dietary deficiencies.
SEE ALSO *anemia*

pertussis The medical term for whooping cough.
SEE *whooping cough*

pessary A device inserted into the vagina to support a displaced uterus; also, a vaginal suppository.

petit mal A mild form of *epilepsy* in which no convulsions occur; the patient may or may not lose consciousness.
COMPARE *grand mal*

phagocyte Any of various cells including certain types of white blood cells *(leukocytes)* that have the ability to surround, absorb, and destroy bacteria and cellular debris in the circulating blood. The process is known as phagocytosis.

pharmacology The branch of science concerned with the study of drugs and other pharmaceutical agents, particularly their effects on living organisms. An expert in this field is known as a pharmacologist.

pharmacopeia Any official or standard publication that lists drugs and their formulas, together with instructions concerning their use. The World Health Organization publishes an international pharmacopeia.

pharyngitis Inflammation of the pharynx; sore throat.

pharynx The muscular, membrane-lined passage (the throat) that extends from the back of the nasal cavities (nasopharynx) to the trachea and the esophagus (oropharynx). The lower part of the pharynx serves as a passageway for both air and food.

pheochromocytoma A disorder caused by a tumor of the *adrenal gland*, characterized by sudden (paroxysmal) or persistent attacks of high blood pressure (hypertension), headaches, a sensation of the heartbeat (palpitations), flushing, cold and clammy skin, chest pains, nausea, vomiting, disturbed vision, shortness of breath (dyspnea), and depression. The incidence and severity of these signs and symptoms vary widely from patient to patient. The treatment of choice is surgical removal of the tumor.

phimosis Abnormal tightness or narrowness of the foreskin so that it cannot be retracted. In severe cases the best treatment is circumcision.

phlebitis Inflammation of a *vein*. It most commonly affects the walls of the veins of the legs, although any vein may be involved. The exact cause is often unclear, but it may be associated with injury to the vein, a chronic infection, obesity, or some problem of the blood circulation. Occasionally it occurs following a surgical operation or childbirth.

A contributing factor in phlebitis is the abnormal slowing of blood flow through the veins. Normal muscular activity helps to pump venous blood back to the heart. When a person is inactive for several days or weeks, the venous blood flow is reduced. For this reason, physicians encourage an early return to walking and moderate exercise following surgery or childbirth.

When a vein near the surface of the body is inflamed there may be intense pain along its course and the skin over it often becomes red, hot, and tender to the touch. The vein itself can frequently be felt as a long, hard cord. In many cases of phlebitis there is a slight fever, rapid pulse, and joint pains that make walking difficult. It is generally not a serious condition.

The physician may prescribe antibiotics and perhaps an anticoagulant to minimize the risk of blood clots forming in the affected vein. If a deeper vein is involved, the condition may become much more serious unless treated promptly. Blood clots that form in the inflamed vein could break off and be carried in the circulation until they reach a narrow vessel in the lungs (pulmonary embolism). In such cases the condition presents a direct threat to life.

phlebotomy The opening of a vein to withdraw blood, as in the treatment of *polycythemia*, or to receive blood from a donor; also called venesection.

phlegm abnormally large amounts of thick (viscid) mucus secreted by the lower parts of the respiratory tract and usually coughed up and expelled through the mouth.
SEE *sputum*

photophobia An abnormal sensitivity of the eyes to light. It can occur in a variety of conditions, including measles, meningitis, inflammation of the eyes, and as a side effect of certain prescription drugs. Until the underlying cause is corrected, the patient can obtain relief by wearing dark glasses.

physiology The branch of science concerned with the function of living organisms and the chemical and physical processes involved in life. An expert in this field is known as a physiologist.

physiotherapy Treatment based on physical and mechanical resources, including voluntary and passive exercise (especially of the limbs), heat, light, and water.

pica An abnormal craving to eat unusual substances, such as coal, clay, plaster, or starch. This condition is occasionally seen in hysteria, mentally retarded children, and in a few women during pregnancy.

piles
SEE *hemorrhoids*

pineal gland A small structure about the size of a pea situated deep within the brain. It secretes the hormone melatonin and may play a role in the synchronization of biological rhythms.

The philosopher René Descartes believed that the pineal gland was the seat of the soul. It has also been claimed to be a vestigial or mystical third eye.

pink eye
SEE *conjunctivitis*

pituitary gland A two-lobed endocrine gland attached to the base of the brain by a stalklike projection called an infundibulum. It is the master gland of the *endocrine* system and secretes several hormones that are essential for normal growth and development.

The pituitary gland (hypophysis) has two basic parts: the anterior (front) lobe and the posterior (rear) lobe. The structure and functions of these two parts are quite distinct. Only the posterior lobe has direct nerve connections with the brain; for this reason it is sometimes referred to as the neural lobe (neurohypophysis). The anterior lobe is much more glandular in structure than its counterpart and is therefore known as the adenohypophysis *(adeno* means "gland").

The posterior lobe releases two hormones: *vasopressin* (also known as ADH, antidiuretic hormone), which regulates the amount of urine secreted by the kidneys, and oxytocin, which aids the secretion of milk from the breasts by causing the milk ducts to contract and helps make the uterus contract during childbirth.

The anterior lobe of the pituitary gland secretes several hormones. These include growth hormone, which controls the rate of growth and development of the bones, muscles, and internal organs; ACTH (adrenocorticotrophic hormone), which controls the development and function of the cortex (outer part) of the *adrenal glands;* FSH (follicle-stimulating hormone), which stimulates development of Graafian (ovarian) follicles; LH (luteinizing hormone), which stimulates the ovaries and induces ovulation and, in the male (where the same hormone is usually known as ICSH, interstitial cell stimulating hormone) controls the secretion of sex hormones by the testicles; TSH (thyroid-stimulating hormone), which controls the functions of the *thyroid gland;* and prolactin, which regulates the flow of milk from the breasts following childbirth.

placebo A chemically inactive substance sometimes given by physicians to otherwise healthy patients who feel that they should receive a drug to cure an imagined illness. Placebos are also used as control substances during blind or double-blind evaluations of an active pharmaceutical product. In the double-blind test, neither the patients nor the prescribing physician know the identity of the substance taken until the conclusion of the test, when the case records are analyzed by a third party. Patients who seem to improve when receiving the inert placebo are said to have experienced a placebo effect.

placenta The vascular structure that develops within the uterus during pregnancy and supplies nourishment to the fetus through the umbilical cord. It is popularly called the afterbirth, as it is usually released, still joined to the infant, shortly after birth.

placenta previa A relatively uncommon condition in which the *placenta* is abnormally situated in the lower part of the uterus. The exact cause is unknown. It is thought to be associated with some fault in the implantation of the ovum at the beginning of pregnancy. The abnormally placed placenta may cover the opening from the uterus to the vagina completely (placenta previa centralis) or partially (placenta previa marginalis).

A placenta implanted in the lower

part of the uterus will be below the fetus's head. The symptoms of placenta previa may be experienced during the seventh or eighth month of pregnancy, usually with slight bleeding (which may gradually become more severe), gradual anemia, pallor, low blood pressure, and a rapid weak pulse. Medical attention is essential at the first sign of bleeding. Hospitalization is usually required to prevent or control further bleeding and prevent complications such as bacterial infection.

In severe cases it may be necessary to deliver the baby by *cesarean section*. In less severe degrees of placenta previa, normal labor is possible; in such cases the placental membranes may be artificially ruptured shortly before the onset of labor.
SEE ALSO *abruptio placentae*

plasma The fluid portion of the blood in which the blood cells are suspended. It contains proteins, salts, hormones, minerals, vitamins, and waste products for excretion from the body in urine. Normal plasma is colorless or has a faint yellow tinge. Blood plasma is often used as an alternative to the transfusion of whole blood (which contains blood cells) to replenish the fluid portion of the blood.
COMPARE *serum*

platelet A tiny round or oval body found in great numbers in blood. Also called thrombocytes, they play an important role in the clotting (coagulation) of blood following cuts or other injuries to the tissues.

pleura A thin, transparent, moist membrane that surrounds each lung and lines the chest cavity and diaphragm, forming an airless space (pleural cavity) between the lungs and the chest wall. A thin film of fluid separates the pleural membranes, allowing the lungs and chest wall to expand smoothly during breathing without rubbing together.
SEE ALSO *pleurisy*

pleurisy Inflammation of the *pleura*, the membrane that covers the outside of the lungs and the inner surface of the ribs, almost always caused by a viral or bacterial infection. If the infection causes only inflammation it is called dry pleurisy; if it begins to weep it is called pleurisy with effusion; and if it exudes pus it is called purulent pleurisy.

Dry pleurisy is nearly always a complication of some other lung disease such as tuberculosis, lobar pneumonia, collapsed lung, or bronchiectasis. It can also follow injuries to the ribs. Pleurisy begins suddenly with an agonizing pain in the side that becomes even worse when taking deep breaths, coughing, or moving. This is caused by the two inflamed walls of the pleural membrane moving against each other. Coughing is dry and very distressing, and slight fever may be present.

If the disease of which the pleurisy is a complication is not serious, then the pain may disappear in two or three days and recovery will be rapid. Severe disease, however, may lead to pleurisy with effusion; when this occurs the pain lessens but only because the presence of fluid in the pleural cavity causes the two membrane walls to separate. Too much fluid may cause pressure on the lungs, resulting in shortness of breath (dyspnea) and possibly a collapsed lung. In moderate effusions the temperature subsides in seven to ten days and the patient is well within a short time.

Treatment of pleurisy is aimed at control of the underlying cause. Accumulated fluid is often drained off in a procedure known as a pleural tap or pleural thoracentesis—surgical entry into the chest cavity, usually with a hollow needle, to remove the fluid. Antibiotics are prescribed to control any associated infection.

pneumoconiosis Any lung disease caused by the inhalation of harmful dust particles. It is an occupational disease found especially in miners and stonecutters.
SEE ALSO *asbestosis*, *siderosis*, *silicosis*

pneumonia An inflammation of the *lungs* typically accompanied by the collection of fluid in the alveoli (air sacs) of the affected lung tissue. Pneumonia is classified by infecting agent—bacteria, viruses, or rarely fungi—and the extent of the infection. Pneumonia that involves one or more of the major divisions (lobes) of a lung is known as lobar pneumonia; when the infection spreads to the lungs from an infected bronchus (major air passage) the condition is known as bronchopneumonia. Bronchopneumonia appears on x-ray film as a series of small solid patches of lung tissue, whereas lobar pneumonia is seen as one large dense area.

Among the more rare causes of pneumonia are the accidental aspiration of food particles or vomit into the lungs, the drawing into the lungs of pus from an infection of the trachea, bronchi, or some other site in the upper part of the respiratory tract, and the inhalation of irritating gases or mineral oils (chemical pneumonia).

Pneumonia can affect people of all ages but is most common in the very young and the elderly. The disease is sometimes a complication of another infection or a debilitating illness that leaves the patient's body defenses at a low ebb. With prompt diagnosis and treatment, most cases of pneumonia can now be successfully treated in a short time. An important factor in the cure of pneumonia is the victim's reporting symptoms to a physician at the earliest possible time.

In lobar pneumonia usually only one lobe is infected and inflamed. There is sudden fever, headache, aching limbs, pain on breathing, and a cough that is at first dry and painful but later produces thick sputum that may be stained with blood. Normally the disease responds rapidly one or two days after the administration of an appropriate antibiotic. However, in the elderly the disease can be extremely serious, especially if a physician is not consulted at the first appearance of suspicious symptoms.

Acute bronchopneumonia is usually a complication of a bronchial infection such as influenza or acute or chronic bronchitis. In children it can be a complication of whooping cough (pertussis) or measles. The disease begins more slowly than lobar pneumonia. The first symptoms are those of the primary infection, but after two or three days the temperature rises even more, breathlessness (dyspnea) and coughing develop, and the sputum may be filled with pus. Pain on breathing is common.

As in all cases of respiratory illness, prompt medical treatment is essential. However, despite the distressing nature of the symptoms, pneumonia today is seldom serious except in infants, the chronically ill, and the elderly.

pneumothorax A condition in which air or gas escapes into the *pleural* cavity, either by rupture of the *lungs* or more commonly by a penetration of the chest wall. The initial effect of both is to cause the lung or parts of the lung to collapse. The consequences depend on the nature of the perforation.

If the lung ruptures spontaneously two conditions can occur. In closed pneumothorax, the hole seals as the lung collapses and does not reopen. The air in the pleural cavity is slowly absorbed and the lung reexpands by itself. In open pneumothorax, usually caused by a ruptured bronchus (major air passage), the air travels backward and forward between the pleural cavity and the mouth without reaching the lung. The lung therefore collapses.

When the pleural cavity is pierced from outside as the result of a wound, pneumothorax can occasionally occur. The air is rapidly absorbed after the wound has been sealed with a dressing; healing then begins.

Pneumothorax begins suddenly and is characterized by breathlessness (dyspnea) and pain or a tight feeling in the affected part of the chest, which is made worse by deep breathing. In closed pneumothorax, the symptoms slowly disappear over a few days.

poliomyelitis A viral infection that attacks the spinal cord and can lead to muscular paralysis, especially of the limbs and the muscles of breathing; also known as infantile paralysis and polio. It has become relatively rare since the introduction of effective *vaccines*.

polyarteritis A disease characterized by widespread inflammation of the smaller arteries, often leading to complications such as kidney disease and high blood pressure (hypertension). A distinguishing feature of polyarteritis is that patches or segments rather than continuous stretches of the arteries are inflamed (segmental lesions); this is noted only under a microscope when a tissue sample is examined. The disease often progresses to the point where small bits of the arterial walls are destroyed. At any time during the course of the disease the lesions may be in various stages of development; some of them tend to heal spontaneously.

The cause of polyarteritis is not perfectly understood; there may be more than one cause. Some researchers have strongly implicated infection or some form of allergic reaction (hypersensitivity) to drugs. The disease attacks men about three times as often as women and may occur at any age, although it is more often seen between the ages of thirty and fifty.

The symptoms and signs of polyarteritis vary enormously, depending on the organs the diseased arteries supply. The disease may involve arteries that supply the heart, brain, kidneys, liver, lungs, digestive tract, testicles, or adrenal glands. In each case the signs and symptoms of the disease may take the appearance of another disease that is specific to the part of the body involved, such as angina pectoris or heart attack (myocardial infarction) if the coronary arteries are involved.

Common early signs and symptoms of polyarteritis are not specific to any one disease. They include fever, weight loss, muscular pain and weakness, high blood pressure (hypertension), skin rash, and firm nodules under the skin. Not all of these are present in any one case. The diagnosis can usually be made only by examining a few small sections of those arteries suspected of being involved.

Treatment of polyarteritis consists mainly in controlling manifestations of disease in the vital organs (especially the heart and kidneys) whose arteries are affected. Corticosteroid drugs may help control the course of the disease for some time.

polycythemia vera A rare condition in which an excessive number of red blood cells *(erythrocytes)* are produced by the bone marrow, causing the blood to become abnormally thick or concentrated. Without treatment there is a risk that the blood may clot and cause a potentially serious obstruction in blood vessels of the brain or lungs. Treatment includes *phlebotomy* (the removal of blood through an opening made in a vein) or the administration of drugs that suppress the production of red blood cells. COMPARE *erythrocytosis*

polyp A small growth *(tumor)* attached to a mucous membrane by a stalk (pedicle). Polyps have a tendency to bleed easily, a factor usually responsible for bringing them to the attention of both the patient and the physician. If they become troublesome, surgical removal is generally indicated.

Polyps are found in such tissues as the lining of the nose (nasal polyps), uterus (uterine polyps), and rectum (rectal polyps). It is thought that polyps sometimes become malignant, especially those in the final section of the intestinal tract (rectal polyps).

The presence of numerous polyps is known as polyposis. Surgical removal of one or more polyps is referred to as polypectomy.

Pontiac fever A usually self-limiting disease caused by infection with bacteria of the species *Legionella pneumophila*. It is characterized by fever, cough, headache, chills, muscular aches, diarrhea, vomiting, pain in the chest, and confusion. Unlike *Legionnaires' disease* (which is thought to be caused by a slightly different strain of the same bacteria), patients with Pontiac fever do not develop pneumonia or potentially serious complications. In most cases the disease seems to run its course within three or four days without specific treatment.

Pontiac fever was first noted in July 1968 during a mysterious outbreak that affected 95 out of 100 people who worked in a single building in Pontiac, Michigan. It was not until almost a decade later, however, that the causative bacteria were indirectly identified by means of antibody tests on serum specimens collected and preserved from some of the original patients.

postmortem Occurring or performed after death; a postmortem examination is another term for *autopsy*.

postpartum Occurring or taking place after childbirth.

preeclampsia A complication of late pregnancy characterized by the development of high blood pressure (hypertension), swelling of the tissues (edema), decreased output of urine, and protein in the urine (albuminuria). The cause is unknown. If untreated, the condition may progress to a much more serious state, *eclampsia*, in which the victim may experience convulsive seizures and coma (unconsciousness).

Preeclampsia develops in approximately 5 percent of pregnant women and is more likely in those with a preexisting disease of the blood vessels or high blood pressure. It can occur any time between about the twentieth week of pregnancy until a week after childbirth. The diagnosis involves urine tests, measurements of the blood pressure, physical examination (especially to detect evidence of tissue swelling), and laboratory blood tests.

Treatment depends largely on the severity of the signs and symptoms, but it basically involves preserving the mother's life and health. Mild forms of preeclampsia may respond well to bed rest, with a medical check by the physician every two days. If the condition does not improve, hospitalization is usually necessary. Severe cases may require the intravenous administration of a balanced salt solution in addition to magnesium sulfate and perhaps a drug such as hydralazine hydrochloride to lower blood pressure.

premenstrual tension A period of emotional or nervous excitability and irritation that precedes *menstruation* in many women. It usually disappears with the onset of the period. Some women may also experience headaches, depression, generalized swelling of the tissues (edema), and painful breasts (mastalgia). In mild cases no treatment is required, with the exception of aspirin or a similar analgesic. Some physicians also prescribe a diuretic to help rid the tissues of excess fluid and a mild tranquilizer to relieve irritability and nervousness. SEE ALSO *dysmenorrhea*

presbyopia Visual impairment characterized by the normal loss of elasticity of the lens of the eye as one ages. As a result it is increasingly difficult to focus on objects close to the eye. The onset typically occurs around middle age and is the change that causes people to need reading glasses even though their vision may have been normal throughout their earlier years.

prescription A written authorization for a drug or pharmaceutical product signed by a licensed physician. It is given to a patient to be filled at a pharmacy or other location where a registered pharmacist is employed to dispense drugs.

The names of most drugs and instructions for their preparation and use are based on Latin (and a few on Greek), a practice retained from the early Middle Ages. By the eighteenth century the art of prescription writing had become extremely complex, and a doctor's instructions to pharmacists for preparing a special concoction might fill several pages. Gradually, many of the instructions were abbreviated to save space. Some of these survive in modern practice: R or R (take); sig. (write; let it be written); b.i.d. (twice daily); non rep. (do not repeat); q.h. (each hour); q.2h. (every two hours); q.i.d. (four times a day); q.s. (as much as is sufficient); t.i.d. (three times a day); c̄ (with); ut dict. (as directed). The general trend today is to reduce Latin abbreviations to a minimum.

The early need for complex instructions about compounding medical preparations has been replaced by the modern pharmaceutical industry, in which hundreds of drugs are already packaged in bulk and need only be transferred to small and labeled bottles for the patient. However, the role of the registered pharmacist is far more important than this might suggest. He or she has studied the chemical nature and function of virtually thousands of potent prescription drugs and frequently spots an error by the prescribing physician in dosage, frequency of administration, or even the name of the drug.

It might seem to many patients that physicians take courses in bad handwriting to be capable of the opaque scribbles that pass for prescriptions. Indeed, a leading professional journal, *Pharmacy Times*, features a monthly section devoted to deciphering atrocious handwriting on actual prescription slips. The serious point for patients is that they know the name of the drug, the *dose*, and any other important information at the time the prescription is written. If the verbal information does not agree with the written prescription, ask the physician for immediate clarification.
SEE ALSO *prescription drug*

prescription drug Any drug or pharmaceutical product that is available only with the written *prescription* of a physician.
COMPARE *over-the-counter drug*

preventive medicine The branch of medicine concerned with preventing physical illness and mental disease, including educating the public about the importance of diagnosis and treatment of minor problems before they cause complications, the need for early *immunization* against a wide range of diseases, and controlling outbreaks of *contagious* diseases.

priapism Abnormal and persistent erection of the penis, usually without sexual desire. The penis is often curved upward because the two cylindrical chambers of erectile tissue on its upper surface (corpora cavernosa) are both rigidly distended with blood while the cylindrical chamber on the lower surface (corpus spongiosum) and the tip of the penis (glans) remain soft. Urination is not affected.

At first the condition is not painful, although it is uncomfortable; because of this, medical treatment is rarely sought during the first twelve hours. After about twenty-four hours the penis becomes extremely painful. The patient does not suffer from a fever or any other discomfort.

If the erection is not treated, it can remain for up to three weeks before gradually subsiding. A possible complication of priapism is *impotence*; thus, it is essential to seek immediate medical attention if the erection lasts more than a few hours.

Since erection is caused by an excess of blood in the penis, priapism is likely related to a disorder of the system that shunts blood in and out

primary care

of the penis. Blood may be removed by means of a syringe, but the effect is only temporary. The causes of priaprism include blood disorders, injuries to the spinal cord, and the effect of some drugs. There may be no apparent underlying cause at all. Treatment is difficult and frequently unsuccessful.

primary care Basic or general health care provided for an individual or family unit. The members of this emerging specialty claim to be offering a new service, although they bear a close resemblance to the fondly remembered family doctors or general practitioners of past years, who assumed total responsibility for the health of their patients from birth through old age. The main difference in modern practice is that the primary-care physician usually treats patients who suffer from the more common general illnesses and diseases; when a problem of *diagnosis* or treatment arises that is beyond the scope of the primary-care physician, the patient is referred to an appropriate medical specialist.

Modern medicine has become greatly fragmented, with many physicians concentrating on only one organ or system of the body; the primary-care physician provides a more broadly based service.

proctology The branch of medical science concerned with the diagnosis and treatment of diseases and disorders that affect the lower part of the large intestine, including the rectum and anus. A specialist in this field is known as a proctologist.
SEE ALSO *proctoscope*

proctoscope A slender illuminated instrument for inspecting the rectum and anus.
SEE ALSO *sigmoidoscope*

progeria A rare condition (approximately 1 in 8 million births in the United States) in which premature aging and senility occur during childhood. The cause is unknown. The signs and symptoms include a face that appears old or shriveled, small stature, skin that is dry and appears thin, scanty hair, and underdevloped sex organs.

Life expectancy is greatly reduced for children with progeria. No treatment exists.

progesterone A hormone produced naturally in the ovaries, adrenal glands, and placenta. It controls the changes that take place in the lining of the uterus during the second half of the menstrual cycle, preparing it for the implantation of a fertilized ovum (egg). It also plays a role in the development of the placenta and the breasts. A synthetic preparation of progesterone is used to treat certain menstrual disorders and threatened miscarriages (spontaneous abortions).
SEE ALSO *estrogen*

prognosis A prediction or evaluation by a physician of the expected duration and severity of a disease or disorder and the patient's chances of recovery.

prolapse An abnormal drooping or downward displacement of an internal organ or part, usually the rectum or uterus. Surgical correction is necessary in severe cases.

prostaglandins A group of chemically related compounds derived from fatty acids and present in semen (where they were first discovered), menstrual fluid, and in many other tissues including those of the brain, lungs, pancreas, kidneys, and prostate gland. They have the ability to lower blood pressure, stimulate contractions of the uterus, regulate body temperature, and regulate the acid secretions of the stomach lining. Prostaglandins are being studied for their possibile therapeutic benefit in a wide range of applications, including those that involve the gastrointestinal, respiratory, and cardiovascular systems. Over twenty prostaglandins have been identified.

prostate gland A gland in the male that surrounds the neck of the bladder and first part of the urethra. The prostate is about the size of a walnut and consists of secretory glands embedded in a mass of connective tissue and muscle tissue. Through twenty to thirty small pores the prostate gland secretes a thin milky fluid into the urethra. This fluid is part of the semen; it dilutes the sperm by thousands to one and makes them move faster by providing energy in the form of sugars and protein. The prostate is the principal storage depot for seminal fluid. When the male reaches puberty, the grapelike clusters of the gland begin to manufacture their fluid.

As men get older they may suffer from an enlargement of the prostate. At the age of fifty, 20 percent of all men are likely to be affected; by eighty, the likelihood increases to 80 percent. Enlargement of the prostate does not in itself mean trouble, but if it enlarges enough to obstruct the flow of urine, the gland may have to be surgically removed (prostatectomy); this does not normally affect sexual activity. The cause of this enlargement appears to have something to do with the secretion of sex hormones.

The prostate may become infected with bacteria. When this occurs, a burning sensation accompanies urination and there is an unpleasant feeling that the bladder has not been completely emptied. This condition is known as prostatitis. Treatment involves the prescription of an appropriate antibiotic.

Cancer of the prostate (prostatic carcinoma) accounts for about 10 percent of all cancer deaths in American males, usually affecting men over the age of sixty. The cause is unknown. Prostatic carcinoma is generally slowly progressive and may cause no symptoms. Late in the course of the disease, however, the victim may note blood or pus in the urine. The condition may be cured with early diagnosis and treatment, often involving surgical removal of both the prostate gland and the testicles (orchiectomy) followed by estrogen therapy. Radiotherapy may also be of value in selected cases.

prosthesis Any artificial organ or part; also, the substitution of an artificial organ or part for one that is missing.

protein Any of a group of nitrogen-containing organic compounds formed by various combinations of *amino acids* that are essential to life and comprise a large part of living plants and animals.

proteinuria
SEE *albuminuria*

prothrombin time (PT) A test often referred to in short as "pro time" that measures the time required for a *fibrin* clot to form in a treated blood sample. It is used to monitor a patient's response to oral *anticoagulant* therapy and to evaluate the general clotting ability of the blood as a diagnostic procedure.

A test for prothrombin time may be performed daily during the initial period of anticoagulant therapy. When the desired medication level is reached, the test is repeated at longer intervals.

pro time
SEE *prothrombin time*

protozoa The smallest and most primitive members of the animal kingdom, consisting of over 30,000 distinct species of microscopic single-celled organisms. Most protozoa live freely on land as well as in water and inhabit nearly every part of the world. A few species are parasites of man and animals; only about thirty species are parasites of man, and not all of them are pathogenic (disease-causing).

Protozoa are generally much larger and more complex than *bacteria* and range in complexity from the relatively simple ameba to forms with tiny hairlike appendages (flagella) that provide movement by means of their whipping action.
SEE ALSO *rickettsia, viruses*

pruritus The medical term for itching. It may occur at any site on the skin or may be generalized over a wide area. It usually results from irritation of the nerve endings in the skin that register pain. When these are slightly stimulated the response is itching rather than pain. It may be mild and of only short duration, or it may be so intense and prolonged that normal activities (including sleep) are totally disrupted.

Common causes of itching include failure to keep the skin (especially the scalp) clean; sensitivity to foods, drugs, or other substances; insect bites; heat rash;

abnormally dry skin; and emotional reactions.

Pruritus accompanies most skin inflammations and several infectious diseases, such as chickenpox. Various bacterial and fungal skin infections can cause intense itching, especially in the anal and genital region. In women, inflammation of the vagina (vaginitis) frequently causes severe itching. When the cause of itching is related to an infection or other disorder, the itching can be relieved by medical treatment of the underlying condition. In other cases the physician may recommend a preparation such as calamine lotion to relieve itching.

If itching is intense, prolonged, and affects a large part of the body it is important to consult a physician so that proper diagnosis can be made. Such symptoms are occasionally the first indication of some more serious problem such as kidney disorders, diabetes, or jaundice. Infestation of the skin and hair with parasites can also cause severe itching.

It is extremely difficult to avoid scratching an itch, but scratching may make the condition worse even though it immediately relieves the sensation for a brief time. Many persons get temporary relief from an itch by pinching the surrounding skin; the resulting mild pain, technically counterirritation, seems to cancel out the itch. All severe and prolonged forms of itching, however, require prompt medical attention.

psittacosis A viral disease transmitted to humans by certain species of infected birds, especially parrots, parakeets, lovebirds, and canaries. The disease is passed mainly by breathing in the dust from the feathers or cage contents of infected birds. Less commonly it may be transmitted by the bite of an infected bird or (very rarely) by the coughs of an infected person. The incubation period is from seven to fourteen days.

The first signs and symptoms of psittacosis include the sudden onset of fever, chills, headache, backache, loss of appetite, and a general feeling of being unwell (malaise). In severe cases there may be a high fever that causes delirium, stiffness and spasm of the muscles in the neck and back, abdominal pain, nausea and vomiting, and a pronounced acceleration of breathing and pulse. A dry cough is common in most cases but may develop into the spitting up of small amounts of mucus (often stained with blood).

Diagnosis of psittacosis includes a recent history of exposure to birds. In its early stages psittacosis often resembles other infections, such as influenza or typhoid fever. The physician will probably recommend a chest x-ray to determine the extent of involvement of the lungs and blood tests that will help identify the disease.

Prompt treatment with antibiotics is usually successful. In severe cases hospitalization may be required until all signs and symptoms of the disease have disappeared. Antibiotic treatment may last for only about one week, during which time the patient is generally isolated.

Once the disease has been confirmed, it may be necessary to kill any bird suspected of carrying the disease to prevent reinfection.

psoriasis A skin disease characterized by the formation of red patches covered with tiny overlapping grayish white or silvery scales. The sites most often affected are the scalp, elbows, knees, legs, chest, and back. It is one of the few skin diseases for which no specific cause is known, although a family history of psoriasis is common.

The onset of psoriasis is usually gradual. The nails sometimes show signs of stippling and other discoloration, and there is often accompanying (and perhaps associated) inflammation of one or more joints (arthritis). In many people the overall condition temporarily improves, although a permanent and complete cure is rare. Itching is occasionally a problem, but it is usually mild. In times of stress and anxiety the psoriasis may worsen.

No specific treatment is available for psoriasis. The condition may be somewhat improved by limited exposure to sunlight. A physician may recommend daily removal of the unsightly scales with soap, water, and a soft brush, and may also prescribe a steroid cream or lotion. More severe forms of the disease are often treated in a hospital, and include such measures as the application of an ointment containing crude coal tar, which is removed the following day with mineral oil. The involved areas are then exposed to sunlight or ultraviolet radiation.

Although psoriasis may be troublesome, the general health is often not affected.

psychiatry The branch of medical science concerned with the diagnosis and treatment of mental and emotional disorders. Unlike *psychologists*, psychiatrists are physicians and can prescribe medication.

psychology The science concerned with normal and abnormal mental processes and behaviors. An expert in this field, who need not be a physician, is known as a psychologist.

psychosis Any of various severe forms of mental illness characterized by the inability to distinguish right and wrong, delusions and hallucinations, and a loss of the sense of reality; popularly and legally referred to as insanity. A psychotic suffers a disintegration of the personality, although there may be periods of lucidity, and usually

requires hospitalization and prolonged psychiatric treatment.
COMPARE *neurosis*

psychosomatic Relating to the mind and body, or to physical disorders caused or aggravated by the patient's mental or emotional state.

psychotherapy A method of treating emotional disorders that involves a prolonged series of interviews with a psychotherapist. Many schools of psychotherapy exist, the earliest and best-known being psychoanalysis, founded by Sigmund Freud (1856–1939). Since then, many others have developed.

The methods of treatment vary greatly from school to school and from therapist to therapist. Some place emphasis on the patient's childhood and later experiences in order to understand the mental attitudes that may account for current emotional problems. Others rely on the interpretation of dreams, paintings executed by the patient, or free association (the patient says whatever comes to mind) in order to discover the patient's unconscious motivations.

ptosis The abnormal drooping or downward displacement of an organ or part, especially of the eyelid. Treatment depends on the underlying cause.

pulmonary Relating to or involving the *lungs*.

pulmonary function tests Any of various related tests of lung function used to determine the cause of breathlessness (dyspnea), evaluate the therapeutic effectiveness of bronchodilators, or to estimate the degree of lung involvement in pulmonary diseases. The tests include tidal volume, expiratory reserve volume, vital capacity, inspiratory capacity, functional residual capacity, forced residual capacity, forced expiratory volume, and maximal voluntary ventilation; all involve the same basic procedure. While the nose is temporarily blocked, the patient breathes into a mouthpiece attached to a spirometer, a device that measures and records the amount of air inhaled and exhaled. Test results are considered abnormal if they are less than 80 percent of the predicted normal value.

Some pulmonary function tests can be performed at the patient's bedside with a portable spirometer.

pulse The regular throbbing or pulsation of the arteries caused by successive contractions of the heart. It can be detected when the tips of the fingers are placed over the inner side of the wrist (radial artery) as well as over other areas, such as the side of the neck (carotid artery), where a major artery is near the skin surface.
SEE *pulse rate*

pulse rate The number of pulsations felt over an artery per minute. For men this is normally between 70 to 72; women average between 78 and 82 per minute. The pulse rate must be taken with the patient at rest, since even mild exercise increases the rate of heartbeat and thus pulse rate. Children generally have higher pulse rates than adults.

pupil The opening in the iris of the eye through which light enters and is focused by the lens on the retina.

pupillary reflex Contraction of the pupil of the eye in response to the stimulation of the retina by light.

purpura A condition characterized by purplish spots formed by bleeding into the skin, mucous membranes, and other tissues. There are several causes, including allergic reactions to food, drugs, and infecting bacteria. Thrombocytopenic purpura is associated with an abnormal reduction in the total number of *platelets* in the blood circulation.

purulent Forming or containing *pus*.

pus A yellowish white collection of viscid fluid that often forms at the site of a wound or infection, containing normal and damaged white blood cells *(leukocytes)* and other cellular debris.

pyelitis Inflammation of the renal pelvis, the part of the *kidney* that forms a funnel-shaped structure for the collection of urine and narrows to form the beginning of the ureter, the tube that conveys urine to the bladder.
SEE ALSO *glomerulonephritis*, *pyelonephritis*

pyelogram The x-ray film made during the process of pyelography.
SEE *intravenous pyelography*

pyelography
SEE *intravenous pyelography*

pyelonephritis Inflammation of both the *kidney* proper and the renal pelvis, its funnel-shaped opening into the ureter. It is caused by a bacterial infection, most commonly one that reaches the kidneys as the result of an infection of the urinary bladder; the bacteria usually gain access to the bladder through the urethra. In contrast to those kidney inflammations caused by bacteria in the blood filtering through the nephrons (the kidney's functional units), pyelonephritis is caused by bacteria traveling up through the urinary tract to the kidney, where the infection can spread and involve large parts of the organ.

The symptoms of acute pyelonephritis develop rapidly and typically include a dull pain in the lower back, tenderness of the region over the kidneys on physical examination (palpation), fever, and often attacks of shivering. Painful and frequent urination is a common problem; in addition, many patients experience nausea and vomiting.

Diagnosis is confirmed by means

of laboratory examinations of the urine, which may reveal pus and cellular debris containing large numbers of bacteria. In the vast majority of cases the prompt administration of an appropriate antibiotic results in the symptoms subsiding within a few days. Periodic urine samples will continue to be taken for several months after all signs of the disease have disappeared and antibiotic therapy has been discontinued to make sure that no bacteria remain in the urinary system.
SEE ALSO *glomerulonephritis, pyelitis*

pyemia A severe form of *septicemia* (blood poisoning) which is associated with the presence of pus-forming microorganisms in the blood and characterized by the formation of multiple abscesses, fever, chills, sweating, and often *empyema*. Without prompt antibiotic treatment, the condition can be fatal.

pyloric stenosis A stricture or abnormal narrowing of the *pylorus*, the muscular ring at the outlet of the stomach. *Stenosis* of the pylorus occurs most often as the result of overgrowth of tissues *(hypertrophy)* in this area; the resulting obstruction is seen especially in first-born male infants. The symptoms typically develop over the first month and a half of life and include forceful vomiting (sometimes resulting in *dehydration*) and visible movements of the intestines caused by strong peristalic waves.

The treatment of choice is pyloromyotomy, the surgical incision through the constricting muscular fibers of the pylorus. Following the procedure the child is usually able to tolerate normal feedings within a few days.

pylorospasm Painful spasmodic contractions of the *pylorus*, the muscular ring at the outlet of the stomach, usually caused by some disturbance in its motor mechanism. It may also be associated with nearby lesions of the stomach or duodenum. Treatment depends on the underlying cause.

Too much caffeine can also cause the pylorus to go into spasm.

pylorus The muscular ring at the outlet of the stomach that opens to permit partially digested food to enter the duodenum, the first part of the small intestine.
SEE ALSO *pylorospasm*

pyrexia The medical term for *fever*.
SEE ALSO *hyperpyrexia*

pyrosis The medical term for *heartburn*.

Q

Q fever An acute disease caused by infection with *rickettsiae* of the species *Coxiella burnetti*. When the disease was first described in 1935 its cause was unknown; Q stood for "query." It is carried by livestock and transmitted to humans by inhaling contaminated dust, contact with infected animals, or by drinking contaminated milk. The disease is usually not serious, especially with early diagnosis and treatment with antibiotics. Patients in occupations where they are exposed to infection may be given a vaccine.

q.i.d. Abbreviation for the Latin phrase *quater in die* ("four times a day"). It is commonly used in the writing of *prescriptions*.

quarantine A period of strict isolation of a patient with an *infectious* disease to prevent its spread to others.
SEE ALSO *communicable, contagious*

quinsy A condition marked by abscess formation in the area of the tonsils, especially behind them. Because of treatment with antibiotics, it is a fairly rare condition today. It was an often-seen complication of tonsillitis.

R

rabies An acute viral disease that attacks the nervous system, transmitted to humans by the bite of an infected animal, including dogs, cats, foxes, raccoons, skunks, and bats. It is traditionally considered the only human disease that is inevitably fatal once the first symptoms have appeared, by which time the virus has reached the nervous system. However, between 1971 and 1977 at least three rabies victims survived the onset of symptoms as the result of emergency tracheotomy and other medical treatment.

The virus of rabies has a paralyzing effect on the muscles of breathing and on the heart muscle, as well as causing painful constriction of the throat muscles following attempts to drink or swallow (hence the alternate name hydrophobia, literally "fear of water"). In the final stages the patient goes into violent convulsions followed by coma and death.

The incubation period varies considerably, but the average appears to be between thirty and sixty days. Anyone who is bitten by an animal suspected of having rabies (regardless of whether it was frothing from the mouth) should immediately clean the wound with soap and water or alcohol and let it bleed a little. Medical attention should then be obtained without delay. If possible, the animal should be held for examination.

The first symptoms of rabies are similar to those of influenza, followed by progressive irritability, anxiety and insomnia, and pain in the area of the wound. This stage is follwed by the more severe symptoms.

No cure exists once the first symptoms are noted. However, several vaccines are quite successful if the course of injections is started before the onset of symptoms—ideally, within a few hours of receiving the wound. The traditional method of treatment involves injection of the vaccine into the skin folds of the abdomen, typically in daily injections for twenty-one days followed by

radiation

two booster shots ten and twenty days later. New vaccines are being developed that will reduce the required number of injections.

The prevention and control of rabies requires not only the immunization of pets against the disease, but the impoundment of stray dogs and restraint of other dogs by their owners. Control of rabies among wild animals is more difficult.

Rabies treatment is rarely justified when a person is bitten by a squirrel, rat, chipmunk, mouse, or rabbit. Wild animals that are particularly suspect as rabies carriers are skunks, foxes, raccoons, and bats. Following a bite from one of these animals (unless its capture proves it free from infection), a course of antirabies treatment is generally essential.

radiation X-rays, ultraviolet light, or *radioisotopes* used in the diagnosis and treatment of disease, especially *cancer*.
SEE ALSO *radiation sickness*

radiation sickness Illness caused by exposure to high-energy radiation, such as that produced by the explosion of a nuclear weapon or chronic overexposure to excessive amounts of therapeutic or diagnostic radiation such as x-rays. Mild cases are characterized by loss of appetite, headache, nausea, vomiting, and diarrhea. Delayed effects, especially with repeated or prolonged exposure, may include a serious disturbance in the formation of blood cells, sterility, leukemia, loss of hair, skin and teeth, and possible genetic changes.

radioisotopes Forms of an element such as iodine that are *radioactive;* they emit high-energy *radiation* and are used in medicine both to diagnose and treat certain diseases such as cancer or disorders such as those that affect the *thyroid gland.*
SEE ALSO *nuclear medicine*

radiology The branch of medical science concerned with the diagnostic and therapeutic use of radioactive materials, x-rays, and other forms of high-energy radiation. A specialist in this field is known as a radiologist.
SEE ALSO *nuclear medicine*

radiopaque Impenetrable to x-rays or other forms of radiation. The term is used to describe substances injected into the blood vessels, swallowed, or given as an enema prior to x-ray examination of specific areas of the body. The radiopaque substance (also called x-ray contrast medium) permits the blood vessels or intestinal tract to be seen clearly (usually as white areas) on x-ray film or a fluoroscope screen.
SEE ALSO *barium sulfate, intravenous pyelogram*

radium A radioactive and fluorescent metallic element used to destroy cancer cells.

radius The outmost of the two bones that form the skeleton of the forearm, the other being the *ulna*. COMPARE *humerus*

rale An abnormal usually rattling sound heard within the chest during examination with a stethoscope. It is produced within the lungs or bronchi (air passages) when they are constricted (dry rales) or contain excessive secretions (moist rales). It is a common finding in cases of bronchitis.

ratbite fever Either of two forms of infectious disease caused by the bite of a rat or other rodent. The microorganisms transmitted, *Spirillum minor* or *Streptobacillus moniliformis*, are common parasites of the respiratory tracts of rats. Symptoms include inflammation of the skin at the site of the puncture, fever, chills, vomiting, headache, and pains in the joints and back. Some patients may also experience a rash on the hands and feet within three days after being bitten. Diagnosis is confirmed by culturing (attempting to grow) the microorganisms from a sample of blood or joint fluid. Treatment involves the administration of an appropriate antibiotic.

Raynaud's disease A condition in which the arteries of the extremities go into spasm and temporarily shut off the blood supply to the affected part. The fingers are most often affected, but the toes, ears, and nose may also be involved. The condition, which occurs most often in young women, usually follows exposure to damp or cold but may be precipitated by a wide variety of factors, including other arterial diseases, infection, emotional upset, injury to the part, blood disorders, and drug poisoning.

When the blood supply to the fingers is cut off by arterial spasm they turn cold, numb, and white. As the fingers are warmed and blood once again flows through the small arteries, two more color changes occur: the affected parts first turn blue and then red or pinkish.

A potentially serious complication of Raynaud's disease is the development of *gangrene* after a long period of continuous or prolonged attacks. However, this is extremely rare.

There is no specific treatment for Raynaud's disease, although in certain severe and chronic forms the nerves that control the diameter of the smaller arteries may be cut to prevent the vessels from going into spasm.

People prone to Raynaud's disease can take various precautions to minimize and limit the frequency of attacks. These include the wearing of gloves and warm socks in cold weather (they should be fairly loose fitting to retain sufficient heat) and general measures to protect the extremities from cold and damp. Smoking is strongly discouraged. Hygiene and general care of the hands and feet should be emphasized. If emotional problems are associated with the condition, tranquilizers or sedatives may be prescribed.

The condition is named after the French physician Maurice Raynaud (1834-1881).

rectum The final portion of the large intestine (colon), ending at the anus.

red blood cell
SEE *erythrocyte*

reflex An automatic or involuntary response to a stimulus. A reflex is any action that is not under conscious control; an example is the sudden withdrawal of the hand the moment it touches something hot. The hand moves away automatically as the result of nerve control at the level of the spinal cord; a split second or so later, associated nerve impulses reach the conscious level of the brain and the experience is sensed as pain.

Some examples of reflex action are used by physicians to test for possible nerve damage. One such test is the knee-jerk response. The physician sharply taps the tendon just below the kneecap of a crossed or suspended leg with a rubber-headed hammer. The normal response is for the leg to jump upward a bit.

A simple type of reflex action requires only three nerve cells and their fibers: a sensory nerve fiber, which sends an impulse from the surface of the body to the gray matter of the spinal cord; a connecting or association fiber, which interrupts the impulse on its way to the brain and directs it to a nearby motor fiber; and the motor fiber itself, which relays the impulse onward to a muscle which causes some part of the body to move. All of this is accomplished in a fraction of a second.

Some normally automatic responses can be modified by the mind, as in quickly setting down a hot dish of food rather than letting it drop.

regression A recurrence of the symptoms of a disease or disorder. In *psychiatry*, the word refers to an abnormal tendency to return to behavior patterns or emotional attitudes that are childlike or otherwise inappropriate in well-adjusted adults.

remission A temporary diminution in the severity of the symptoms of a disease; the period during which this occurs.

renal Relating to or involving the *kidneys*.

renal calculus The medical term for kidney stone.
SEE *nephrolithiasis*

renal failure
SEE *kidney failure*

resection The surgical removal or excision of an organ or part. The surgical removal of part of the stomach is known as a gastric resection (or partial gastrectomy).

respiration The physical and chemical processes whereby gases are exchanged between the living cells of an organism and its environment. In man this involves the inhalation of oxygen and its exchange in the *lungs* for the waste product carbon dioxide. Oxygen enters the blood and is carried to all the organs and tissues. They in turn give up carbon dioxide, which returns in the venous circulation to the lungs where it is expelled in the breath.

resuscitation The restoration to breathing or consciousness after apparent death, especially by means of artificial respiration.
SEE *cardiopulmonary resuscitation, resuscitator*

resuscitator A mechanical device that aids in *resuscitation* by forcing oxygen or an oxygen mixture into the lungs under the appropriate pressure.

retention The abnormal holding in the body of waste products that should be excreted. Retention of urine demands prompt medical attention to diagnose the cause and initiate treatment.
COMPARE *incontinence*

reticular activating system A complex system of nerve cells and fibers in the brain stem, hypothalamus, and adjacent areas. It has direct connections with the cerebral cortex and plays an essential role in maintaining alertness or wakefulness. It is thought that some sedatives and tranquilizers act on this system by blocking or impairing the normal flow of nerve impulses. A serious injury to this part of the brain can result in prolonged coma.

reticuloendothelial system All the cells dispersed throughout the body in various tissues and organs that can surround, absorb, and destroy bacteria and other foreign invaders. They also produce specific antibodies and thus play an essential role in the body's general defense mechanism, the immune system.

retina The light-sensitive structure at the back of the eyeball on which incoming light rays are focused. The retina contains millions of specialized nerve endings called rods and cones that convert light into electrical impulses. These impulses are relayed to the brain by means of the optic nerves, a bundle of nerve fibers originating at the back of the retina. When the nerve impulses reach the *occipital lobe* of the brain, sensation of vision is experienced.
SEE ALSO *detached retina, diabetic retinopathy, ophthalmoscope, retinopathy*

retinal detachment
SEE *detached retina*

retinitis pigmentosa A slowly progressive disease beginning in early childhood, characterized by degeneration of the retina, widespread changes in the pigmentation of the retina, atrophy (wasting) of the optic nerve, and defective night vision. By middle age the central vision may be seriously impaired; eventually the condition may lead to total blindness.

Some patients with retinitis pigmentosa may also develop cataracts and, for unknown reasons, experience a gradual impairment of hearing, occasionally to the point of total deafness.

The specific cause of the disease is unknown, although hereditary factors are strongly implicated. No curative therapy exists. Vocational guidance and genetic counseling can be offered.

retinopathy Any disease or disorder of the retina.
SEE *diabetic retinopathy, retinitis pigmentosa*

retractor A surgical instrument used to hold back the edges of a wound, thus permitting the surgeon better access to the underlying areas.

Reye's syndrome A potentially fatal disorder that mainly affects children under the age of eighteen (especially those between the ages of five and fifteen) who have recently had a viral infection such as type B influenza or chickenpox. It is characterized by acute disturbances of brain function (encephalopathy), increased pressure on the brain, and fatty degeneration of the liver. The symptoms include severe continuous and persistent vomiting, high fever, headache, disorientation or delirium, and fainting. The child may become progressively unresponsive and lapse into a coma.

The cause of Reye's syndrome is unknown, and thus no specific therapy or preventive measures now exist. However, because the disease typically follows a viral infection, research continues to attempt to identify the nature of this association. Various drugs have been prescribed to help reduce the increased pressure within the brain; one of the most useful of these is mannitol, an intravenous *diuretic.*

The results of some studies reported in 1982 suggest that giving a child *aspirin* during the fever stage of a viral disease such as influenza or chickenpox may increase the risk of Reye's syndrome. This association is far from clear; but until the question is clarified, it is a wise precaution not to give children aspirin during the fever stage of any viral illness.

The prognosis depends largely on the extent of brain involvement and the severity of symptoms. In severe cases a child may eventually experience convulsions and then lose consciousness as the pressure within the brain increases. In such cases immediate medical treatment is essential to prevent permanent brain damage or death.

The diagnosis of Reye's syndrome typically involves a careful physical examination, biopsy of the liver, and various blood tests including those that measure the blood levels of ammonia and liver enzymes.

Treatment is not specific and several approaches have been used; intravenous fluids including glucose and various *electrolytes* are usually given to prevent or correct any disturbances in the body's own supply.

Reye's syndrome is named after the Australian pathologist R.D.K. Reye, who together with his associates first described the condition in 1963.

Rh factor (Rhesus factor) A substance in the blood of approximately 82 percent of the population of the United States and Great Britain, who are said to be Rh positive; those without the factor are Rh negative. Its presence or absence, which is inherited, makes no difference to the health of the individual. However, difficulties can accompany transfusions if blood of the wrong group is given.

An Rh-negative person who receives Rh-positive blood reacts by producing anti-Rh *antibodies*. The antibodies might not be strong enough to have great effect, but if the same person receives another Rh-positive transfusion, those same antibodies could be active enough to destroy the foreign red cells that had been introduced.

A pregnant Rh-negative woman may be carrying an Rh-positive fetus. Some of the fetus's blood may cross the placental barrier between maternal and fetal circulation; this could easily happen during the mechanical stress of labor. The mother then develops anti-Rh antibodies. With the first pregnancy in which this happens the effect is likely to be slight, but should she become pregnant with another Rh-positive fetus, the effect could be greater. During labor some of the maternal blood could pass across the placental barrier into the baby's circulation, where the antibodies would damage the baby's red blood cells (erythrocytes), causing anemia and jaundice.

Only an extremely small number of the babies who are theoretically at risk are likely to have any trouble; the vast majority are normal babies. Routine blood tests during pregnancy will detect any likelihood of Rh incompatibility, and steps can be taken to minimize the effects. Even if the baby is born with this kind of anemia, there is definitive treatment to counter it. (The majority of cases of anemia and jaundice in the newborn is due to other quite simple and nonalarming factors.)

Any mother who has been found to develop anti-Rh antibodies during pregnancy can, immediately after the birth of the baby, be given injections to prevent the difficulty from arising in subsequent pregnancies.

rheumatic fever A disease of unknown origin but associated with a recent bacterial infection of the throat. It is primarily a disease of childhood and adolescence, characterized by pain, stiffness and swelling of one or more large joints, and (if untreated) potentially serious complications that could lead to permanent heart damage. The majority of cases of rheumatic fever occur between the ages of eight and fifteen.

The onset of rheumatic fever usually follows within two to three weeks of a sore throat or other bacterial infection caused by the Group A beta-hemolytic streptococcus, the species responsible for "strep throat." It is believed that the disease represents an allergic reaction caused when the bacteria release their poisonous substances (toxins) in the body. The delicate membrane lining of the heart and its valves (endocardium) may become inflamed (endocarditis). If any scars remain on the valves after the inflammation has healed, they can cause serious impairment of the heart's functions, a condition known as rheumatic heart disease.

The first symptoms of rheumatic fever include pain, stiffness, and swelling in the shoulder, elbow, wrist, hip, knee, or ankle. The smaller joints are rarely affected. The pain normally lasts only a day or so in the particular joint and then flits to another; this seems to be a characteristic symptom. Other common symptoms and signs include fever, rapid pulse, sweating, and occasionally a skin rash. Sleeping may be difficult due to pain in the joint.

Not all children suffer serious symptoms from rheumatic fever. In fact, some cases are so mild that the disease is never diagnosed. About half of the patients who are found to have some form of chronic rheumatic heart disease do not have a history of rheumatic fever.

Any child suffering from rheumatic fever should be put to bed at once; bed rest puts less strain on the heart and helps to minimize the possibility of complications. Meals should be light and liquids offered generously. The physician will probably prescribe aspirin or a similar drug to relieve pain, lower fever, and reduce inflammation. If the child complains of a ringing sensation in the ears (tinnitus), a loss of hearing, or starts to vomit, consult the physician at once; he or she may wish to modify the treatment. It is absolutely essential to keep the child from any strenuous activity, and to follow exactly the physician's instructions, especially regarding the term of antibiotic treatment.

rheumatism A rather nonspecific term, rarely used in medical practice, that refers to any condition characterized by muscular aches and pains and inflammation of the joints.
SEE *gout, osteoarthritis, rheumatic fever, rhematoid arthritis*

rheumatoid arthritis A chronic and usually progressive inflammatory disease that affects the joints. It is characterized by pain and swelling of the joints with consequent restriction of movement. In more severe forms it may produce crippling deformities, particularly in the hands and fingers. In some cases the onset may be abrupt (acute rheumatoid arthritis) and be accompanied by a high fever and the rapid development of joint deformities. The cause of rheumatoid arthritis is unknown, although it is strongly suspected to be an *autoimmune disease*. It affects women nearly three times more frequently as men.

Early signs and symptoms are not specific for this disease. They include fatigue, weight loss, moist skin (often with sweating of the palms and soles), and general stiffness and pains in the joints. The common sensation of coldness of the hands and feet is the result of a disturbance of blood circulation. The disease may affect persons at any age, although the onset is usually between thirty and fifty.

The affected joint is usually red, hot, and tender to the touch. In severe and prolonged cases there may also be a wasting away (atrophy) of the muscles surrounding the joint. To prevent or minimize atrophy, the physician may recommend that the joint be exercised as soon as partial relief of pain permits, which will help prevent the joint from becoming stiff. Acutely painful joints should not be exercised.

There is no specific treatment for rheumatoid arthritis. The best that can be done is to provide relief of pain with appropriate doses of aspirin or another analgesic. In some cases corticosteroids will also be prescribed to control severe inflammation and swelling.

SEE ALSO *Still's disease*

rhinitis Inflammation of the mucous membrane that lines the nasal cavity. It is generally caused by a viral infection (typically the common cold) or hay fever (allergic rhinitis).

rickets A childhood disease caused by an inadequate amount of vitamin D, either through dietary lack or insufficient exposure to sunlight or both. Rickets interferes with the normal deposition of calcium, the mineral that makes the bones rigid and strong. In severe cases the bones become soft and yield under the weight of the body, causing bowing of the legs, downward compression of the vertebrae of the spine, and a flattening of the pelvis.

Rickets is now relatively uncommon in developed countries, largely as the result of a better understanding of nutrition and the fairly routine addition of vitamin D to the diet given infants during and after weaning.

SEE *osteomalacia*

Rickettsia A group of microorganisms intermediate in size between *bacteria* and *viruses*. Unlike bacteria, they must inhabit (parasitize) living cells in order to survive; unlike viruses, they are too large to pass through a Berkefeld filter, an identifying test for all particles of viral size. Rickettsiae cause several human diseases, including Rocky Mountain spotted fever, Q fever, and typhus. The microorganisms are usually transmitted by infected lice, fleas, ticks, and mites.

This group of microorganisms is named after the American pathologist Howard T. Ricketts (1871-1910).

ringworm A *fungus* infection of the skin, hair, or nails; in medical terms, *tinea*. It has nothing to do with worms; it is named after the ringlike lesions often produced.

risus sardonicus An acute spasm of the facial muscles occasionally seen in *tetanus* that results in a grotesque or distorted grin.

Rocky Mountain spotted fever An infectious disease caused by a species of *rickettsia*. It is transmitted to humans by infected ticks and is characterized by sudden fever, chills, headache, pain in the muscles and joints, and (after about the fourth day of fever) a rash, which appears first on the wrists, ankles, palms, soles, and forearms and extends quickly to other parts of the body. The disease was once thought to be limited in the United States to those states near the Rocky Mountains; it is now known that other geographical areas such as the Atlantic seaboard also harbor the microorganisms.

Prompt cure of Rocky Mountain spotted fever is usually possible with the administration of antibiotics.
SEE *typhus*

root canal The part of the root of a tooth that contains the soft vascular tissue (dental pulp) that keeps the tooth alive. Root-canal work is a dental procedure that involves drilling into the pulp cavity of a tooth, cleaning and sterilizing it, and filling the cavity with a material to prevent future infection.

roseola Any rose-colored skin eruption, such as the rash typical of measles or German measles.
SEE ALSO *roseola infantum*

roseola infantum A noncontagious skin rash that sometimes affects infants, characterized by fever and enlargement of the *lymph glands* in the neck. It is thought to be caused by a viral infection, usually runs a relatively mild course, and is most commonly seen in the spring and fall. The incubation period is between four and seven days. The rising fever (which may occasionally reach 105°F/40.5°C) may lead to convulsions; after about the fourth day the fever usually falls and the skin rash appears, most prominently on the chest and abdomen. By the time the rash appears the child should have a normal body temperature and feel no discomfort.

Treatment of roseola infantum

(also known as exanthem subitum and pseudorubella) is aimed at relief of symptoms: control of possible convulsions and reduction of fever with aspirin or another antipyretic.

roughage The nondigestible element in plant foods, also called fiber, considered an essential part of the diet for the prevention and treatment of intestinal disorders such as *diverticulitis*.

rubella The medical name for German measles. It is a much milder childhood illness and is not as contagious as true *measles*. It is caused by a virus spread from the nose and throat of an infected person; the incubation period is from fourteen to twenty-one days.

The first signs of rubella may be a sore throat and a slight fever. The rash consists of small flat pink spots that first appear on the face and neck and then spread to the body and limbs. Generally the glands behind the ears become swollen. It is best to keep the child in bed until the rash and fever have disappeared, for until that time the disease is contagious.

In most cases no special treatment is required. The child should have plenty of rest, eat lightly, and be given cooling drinks. One attack of rubella usually provides *immunity* for life.

Adults who have not had rubella may get the disease if exposed to an infected child. This is potentially dangerous for pregnant women, since rubella during the first three or four months of pregnancy may lead to serious complications in the fetus.

Rubin's test A test to determine if a Fallopian tube is obstructed by blowing a gas such as carbon dioxide into the tube, a procedure known as insufflation. If the tube is open, the gas will pass through it and enter the peritoneal cavity, where its presence can be detected on an x-ray film or fluoroscope screen.

The test is named after the American physician Isidor Clinton Rubin (1883–1958).

S

saline Relating to or containing salt; salty.

saliva The tasteless clear fluid secreted by the *salivary glands* of the mouth. It moistens food particles (making them easier to swallow) and initiates the first stages of digestion. Saliva also contains the enzyme ptyalin, which aids in the breakdown of starchy foods.

salivary glands Various *saliva*-secreting glands located in the cheeks and below the angle of the jaw. The largest of these are the parotid glands, which become infected and swollen in mumps (epidemic parotitis).

salmonellosis The most common form of *food poisoning*, caused by eating food contaminated with bacteria of the genus *Salmonella*.

Salmonellosis results in severe inflammation of the lining of the stomach and intestines (gastroenteritis). The bacteria multiply in food that has been improperly canned or preserved or in food that has been left in an opened can or container. The bacteria may also multiply in meat or other food that has been left too long in a warm or hot environment, which favors rapid bacterial development.

The incubation period from eating the contaminated food to the first symptoms of the disease is between six and forty-eight hours. In most cases the illness lasts only one or two days and may even be so mild that bed rest or medical treatment is not required.

Diarrhea and vomiting may drain the body of fluid and mineral salts; to replace them, the patient should drink meat or vegetable extracts or citrus fruit juices after starting with cola, tea, and bland foods. The liquid should be tepid and sipped very slowly, using a teaspoon if necessary, to prevent further vomiting.

Antibiotics are rarely necessary in the treatment of uncomplicated cases of salmonellosis—in fact, their use tends to delay the excretion of the bacteria from the intestinal tract. In some cases a physician may prescribe antispasmodic drugs to relieve associated intestinal spasm.

salpingectomy Surgical removal of a Fallopian tube.

salpingitis Inflammation of a Fallopian tube. It usually occurs as the result of a bacterial infection that spreads upward from the uterus, cervix, or vagina. The symptoms include severe abdominal pain (which may at first be felt on only one side and, if on the right side, may mimic an attack of appendicitis), vaginal discharge, fever, and a rapid pulse. Early diagnosis and treatment with antibiotics will be effective; delay in seeking medical attention can result in serious complications, including sterility if both tubes are involved.

sarcoma The general name for any malignant growth *(cancer)* composed of cells that arise from the connective tissue of the body, such as muscle or bone. Sarcomas can involve the bladder, kidneys, lungs, liver, spleen, and nearby tissues. A sarcoma is often named after the tissue in which it originated, such as osteosarcoma (sarcoma of bone), chondrosarcoma (sarcoma of cartilage), and lymphosarcoma (sarcoma of lymphatic tissue). It may also be named for the type of cell it contains (giant-cell sarcoma, Kupffer cell sarcoma, mixed-cell sarcoma).

Sarcomas are less common than *carcinomas;* they can be very malignant and difficult to treat.

scabies A skin disease caused by the irritating effects of the female itch mite, *Sarcoptes scabiei*. The mite can just be seen with the unaided eye. It burrows into the upper part of the skin (epidermis) and deposits its eggs, leaving irregular track marks. The sites most often affected are the hands and wrists, elbows, genitals, and lower back. The eggs hatch within the burrows and after about two weeks produce mature mites. The infected person becomes sensitized to the mites and their irritating secretions, which cause intense itching that is often much worse at night, the period of greatest mite activity.

The disease is spread by close contact with infected persons. Prompt medical attention is effective in curing scabies, especially if other members of the family and close contacts are also treated.
COMPARE *pediculosis*

scarlet fever An acute contagious disease caused by a bacterial infection spread by the breath or cough of an infected person or by handling contaminated objects. The incubation period is from one to four days. Not all persons infected with the bacteria (any one of more than forty strains of type A hemolytic toxin-producing streptococci) break out in the typical bright red rash of scarlet fever. The disease is more common in childhood, although adults may also be affected.

The first signs of scarlet fever are

common to many other illnesses—sore throat, chills, fever, cough, and sometimes nausea and vomiting. The tongue is occasionally covered with a white coat that gradually peels off to reveal bright red areas ("strawberry tongue"). On about the second day the rash breaks out on the skin, starting on the neck and behind the ears. It rapidly spreads over the entire body with the usual exception of the area around the mouth. The skin has a bright red color and is covered with many tiny red spots. In about a week little round dead patches of skin flake off; by this time the rash will have disappeared.

Penicillin is the most effective antibiotic used to treat scarlet fever; it must be taken for a minimum of ten days to prevent the possible complications of *rheumatic fever* and acute *glomerulonephritis*. The child should be kept isolated and comfortable until all symptoms disappear. Cool drinks may be offered to help soothe the sore throat.

Schick test A test to determine immunity or susceptibility to diphtheria in which a tiny amount of diluted diphtheria toxin is injected into the skin. The results are available within three to four days. Susceptibility to diphtheria is shown by the development of redness and slight swelling at the point of injection. If the patient is immune to diphtheria because of the presence of specific antibodies in the blood there will be little or no reaction to the injection.

The test is named after the Hungarian-American pediatrician Béla Schick (1877-1967).

schistosomiasis A parasitic disease also known as bilharziasis caused by infestation of the body with blood flukes (a type of worm) of the genus *Schistosoma*. Three species infect humans: *S. haematobium*, *S. mansoni*, and *S. japonicum*; the disease is widespread in Africa, the Middle East, the Caribbean, and parts of Central and South America. The japonicum form is restricted to Southeast Asia, especially Japan, the Philippines, and parts of China.

The blood fluke requires a freshwater snail to complete its life cycle. The eggs are passed in the feces or urine of infected people; if they are allowed to reach water they hatch and release free-swimming larval forms (miracidia) that penetrate the snail. Inside the snail they develop into thousands of infective larvae that are eventually released into the surrounding water; there they can penetrate the skin of anyone wading, swimming, or otherwise coming into contact with the infested water.

The larvae (also known as cercariae) make their way through the blood vessels to the lungs and liver and sometimes to other parts of the body, where they mature into adult worms. These can move to the intestines and bladder. Although the worms can cause damage themselves, the main problems are caused by the eggs they lay: for example, eggs deposited in the urinary bladder can cause irritation, and blood is then seen in the urine. A hypersensitivity (allergic) reaction to the presence of the eggs has been implicated as one cause of tissue damage. In untreated chronic cases, malignant changes may occur in the affected organs and tissues.

Definitive diagnosis involves the identification of eggs in stool samples or by means of serological tests. Treatment with drugs such as tartar emetic, stibophen, and stibocaptate is effective against all three forms of schistosomiasis, particularly when administered as soon as the diagnosis has been confirmed. As a sensible precaution, visitors to areas where the disease is prevalent should not swim in water unless it has been judged safe by the local authorities.

sciatica A condition characterized by pain along the course of the sciatic nerve, the body's largest nerve, which extends down the leg. A symptom of a disorder and not a disease, sciatica is typically experienced as a sharp, shooting, or occasionally dull and aching pain from the buttocks or thigh down the back of the leg. (Some patients have pain to the sole of the foot.) The pain is usually constant and more intense when standing, although in some patients it is intermittent. In addition, the back of the leg is frequently very sensitive to pressure. Because of this, the pain may be aggravated by sitting with undue pressure on the back of the legs or the buttocks.

The cause of sciatica in the vast majority of cases is a *slipped disk* or other cause of compression of the spinal roots of the sciatic nerve. Less commonly the cause may be an inflammation of the nerve or pain impulses referred from another part of the body.

Treatment includes analgesics to reduce the pain, the application of heat along the course of the nerve, and rest on a firm mattress. In those particularly severe cases caused by the compression of the spinal root where the patient fails to respond to such treatment, surgical correction may be necessary to relieve the pain.

sclera The tough white fibrous tissue that forms the outer coating of the eyeball.

sclerosis An abnormal hardening of an organ or part, as by the overgrowth of fibrous tissues.
SEE *multiple sclerosis*

scoliosis An abnormal sideways curve of the spine. The adult vertebral column has four natural curves. A congenital defect, injury, disease, or chronic bad posture may result in the formation of one or more abnormal curves. If bad posture alone is responsible, the curve can usually be corrected by appropriate exercises professionally prescribed and directed. Such exercises are of greatest benefit during childhood, when the bones are still growing at a relatively rapid rate.

If incorrect posture in childhood is maintained for some time, a postural deformity (one that can be corrected voluntarily) may become gradually transformed into a structural deformity (one that cannot be corrected voluntarily). Surgical correction may then be required.
SEE *spinal curvature*

screening Examination of large groups of the general population to detect early evidence of any particular disease or disorder, such as diabetes, tuberculosis, or cancer of the cervix, or to reveal health-risk factors such as high blood pressure (hypertension). Many communities provide periodic mass screening by offering chest x-rays, Pap tests, and blood-pressure measurements.

The term also refers to the use of several diagnostic tests during the same period of time (multiphasic screening) to determine the presence in an individual of one or more diseases or disorders.

scrotum The pouch of skin hanging behind the penis and containing the *testicles* (testes). It is composed of darkish skin arising from the area between the legs known as the perineum. In the adult male it is sparsely covered with fairly long hairs. When the skin is gently stretched, a large number of sebaceous (oil-secreting) glands that look like small white pimples can be seen.

Inside the scrotum is a wall (septum) which divides it into two halves, each containing a testicle. The scrotum is rich in sweat glands, which cool by evaporation of moisture. These glands enable the scrotum to carry out its main function—to regulate the temperature of the testicles, the manufacturers of sperm cells (spermatozoa). Sperm cannot be produced if the temperature of the testicle is the same as that of the body; it must be two degrees below this point.

The scrotum is very sensitive to temperature changes and it raises or lowers the testicles mechanically to maintain their temperature. For example, in hot weather the muscles that form the wall of the scrotum relax and the testicles hang loosely between the legs. The distended scrotum can thus give off more heat since a larger skin area is exposed. In cold weather the muscles become tense and draw the scrotum closer to the body.

Itching sensations are experienced in the scrotum from time to time; this may be due to variations in the state of contraction of the muscle fibers, which are also influenced by emotional factors. If the skin of the scrotum is cut or injured, it ordinarily heals very quickly.

sebaceous cysts Cysts just beneath the skin (especially on the scalp) formed by distension of the *sebaceous glands*. They contain modified particles of keratin (a tough protein substance found in hair) and small amounts of *sebum*, a greasy substance that may turn rancid. Surgical removal of the cysts under local anesthesia is not always desirable, since the cysts are frequently reabsorbed spontaneously and may reform even if removed.

sebaceous glands The oil-secreting glands of the skin. Each gland is usually associated with a hair follicle. The greasy lubricant the glands secrete is known as *sebum*.
SEE ALSO *sebaceous cysts*

seborrhea A disorder of the sebaceous glands characterized by an abnormal increase in their secretion of *sebum*. There is no effective treatment for seborrhea, although associated conditions, such as acne or dandruff, may respond to specific therapy.

sebum The greasy material secreted by the *sebaceous glands* that lubricates the skin. This thick, semifluid substance is composed largely of fat and epithelial debris from certain skin cells.
SEE ALSO *sebaceous cysts, seborrhea*

sedative Any drug or agent that induces calming or sleep, such as barbiturates and certain *tranquilizers*.
SEE ALSO *hypnotic drug*

sedimentation rate
SEE *erythrocyte sedimentation rate*

semen The whitish or slightly yellow viscous secretion produced by the testicles and supplemented by secretions from the seminal vesicles and the prostate gland. It contains the spermatozoa (sperm cells).

senile dementia A general term used to describe a wide variety of mental and emotional changes that often occur in the elderly, especially in those over the age of seventy. The condition, also known as senility or senile psychosis, is characterized by various degrees of impairment of intellectual function, memory loss (particularly for recent events), disorientation for time and place, impaired ability to handle numerical calculations, short attention span, irritability, loss of humor, and other evidence of a dramatic personality change.

The cause of senile dementia is associated with a gradual degeneration of various areas of tissue in the cerebral cortex (outer layer of the brain) and the substantial loss of brain cells. The brain also shows evidence of marked *atrophy*. The condition appears to be more common in women than men and tends to progress steadily. The individual may become extremely depressed and fail to pay adequate attention to basic hygiene and nutrition. Severe *atherosclerosis* may also play a role in the development of symptoms.

sensitization

Senile dementia is an irreversible condition and no specific treatment exists.
SEE ALSO *Alzheimer's disease*

sensitization The process of becoming abnormally reactive (hypersensitive) to antigens or allergens, such as pollens, feathers, or serums.
COMPARE *desensitization*
SEE ALSO *allergy*

sepsis The presence in the tissues or the bloodstream of various pathogenic (disease-causing) bacteria or their toxic (poisonous) products.
SEE ALSO *septicemia*

septicemia A systemic (involving the entire body or large parts of it) disease caused by the presence in the blood of large numbers of rapidly multiplying bacteria; popularly called blood poisoning. Treatment involves the administration of an appropriate antibiotic.

serum The fluid portion of the blood (plasma) without clotting (coagulation) factors. It contains *antibodies* and is used in the treatment of conditions in which specific antibodies can exert a therapeutic effect.

serum sickness A condition characterized by fever, skin rash, enlarged spleen, painful joints, and swollen lymph glands. It may occur eight to twelve days following an injection of a foreign serum and is thought to represent a relatively mild form of *anaphylactic reaction*.

shingles
SEE *herpes zoster*

shock A clinical condition in which there is a dangerous disturbance of blood circulation (circulatory collapse) and a consequent lack of oxygen to the tissues. Prompt medical attention is usually essential to prevent death from reduced blood flow to the brain, which cannot survive such deprivation.

Shock may result from serious bleeding, damage to the heart muscle, or a sudden dilation (widening) of blood vessels after injury.
SEE ALSO *hypotension*

shortness of breath
SEE *dyspnea*

sickle-cell anemia A hereditary form of *anemia* characterized by a genetic abnormality of the red blood cells (erythrocytes) in which they become crescent-shaped. It is associated with the presence of an abnormal type of *hemoglobin* (hemoglobin S) in the red blood cells. The gene responsible for this abnormality is seen mainly in people from the Mediterranean area and certain parts of Africa.

side effect Any effect of a drug or pharmaceutical product on the body other than that intended. Most prescription and over-the-counter drugs are capable of producing unpleasant or adverse reactions in a few people who take them. The very fact that a drug can modify the body's physiology to produce a beneficial effect means that it can also interfere with other organs or tissues to produce unwanted effects.

Possible side effects depend on many factors, such as the type and dose of drug and the susceptibility of the individual patient. Typical side effects include nausea, vomiting, blurred vision, ringing in the ears (tinnitus), diarrhea, constipation, skin rashes, itching, weakness, loss of appetite (anorexia), impaired muscular coordination (ataxia), sensitivity of the eyes to light (photophobia), insomnia, drowsiness, excitability, and nervousness. Some people may experience more severe side effects, including those that are a direct threat to life. For example, some drugs may affect the normal ability of the bone marrow to produce healthy blood cells. Other drugs may have an adverse effect on the liver and kidneys, especially in those who already suffer from a disease of these organs. The most dramatic example of a potentially fatal side effect to drugs is an *anaphylactic reaction*, as in those allergic to penicillin.

The possibility of side effects from a particular drug can be greatly reduced by paying strict attention to the instructions of the physician or the dosage instructions and warnings printed on the label.

In a very few cases a drug's side effect can become a desirable effect in another therapy. For example, antihistamines are available over-the-counter to relieve the symptoms of various common allergic conditions and they have the characteristic side effect of causing drowsiness. This can be a beneficial effect to insomniacs, and antihistamines are often used in products designed as sleep aids.

If a troublesome side effect occurs while taking a nonprescription drug, its use should be discontinued. If side effects occur while taking a prescription drug, it is essential to tell the physician at once; he or she may modify the dosage or prescribe another drug that may be more successfully tolerated by the patient.

siderosis A lung disease caused by the inhalation of dust or vapors that contain iron particles. It is a form of *pneumoconiosis*.

SIDS Abbreviation for *sudden infant death syndrome*.

sigmoidoscope An illuminated instrument used to examine the S-shaped (sigmoid) part of the large intestine (colon), just above the rectum.
SEE ALSO *proctoscope*

sign Any objective evidence of a disease or disorder, such as an enlarged organ or a heart murmur, representing what the physician finds on examination rather than what the patient feels.
COMPARE *symptom*

silicosis A lung disease caused by the inhalation of silica dust (quartz dust). It is a form of *pneumoconiosis*

sinus

and an *occupational disease* of miners and quarry workers.

sinus A recess or cavity; in particular, the drainage channels of the frontal bones of the skull (nasal sinuses), a large channel containing venous blood (venous sinuses), or a tract or passage leading to an abscess.
SEE ALSO *sinusitus*

sinusitis Inflammation of the mucous membrane that lines the nasal sinuses. It most commonly occurs as an extension of nasal infections, but any condition within the nose that interferes with sinus drainage renders that sinus liable to infection. A deviated septum or foreign bodies or growths in the nose may make a patient susceptible to sinusitis.

Because of the close anatomical relationship between the upper teeth and the floor of the maxillary sinus (the largest sinus, situated between the nose and the cheekbone), root abscesses of the teeth can produce chronic maxillary sinusitis. Excessive nose blowing that increases the pressure within the nose may drive infected material into a sinus rather than out of the nose. The same problem can be caused by underwater swimming and diving when a cold is developing or already established.

A healthy sinus contains some air in addition to slight secretions from its mucous membrane lining. The sinus opens into the nose through a narrow aperture, and an inflamed lining may swell sufficiently to block this. Once this normal drainage channel to the nose has become blocked, the secretions build up and cause pain by exerting pressure against the sinus's bony walls. The pain may be experienced as a headache or felt directly over the affected sinus, and is often made worse by coughing or bending down.

X-rays may help identify a blocked sinus, which will appear denser than nearby healthy sinuses because it is filled with fluid. In severe chronic cases a minor surgical incision may be made to permit the sinus to drain, without which healing is impossible. Pain is often relieved with aspirin and the application of heat to the area above the affected sinus. Antibiotics may also be prescribed to control bacterial infection.

skin graft Transplantation of pieces of skin from one part of a patient's body to another, as in the treatment of severe burns or other disfiguring injuries to the skin. The damaged area is usually covered with a small amount of skin removed surgically from the thigh, back, or abdomen. The depth of the skin graft depends largely upon the severity of the damaged area. The area from which the transplant tissue is taken repairs itself naturally with the regrowth of new skin.

When severe burns over a large

part of the body or other extensive skin injuries make it impossible to borrow skin for transplanting from the patient's own body, it is sometimes possible to make use of grafts from donors. This is more difficult, since unless the donor is an identical twin of the patient the graft may be rejected. In many cases, however, the graft will "take" long enough for the patient's own skin to start regrowing and filling in the damaged areas.

Grafts are essential when wide areas of the skin are damaged. Without the protective covering of the skin the patient is not only susceptible to bacterial infection but would lose body fluids that are necessary to maintain life.

Modern surgical methods and advanced medical treatment have made skin transplantation or grafting a relatively safe and uncomplicated procedure.

SEE ALSO *graft*

skull The complete bony framework of the head, consisting of the *cranium* (the fusion of eight separate bones that encloses the *brain*) and the fourteen facial bones. The thickness of the skull varies considerably over different parts of the brain; it is generally much thicker at the top than at the sides. The skull contains several openings through which nerves and blood vessels pass; the largest of these, the foramen magnum, is at the base of the skull and is the opening through which the spinal cord enters the brain. In certain places the skull contains small cavities known as air sinuses, most of which are connected to the nasal cavity.

From birth until about twelve to eighteen months, soft areas where the bone is as yet absent can be felt through the skin at the top and sides of the head; these are called *fontanels*. There are usually six: a large one at the top of the head, one toward the rear, and one behind and one over each ear. The fontanels gradually become replaced by bone.

sleep The normal periodic loss of consciousness during which the body is in a state of physiological rest. In adults it lasts an average of six to eight hours each day, although the elderly may require less. Sleep is characterized by typical modifications in the brain's electrical activity that can be detected by electroencephalograms and by dreaming, recognized by rapid movements of the eyes under closed lids (REM sleep). Most people dream four to five times during normal sleep, although the subject matter of all but the final dream is rarely recalled in detail.

Despite many interesting theories about sleep and dreaming and ongoing research in these areas, surprisingly little is known about the reasons for either or the mechanisms involved.

Prolonged lack of sleep (sleep deprivation) influences the nervous system, resulting in progressive changes in mood and behavior and the inability to concentrate. It is believed that the *reticular activating system* plays an essential role in maintaining alertness or wakefulness. During sleep this system is somehow closed down temporarily.

Normal sleep differs from other states of unconsciousness such as coma in that arousal is usually possible with only slight stimulation.
SEE ALSO *narcolepsy*

sleeping pill
SEE *hypnotic drug*

sleeping sickness Another name for African *trypanosomiasis*, a parasitic infectious disease caused by invasion of the body with either of two distinct species of *protozoa*. The term is also used to describe the viral disease *encephalitis* lethargica characterized by a severe inflammation of the brain; a pandemic occurred during 1916–1917.

slipped disk A herniation (slipping out) of part of the intervertebral disk, the protective cushion of firm elastic tissue between two adjacent vertebrae of the spinal column. The condition is also known as a herniated disk, ruptured disk, or prolapsed disk.

An intervertebral disk is normally held in position by a ring of fibrous tissues. Gradual weakness of these constraining fibers may result in the disk's protruding or slipping out a bit from between the vertebrae. When this occurs it often causes intense pain and severely restricts movement because the protruding disk exerts pressure against a spinal nerve. Occasionally the protruding disk may cause a partial or total loss of sensation in a part of the body supplied by the compressed nerve.

The pain caused by a slipped disk may not appear to come from the spine but may be felt in another part of the body (referred pain). Often intense pain is felt down the leg (*sciatica*). In other cases the slipped disk may cause an acute attack of lower back pain or muscle spasms.

The condition is likely if there is a congenital weakness in the disk or a gradual deterioration of the ligaments that hold the disk in position (sometimes seen in middle or old age). The actual displacement may be caused by an injury or, more commonly, by sudden strain on the vertebral column.

Treatment depends largely on the nature and severity of the injury. The problems can be minimized and the disk may return to its normal position if the back is kept straight. Good posture is important and bending the spine should be avoided; when picking up a heavy object, one should always bend the knees and keep the back straight.

Severe cases of slipped disk may require a surgical procedure known as a *laminectomy*, in which part of one or more vertebrae is removed in order to reach and remove the disk fragment that is causing pressure on the spinal cord.

small intestine The part of the *digestive tract* between the *stomach* and the *large intestine*, consisting of the *duodenum, jejunum,* and *ileum.* The small intestine forms a coiled loop about 20 feet (6 meters) long. During the first stage of the digestive process, which takes place in the stomach, food becomes liquid (chyme); the pylorus, the muscular ring at the outlet of the stomach, opens to permit the chyme to enter the first part of the small intestine, where the bulk of digestion takes place.

Food leaving the stomach enters the duodenum in a series of brief spurts. There it is subjected to additional digestive juices conveyed by ducts from the *pancreas* and *gallbladder.* The pancreatic juice contains enzymes that continue to break down starch, fats, and proteins. Bile enters the duodenum through a duct from the gallbladder; this helps emulsify fats, making them easier to digest. The ducts from the pancreas and the gallbladder join just as they reach the duodenum and their secretions enter by a common duct.

Food products are completely digested and their nutrients absorbed into the bloodstream during their passage through the final two portions of the small intestine. Absorption occurs through thousands of villi, tiny projections on the intestinal walls.

smallpox An acute and highly contagious disease caused by a viral infection. At one time smallpox was a major cause of death throughout the world. In 1967 the World Health Organization launched a worldwide campaign to vaccinate as many people as possible against the disease; as a result, by 1982 the disease was officially considered eradicated.

smear A preparation of material such as blood, bodily secretions, cellular specimens, or microorganisms spread out on a glass slide for examination under a microscope. A *cervical smear* is a test for cancer of the cervix.

smegma The cheeselike sebaceous secretions that can collect beneath the foreskin of the penis or around the clitoris.

sonogram A record or display obtained during *ultrasonography.*

spasm Involuntary contraction of muscles. It can be caused by irritation or inflammation of adjoining tissues or nerve damage.

spastic Afflicted with muscular *spasms;* especially those of cerebral palsy (spastic paralysis).
SEE *spastic colon*

spastic colon
SEE *irritable bowel syndrome*

species A biological classification of living organisms subordinate to *genus*. Members of the same species can usually breed and produce fertile offspring, while those of the same genus can not.

speculum An instrument for holding back the walls or normally closed entrance of a bodily passage or cavity so that its interior can be inspected.

sperm cell
SEE *spermatozoa*

spermatozoa Male sex cells; sperm cells. Spermatozoa are the smallest cells in the body of sexually mature males and they look like tiny tadpoles when examined under a microscope. They are produced within the *testicles* in an area called the seminiferous tubules and are released through the tip of the penis during ejaculation. Sperm cells have a broad oval flattened head, a middle section (neck), and a long tail. The tail (flagellum) provides movement for the sperm by means of a constant whiplike action.

All body cells have forty-six *chromosomes* (the carriers of *genes*, which determine hereditary characteristics) except for the sperm cell and the ovum (female sex cell), which contain only twenty-three. The sperm contains both Y *chromosomes* and X *chromosomes* and thus determines whether the baby will be a girl or a boy.

Spermatozoa are able to swim at a rate of several inches per hour. Each sperm cell is equipped with an enzyme that helps dissolve part of the tough coating of the ovum so *fertilization* can take place. The opening in the coat of the ovum immediately seals itself after one sperm cell enters, thus prohibiting more than one sperm cell from entering.

It takes from seven to ten weeks for the sexually mature male body to make a sperm cell, and approximately 200 million mature spermatozoa are produced each day in the testicles. Should sexual activity not occur for prolonged periods, these cells disintegrate, become liquid and are reabsorbed by the body. Following ejaculation, the lifespan of spermatozoa is limited. Within the uterus they may survive for two or three days; those that remain in the vagina cease to move after an hour or so.
SEE ALSO *scrotum, semen*

sphincter A circular muscle that controls the opening and closure of some bodily passages (for example, the anal sphincter).

sphygmomanometer An instrument for measuring blood pressure, consisting in its basic form of a hollow rubber cuff which is wrapped around the upper arm and inflated with a hand bulb. When the pressure inside the cuff is greater than the pressure inside the artery beneath it, the blood flow is temporarily interrupted.

The physician or nurse usually places a *stethoscope* over an artery just below the cuff and inflates the cuff until the arterial flow has been stopped. Then air is slowly released from the cuff by means of a valve. The moment the pulse beat is heard to return to the artery, this figure is noted on a column of mercury or other method of measurement. This figure represents *systolic* pressure, the greatest pressure exerted on the artery by the circulating blood. The air in the cuff is gradually released until the sound of the pulse beat disappears. The figure noted at this point indicates *diastolic* pressure, the minimum pressure exerted on the arteries during each heartbeat cycle.

spina bifida A congenital defect (*neural-tube defect*) in a section of the vertebral column, which fails at some point during embryonic development to close normally around the spinal cord. The gap that results, usually in the lumbar region (lower back), may be covered with skin and present no special problems (spina bifida occulta). In some children, however, the membranes surrounding the spinal cord or part of the cord itself may protrude through the opening. In more severe cases the defect may result in the exposure of up to several inches of cord.

Any disruption of the spinal cord and its nerves results in a loss of sensation and movement in the part of the body the affected spinal nerves supply and control. It is not uncommon for the entire lower half of the body to be paralyzed.

The treatment of spina bifida depends on the extent of the damage to the spinal cord and how early the surgical correction of the defect is undertaken. Some surgeons operate within a few hours of birth in severe cases. New surgical techniques and antibiotics have played a major role in prolonging the children's lives, but it is not possible to restore functions lost as the result of nerve damage. Even after surgical closure of the vertebral column, the child will require frequent attention to make sure that no complications arise. (Some children with spina bifida also have congenital *hydrocephalus*.)

The diagnosis of spina bifida can be made while the fetus is in the uterus by *amniocentesis* to measure the amount of *alphafetoprotein* in the amniotic fluid and *ultrasonography*.

spinal column The backbone or spine; also called the vertebral column. It contains thirty-three irregularly shaped bones called *vertebrae*, the majority of which form a hollow ring through which the *spinal cord* passes.

spinal cord A slightly oval-shaped column of nerve tissue that extends from the base of the *brain* down the central cavity of the backbone or spine. In adults it is approximately 17 inches (43 centimeters) long and about the diameter of a pencil. It contains nerve cells and fibers that act as connecting links between the brain and nerves of the trunk and limbs.

A horizontal section of the spinal cord reveals a central mass of gray tissue shaped like the letter H. The projecting masses of gray matter that form the legs of the H are known as horns: two in front (anterior horns) and two at the back (posterior horns). The gray matter consists of nerve tissue that extends throughout the length of the spinal cord. The white matter that surrounds gray columns is composed largely of nerve fibers covered with a protective fatty *(myelin)* sheath that provides electrical insulation for nerve impulses. The entire cord is surrounded by three protective membranes called *meninges* and by *cerebrospinal fluid*, as is the brain.

The spinal cord contains thirty-one pairs of nerves (spinal nerves) that branch out to supply nearly all parts of the body. They are classified according to their original (fetal) position on the *spinal column* or backbone: cervical (eight pairs); thoracic (twelve pairs); lumbar (five pairs); sacral (five pairs); coccygeal (one pair). These nerves are further classified as sensory (conveying impulses of feeling toward the spinal cord or brain), motor (conveying impulses to muscles) or mixed.

Each segment of the spinal cord contains nerves that control specific muscular movements or receive sensations from one particular area. The loss of sensation or impairment of movement in a specific part of the body is usually related to disease or injury of a specific spinal nerve or a group of nerves connected to it.

Motor nerves originate in the anterior horns of the gray matter of the spinal cord; sensory nerves originate in the posterior horns. Some incoming nerve impulses are acted on at the spinal cord and are not passed on to the brain; this is called a *reflex* reaction.

SEE *central nervous system*

spinal curvature One or more abnormal curves of the spine; for example, *scoliosis*, an abnormal spinal curve to one side. Kyphosis is a backward angular curve of the spine, popularly known as hunchback or humpback.

spinal tap
SEE *lumbar puncture*

spirometer A device or apparatus for measuring the air inhaled and exhaled from the lungs. It is used in the diagnosis of various lung disorders.
SEE *pulmonary function test*

spleen A dark red elongated organ on the left side of the abdomen just beneath the rib cage. It is approximately the size of the hand and, unless enlarged by disease (splenomegaly), cannot be felt by the examining physician because of its position behind the ribs.

The spleen is part of the lymphatic system and is in effect a large *lymph gland*. It produces two types of cells: lymphocytes, which are concerned with immunity and the production of antibodies, and macrophages (scavenger cells), larger cells capable of removing from the circulation bacteria or other foreign material and worn or damaged blood cells.

In a number of diseases the spleen removes cells from the bloodstream so effectively that a shortage of circulating cells results. In certain inherited disorders of the red blood cells, for example, the abnormal cells may be removed from the blood long before their normal lifespan is over. In other conditions, enlargement of the spleen occurs as a complication of disease; an enlarged spleen may remove red and white blood cells and platelets in excessive amounts.

If the spleen is damaged by injuries to the abdomen, it may have to be surgically removed (splenectomy). The lack of harmful effects from such an operation suggests that the function of the spleen is not absolutely essential to health. It is often removed surgically from patients in whom it is overactive or malfunctioning; the consequent improvement in the patient's condition is often dramatic.

spondylitis Inflammation of the vertebrae, the bones that form the spinal column.
SEE *ankylosing spondylitis*

spondylosis Abnormal stiffness or rigidity of the joints between the vertebrae.

spotted fever The general name for any of various eruptive diseases, especially those caused by infection with *rickettsia*.
SEE *Rocky Mountain spotted fever*

sprue A disease characterized by a failure of the digestive system to absorb and make proper use of nutrients, characterized by chronic diarrhea and anemia. The exact cause is uncertain. Tropical sprue is associated with malnutrition and lack of B vitamins. Nontropical sprue or *celiac disease* is related to a hypersensitivity to gluten.

sputum Matter brought up from the lungs and upper respiratory system and expelled during coughing or clearing the throat; some sputum is inevitably swallowed. Sputum may contain cellular debris, mucus, pus, blood, and microorganisms. Laboratory examination of a sputum sample can be of diagnostic value in various diseases of the lungs and respiratory tract.
SEE *phlegm*

stapedectomy A surgical procedure to correct a form of conduction deafness known as *otosclerosis*, caused by an abnormal overgrowth

stenosis

of bone around the stapes, one of the tiny sound-conducting bones (ossicles) of the middle ear.

stenosis An abnormal narrowing or constricting of a bodily opening or passage; stricture. For example, pyloric stenosis is a constriction between the outlet of the stomach *(pylorus)* and the beginning of the small intestines *(duodenum)* and usually demands immediate surgical treatment.

sterilization The technique or act of destroying all the living microorganisms on a substance, as by immersing it in chemicals or subjecting it to radiation or intense heat.

The term also refers to the act or procedure of rendering a male or female incapable of producing children.
SEE *tubal ligation, vasectomy*
COMPARE *fertilization*

steroid hormones The hormones produced by the sex glands (ovaries and testicles), including *estrogen*, *progesterone*, and *testosterone*, and those produced by the cortex of the *adrenal glands.*
SEE *corticosteroids*

stethoscope An instrument for listening to sounds that originate within the body. It typically consists of a Y-shaped piece of rubber tubing; the upper arms of the tubing are fitted with earpieces and the end is fitted with a metal diaphragm. When placed over the chest or back, the diaphragm conveys the sounds made by the action of the heart and the blood flowing through it and the sounds produced within the lungs during breathing. The interpretation of these sounds is of diagnostic value to the physician. More sophisticated forms of the stethoscope use electronic amplification.
SEE *auscultation*

Still's disease A condition also known as juvenile rheumatoid arthritis that is similar to *rheumatoid arthritis* in adults. It occurs most often in early childhood, with girls more commonly affected than boys. Although the disease can be severe, the prognosis (outlook) is generally good. As in adult rheumatoid arthritis, the cause of the disease is unknown.

In the early stages of the disease the common signs and symptoms are painful and swollen joints (especially the larger joints, unlike the adult form of the disease), skin rashes, and abnormal enlargement of the liver and spleen. The lymph glands may also be swollen.

A striking difference between the juvenile and the adult forms of rheumatoid arthritis is that children are often affected much more severely during the development of the disease. The body temperature may rise to about 105°F (40°C) and remain there for several weeks. In some cases there is an associated inflammation of the lungs and the covering membrane of the heart (pericarditis).

In the majority of juvenile cases the disease takes a much milder form in its later stages than its equivalent in adults. Total recovery is the rule. However, in severe and prolonged cases there may be an associated interference with normal growth and development. A characteristic feature in such cases is involvement of the lower jaw, which may result in a receding chin.

Other than analgesics, there is virtually no treatment.

The condition is named after the British physician Sir George Frederick Still (1868-1941).

Stokes-Adams syndrome A condition characterized by lightheadedness or sudden loss of consciousness, caused by a temporary reduction in the amount of blood that reaches the brain. It is associated with any of various disorders of the heart that interfere with its normal pumping action and consequent output of blood. The patient may suffer only a transient interference of consciousness in milder forms. In some cases the patient may also experience convulsions. Treatment of severe forms generally involves the injection of *epinephrine* into the heart and the use of an external electric *pacemaker*.

The condition is named after the Irish physicians William Stokes (1804-1878) and Robert Adams (1791-1875).

stomach The widest part of the *digestive tract*, consisting of a muscular distensible sac between the *esophagus* and *duodenum*, the beginning of the *small intestine*. In the stomach, food particles are subjected to the chemical action of the *gastric juice*, a fluid containing various acids and enzymes that digest protein. Food often remains in the stomach for three or four hours, although it may leave after only thirty minutes.

stomach pump A term loosely given to any device with a tube that is inserted through the mouth into the stomach to extract its contents. It is used to remove toxic material in cases of food poisoning (where much of the contaminated food is still in the stomach) or drug overdose. To be effective, a stomach pump must be used before the toxic material has been absorbed in large quantities through the stomach wall or passed into the small intestine, ideally less than half an hour after the toxic material has been ingested.

stomatitis Inflammation of the mucous membrane of the mouth.
SEE ALSO *glossitis*

stools
SEE *feces*

strabismus A condition in which the eyes fail to point in the same

243

direction; cross-eye or squint. It is caused by a disorder of one or more of the muscles that control movement of the eyeballs.

Strabismus is fairly common in babies at about the age of six months, when it is usually only a momentary deviation of one or both eyes from the direction of vision. The child appears to be looking in two directions at once. Cross-eye (convergent strabismus) is when both eyes appear to look toward the nose; divergent strabismus is when both eyes appear to look away from the nose. Most often only one eye is involved.

In babies the muscles that control eye movements are not yet fully developed. The eyes are learning to cooperate in the task of focusing on an object together. If the eyes are constantly crossed or if one or both eyes constantly look outward or inward, a physician should be consulted at once. He or she may arrange for the child to be seen by an eye doctor (ophthalmologist). In many cases a simple operation will correct the fault.

As a general rule, intermittent strabismus before the age of six months is not serious and requires no special treatment. However, this decision must not be left to parents, since potentially serious disease of the eyes or nerves may be the underlying cause and a thorough examination of the child is essential at the earliest time. Any deviation of the eyes should be investigated by a physician shortly after birth.

strep throat A sore throat caused by infection with bacteria of the genus *Streptococcus*, specifically, Group A beta-hemolytic. If the infection is not promptly treated with an appropriate antibiotic, especially in children, there is a danger that *rheumatic fever* or *rheumatic heart disease* can develop.

stroke A condition also known as a cerebrovascular accident (formerly called apoplexy) caused by dramatic disturbance to the blood supply of the brain, such as the blocking of a cerebral artery by an *embolus* or *thrombus* or the rupture of a blood vessel in the brain. This results in localized destruction of brain tissue due to lack of oxygen in the part deprived of blood.

The immediate effects of a stroke depend on the extent and location of the damage. The typical results of sudden massive bleeding of a cerebral artery deep within the brain are immediate loss of consciousness, paralysis on the side of the body opposite the damage, and disturbance of speech. The patient may remain in a coma for some time following the stroke and recovery may be incomplete. Severe bleeding within the brain may prove fatal within forty-eight hours or after several days, and sometimes as long as two weeks after the stroke. In milder cases the patient may remain conscious and alert or have an impression of slightly dim or clouded awareness. Paralysis or some disorder of speech may also occur.

Following a stroke it is essential to seek immediate medical attention. The period of convalescence after milder cases may be up to six months, the time required for physicians to confirm the extent of permanent neurological damage; some impairment of speech or movement may persist. In such cases, speech therapy and physiotherapy may improve the outlook considerably.

subacute Relating to the course or symptoms of any disease or disorder between *acute* and *chronic*.

subcutaneous Beneath the skin or designed for introduction beneath the skin, as an injection.
SEE *hypodermic*

sudden infant death syndrome (SIDS) The unexpected and unexplained death of an apparently well or virtually well infant, most often between the second week and the first year of life; also called crib death. The distribution of SIDS is worldwide and its occurrence over the years has been constant. It occurs most frequently in the third and fourth months of life, in premature infants, in males, and in infants living in poverty. Almost all infants who are victims of SIDS die in their sleep, especially during the winter months.

The cause is unknown, although in approximately 10 to 15 percent of cases it is associated with some disorder of the *cardiovascular* or *central nervous systems*. Over 10,000 infants die in the United States each year from SIDS.

Parents who have lost a child from SIDS frequently suffer guilt feelings; counseling and other forms of support may be advisable.

sulfonamides A class of chemically based drugs also known as sulfonilamides and popularly called sulfa drugs, once widely used to treat bacterial infections. Sulfonamides suppress the growth and multiplication of bacteria (bacteriostasis) rather than kill them outright. Sulfonamides were discovered around 1910, but not used in medical practice until the early 1930s.
SEE ALSO *antibiotic, penicillin*

sunstroke A severe reaction caused by exposure to excessive heat from the sun; also called heatstroke. It is characterized by high fever, delirium, and usually collapse. The body temperature may go above 105°F (40.6°C); the victim usually sweats profusely and experiences headache and confusion before becoming delirious or lapsing into coma. The pulse and respiratory rate increase and blood pressure may be elevated. Without immediate attention the condition can be fatal.

Emergency treatment involves

superinfection

placing the victim in a bathtub filled with ice water; should a tub not be available, wet sheets can be placed on the victim's nude body, accompanied by vigorous fanning and skin massage. A physician should be consulted immediately; he or she may prescribe sedatives to control convulsions and will want to observe the patient for several days for signs of fluid imbalance and possible *kidney failure*.

superinfection Any new infection that follows an earlier one and is (usually) caused by a different species of microorganism. Superinfection is a possible side effect of prolonged antibiotic therapy, which can cause a disturbance of the normal bacterial population of the digestive tract. This promotes an overgrowth of one or more species of microorganisms.

suppository A medicated mass of various shapes and sizes for introduction into a bodily opening, such as the vagina (vaginal suppository) or rectum (rectal suppository). Once the suppository has been inserted, the normal body temperature dissolves the substance and the medication is absorbed through the mucous membranes.

suppuration The process of *pus* formation or discharge.

suprarenal gland
SEE *adrenal gland*

suture The surgical joining of the edges of a wound by stitching them together; a stitch (or the material) used to join the edges of a wound.

symptom Any evidence of a disease or disorder, such as nausea, pain, or headache, experienced or noticed by the patient rather than a physician.
COMPARE *sign*

syncope A temporary loss of consciousness (fainting) caused by an inadequate blood supply to the brain.
SEE *Stokes-Adams syndrome*

syndrome A group of *signs* and *symptoms* that characterize or are frequently associated with a particular disease or disorder. A syndrome can be named after the medical specialist who first described or recognized it (such as *Down's syndrome*), or expressed in medical terms (such as *adrenogenital syndrome*).

By recognizing that some diseases are typically characterized by a given syndrome, a physician can arrive at a correct *diagnosis*.

syphilis A *venereal disease* caused by infection with bacteria of the species *Treponema pallidum*, a spiral-shaped (spirochete) and highly active microorganism that requires a moist environment to survive. The infection is spread almost exclusively by sexual intercourse with an infected partner. The disease can also be transmitted by an infected mother to her unborn child during the later stages of pregnancy.

Congenital syphilis is very rare today, largely as the result of early diagnosis and treatment before pregnancy and by the use of routine blood tests at many prenatal clinics.

The first sign of syphilis is a hard painless sore (chancre) at the site of the initial infection—usually on the penis or the vaginal labia, although it may appear within the vagina or on the cervix. These sores represent the primary or first stage of syphilis and appear within about three weeks of infection. The incubation period may vary, however, from about ten to ninety days. The hard sore heals slowly and leaves a scar.

The secondary stage of syphilis usually develops about six weeks after the appearance of the hard sore. By now the bacteria have entered the bloodstream and begun to affect all parts of the body. The most common occurrence at this point is the appearance of various types of skin rash, sore throat, low fever, and generalized enlargement of the lymph glands. The moist sores that may develop on the skin and the inside of the mouth are highly infectious, and during this stage the disease can be passed to others by nonsexual contact. In time all the sores heal, usually without leaving scars, and other signs and symptoms of the disease completely disappear.

If the disease is untreated, however, the bacteria may remain inactive (latent) in the body for many years even though no outward sign or symptom of the disease is noted. The bacteria nevertheless are invading the organs and tissues of the body and may cause serious complications many years from the time of the original infection. When this occurs, the disease is said to be entering its third (tertiary) stage.

During the third stage of syphilis, rubbery growths (gummas) may appear anywhere in the body. They contain no bacteria and therefore cannot cause infection in others. When they eventually soften and break they release a viscous, gummy material. They can occur just underneath the skin, in the membranes of the nose and throat, and internally (in the liver, lungs, or stomach). Serious complications during the third stage include inflammation of the bones, blindness, syphilitic heart disease, degeneration of the spinal cord resulting in a loss of muscle control, and inflammatory and degenerative changes in the brain and its covering membranes resulting in physical, emotional, and intellectual deterioration.

With modern diagnostic techniques and treatment with antibiotics early in the disease, it is extremely rare for syphilis to reach the tertiary stage.

Clinics exist in most large hospitals where information and treatment can be obtained in confidence. In addition, venereal disease centers are available in many cities to provide similar help and advice.

SEE ALSO *gonorrhea, tabes dorsalis, Wassermann test*

syringe A piston-action device or instrument for injecting fluids into cavities, blood vessels, or tissues or for removing fluids from them.
SEE ALSO *hypodermic*

systemic Relating to or involving the entire body rather than one of its parts.

systolic Relating to the blood pressure when the chambers of the heart are in their brief period of contraction (systole) between beats. The systolic pressure is given before the *diastolic* pressure when a measurement is made. Normal systolic pressure in a young person is about 120.

T

tabes dorsalis A late manifestation of *syphilis* that involves the spinal cord. It occurs from about ten to twenty years following the original infection in patients who received inadequate or no treatment during the early stages of the disease. Tabes dorsalis attacks certain nerve fibers at the back of the spinal cord and causes atrophy (wasting) of their fatty insulation (myelin) and a hardening of the cord. Eventually the disease spreads to involve all the spinal nerve roots and their extensions (axons).

The early symptoms of tabes dorsalis (also known as just tabes or locomotor ataxia) include visual disturbances, loss of bladder control (incontinence), impotence, impaired muscular coordination, and unsteadiness when walking. As the nerve fibers continue to degenerate the ability to walk becomes progressively impaired; eventually, a conscious effort must be made in order to walk at all. Joints may become injured accidentally because the nerves are no longer able to convey the sensation of pain.

Treatment of tabes dorsalis is aimed at relief of symptoms, protecting the joints from injury, and the intramuscular injection of antibiotics to control the progression of the disease. Because of modern methods of diagnosing and treating syphilis, tabes dorsalis has become relatively rare.

tachycardia An abnormally fast heartbeat, especially over 100 beats per minute. Some attacks of tachycardia may be associated with conditions such as an overactive thyroid gland (hyperthyroidism) or other bodily disorders, including some form of heart disease. In a condition known as paroxysmal tachycardia the heart suddenly starts to beat rapidly, a fluttering sensation is felt in the chest, and the individual may feel faint. Often the attack ends abruptly after a few minutes. These symptoms can occur in a person with a healthy heart,

talipes

although a physician should be consulted in such cases to evaluate the condition and perhaps initiate treatment.
COMPARE *bradycardia, palpitation*

talipes The medical term for *clubfoot*.

tampon A plug of cotton or other absorbent material for insertion into a body cavity such as the nose (to control nosebleed) or the vagina (to absorb the menstrual flow).
SEE ALSO *epistaxis, toxic-shock syndrome*

tartar The hard deposit of calcium and other minerals that forms on the teeth, especially in the absence of regular brushing and oral hygiene; also called dental calculus.

taste buds The oval or flask-shaped nerve endings responsible for the sense of taste. They are embedded in the tongue, in the soft palate, and the epiglottis and can distinguish four basic qualities of taste: sweet, sour, salty, and bitter.

The sensation of taste depends more on smell and visual clues than on the taste buds.

Tay-Sachs disease An inherited disease caused by the transmission of an abnormal gene which results in the deficiency of the enzyme hexosaminidase. It primarily affects Jewish children of Eastern European background. Tay-Sachs disease is characterized by progressive mental and physical retardation, paralysis, blindness, spasticity, convulsions, red spots on the retina, and often early evidence (from the age of four to six months) of abnormal enlargement of the head. Death can occur during the first eighteen months of life or the fatal outcome may be prolonged until the child is three or four years old.

The diagnosis of Tay-Sachs disease can be made while the fetus is in the uterus by *amniocentesis*, the examination of a sample of the amniotic fluid that surrounds the fetus. The disease can also be diagnosed soon after birth by examining a blood sample, usually taken from the baby's arm, neck, or umbilical cord. The possibility of giving birth to a child with Tay-Sachs disease can also be determined prior to pregnancy by examining blood samples from the prospective parents; both must be carriers of the defective gene for the child to have the disease.

Tay-Sachs disease is named after the English physician Warren Tay (1843–1927) and the American neurologist Bernard Sachs (1858–1944).

telangiectasia Dilation of capillaries or a group of small blood vessels, causing a small dark-red elevation on the skin. It may appear as a birthmark or become noticeable in young children.

Hereditary hemorrhagic telangiectasia refers to an inherited disease characterized by abnormal thinness

or fragility of the walls of the blood vesssels of the nose, skin, and digestive tract leading to the tendency to bleed. This condition is also known as Osler-Weber-Rendu or Rendu-Osler-Weber disease.
SEE ALSO *angioma*

temporal arteritis An inflammation that mainly involves the arteries that supply the sides of the scalp (temporal arteries), with branches and twigs extending to areas around the lower jaw and the socket of the eye. In some cases other arteries may be involved. The exact cause of the disease is not known. It occasionally seems to follow a severe infection of the respiratory tract or to be associated with some other disease of the blood vessels. The condition, which is rare in people under the age of sixty, is becoming increasingly recognized in the elderly.

Among the general signs and symptoms (which are not specific to this disease) are severe headaches, fever, sweating, fatigue, weakness, anxiety, depression, loss of appetite, weight loss, and muscular or joint pains. Involvement of certain arterial branches may lead to visual disturbances or even temporary or permanent blindness. In some cases the patient may suddenly become blind in one eye.

Often there are no obvious signs or symptoms of temporal arteritis, which may progress slowly and quietly until some dramatic change alerts the patient and physician (the most dramatic being sudden blindness). The disease may run its course for a few months and present no further problems, although visual changes are rarely reversible. In other cases it may persist for several years. Exact diagnosis is possible only by examining a tiny piece of the affected arterial tissue.

Treatment consists in prescribing *corticosteroids* to control the course of the disease. Relief of symptoms often occurs within a few days, but complete eradication of the inflammatory process is rare. The prognosis is generally good, especially if treatment is started before the onset of serious complications.

tendon Fibrous cords that connect muscles to bone. Tendons can be strained by excessive effort and can even be torn from the bone or otherwise damaged by direct injury. Unaccustomed and prolonged physical exercise can produce degeneration of the tendon tissue. This causes inflammation and swelling of the tendon and its covering sheath (tenosynovitis), with consequent pain during movement.

Severe lacerations that sever tendons require surgical repair.

tennis elbow Pain or stiffness in the elbow often radiating to the outer side of the arm and weakness of the wrist, making grasping difficult. The condition can occur as the result of muscle tears after excessive or unaccustomed twisting movements of the hand, as in playing tennis.

teratogenesis The development of malformations or abnormal structures in an embryo or fetus. The branch of science concerned with the study of abnormal embryonic or fetal development is known as teratology.

testicle Either of two oval organs contained in the *scrotum*, the sac which hangs behind the penis. Each testicle (testis) is suspended from the body by a fibrous tube called the spermatic cord, which contains blood vessels, nerves, and ducts leading to and from each testicle.

The testicles have two functions. They produce the male hormone *testosterone*, which is responsible for the development of the secondary sexual characteristics at puberty and is essential for normal sexual behavior. The testicles are also responsible for the formation of *spermatozoa* (sperm cells), the male reproductive cells.

Each testicle is divided into approximately 250 compartments or lobules. Each lobule contains one to three fine tubules where the spermatozoa are manufactured; the sperm are passed to the *epididymis*.

Orchitis is the name given to inflammation of the testicles. It may follow an acute bacterial infection of the epididymis or urinary tract; the condition responds well to antibiotic treatment. Orchitis as a consequence of mumps is now rare in young boys and infrequent in adult males, due to modern medical care. Orchitis can lead to sterility only if the infection is severe and both testicles are involved. The cells that produce testosterone are rarely affected, but sperm manufacture is impaired.

testosterone The male sex hormone (also called androgen) produced by the *testicles* and (in both men and women) the cortex (outer part) of the *adrenal glands*. It is responsible for the development of the secondary sexual characteristics in men, such as deepening of the voice and growth of facial and pubic hair. Testosterone also affects and influences many physiological and metabolic processes. The hormone can be prepared synthetically in the laboratory for replacement and other therapeutic use.

test-tube baby
SEE *in vitro fertilization*

tetanus A disease caused by infection with the bacteria *Clostridium tetani*, which live in soil, dust, and the intestinal contents of both man and animals. They can survive for years in animal feces.

The tetanus bacteria enter the body through a scratch or wound; the disease is caused by the poison (toxin) they release during growth and multiplication. Unless the bacteria are in an environment with little or no oxygen (such as a pus-filled wound or areas with extensive tissue damage) they will not release their toxin. The first sign of the disease is stiffness of the jaw, which becomes so severe that it is difficult or even impossible to open the mouth; this gives tetanus its popular name, lockjaw.

As the toxin is carried from the wound through the bloodstream it begins to affect the nervous system. This usually results in spasm of the facial muscles sometimes so severe that it causes a fixed hideous smile *(risus sardonicus)* and raised eyebrows, as well as rigidity or spasm of the muscles of the abdomen, neck, and back. Painful convulsions may occur and the chest wall may become so rigid that breathing is extremely difficult. During severe spasms of the back muscles the entire body may be violently arched backward.

Protection against tetanus is possible with an injection of tetanus *antitoxin*, which generally provides immunity against tetanus toxin for several years. Most physicians recommend a booster injection every few years to maintain the proper level of protection. A wound inflicted with a dirty implement or contaminated by soil or dirt demands prompt medical attention; the physician will determine if an injection is necessary. Penicillin or another antibiotic may be given to kill the bacteria that have entered the wound.

tetany A condition that can occur following a critical drop in the amount of calcium in the circulating blood. It is characterized by restlessness and overexcitability of the nerves, causing the limbs to twitch or go into spasm. Treatment basically involves the injection of parathyroid hormones. The physician may also prescribe the infusion of calcium salts and recommend supplemental amounts of vitamin D.
SEE *parathyroid glands*

tetracyclines A group of broad-spectrum *antibiotics* that can destroy several species of bacteria. The group includes tetracycline, oxytetracycline, and chlortetracycline. Tetracyclines are also used to control some infections caused by *protozoa* and *rickettsiae*. At the recommended dosage levels, all tetracyclines have a relatively low incidence of side effects.

The use of tetracycline in children under the age of eight years may cause permanent discoloration of the teeth.
SEE *superinfection*

thalamus A neural (nerve) relay center deep within the brain. It receives incoming sensory impulses from the spinal cord and distributes them to various areas of the cerebral cortex, (from which it also receives and relays impulses).
COMPARE *hypothalamus*

thalassemia A form of *anemia* characterized by the development of abnormally thin and fragile red blood cells. There are several variants of the disease, which is most common among people of the

thermography

Mediterranean regions, the Middle East, and the Far East.

thermography A diagnostic technique that records the heat given off by an area of the body. Infrared sensors are used to measure and record heat patterns from two adjacent areas of skin surface as an aid, for example, in diagnosing irritation of a nerve root, which typically produces an abnormal heat pattern along the overlying area of skin.

It is also used to record heat patterns within breast tissue and was once widely used as an aid in the diagnosis of breast cancer; a cancerous growth gives off more heat than normal tissues. However, because of the relatively high incidence of false-positive test results, many physicians discount its value in this application.
See *mammography, ultrasonography*

thoracic Relating to the chest *(thorax).*

thorax The medical term for the chest. It contains all the organs and other structures between the base of the neck and diaphragm, including the lungs, heart, ribs, trachea, and esophagus.
COMPARE *abdomen*

thrombocytopenia An abnormal reduction in the total number of *platelets* (thrombocytes) in the circulating blood. The signs include bruising and bleeding from mucous membranes of the nose, vagina, stomach, and intestines. A reduction in the number of platelets means that the blood is no longer able to clot efficiently. Treatment depends on the diagnosis of one of the several underlying causes of reduced platelet production, such as damage to the *bone marrow* (where blood cells are manufactured) or liver disease. Uncontrolled thrombocytopenia can lead to anemia as the result of undetected internal bleeding, which leads to symptoms such as weakness, fatigue, and signs of congestive heart failure.

thrombophlebitis Inflammation of a vein *(phlebitis)* associated with the formation of a *thrombus.*

thrombosis The formation of a blood clot *(thrombus)* in a blood vessel.
COMPARE *embolism*

thrombus A blood clot that forms within a blood vessel or a chamber of the heart.
COMPARE *embolus*

thymus A two-lobed organ behind the sternum (breastbone) in children that gradually shrinks until it virtually disappears in adults. It plays an early role in the body's immune mechanism and was once believed to secrete a hormone.
SEE *autoimmune diseases, myasthenia gravis*

thyroidectomy Surgical removal of all or part of the *thyroid gland,* especially in the treatment of severe cases of *hyperthyroidism.*

thyroid gland An *endocrine gland* situated at the base of the neck. It consists of two vertical lobes (one on each side of the trachea) connected by a horizontal lobe, and somewhat resembles the letter H. The thyroid gland is essential for regulating the rate of the body's *metabolism*.

The thyroid gland secretes three *hormones* necessary for growth and development: thyroxine, triiodothyronine, and calcitonin; the first two of these, by convention, are known as the thyroid hormones. Their release into the bloodstream is under the direct influence of the *pituitary gland*. Thyroxine plays the major role in the body's metabolism, and like triiodothyronine requires minute amounts of *iodine* for its manufacture. Iodine is normally supplied to the body in adequate quantities in the diet or is added to table salt (so-called iodized salt). More than half of the iodine found in the body is concentrated in the thyroid for use in synthesizing thyroid hormones.

Calcitonin, together with a hormone secreted by the *parathyroid glands*, plays an important role in maintaining the blood level of *calcium*, an element necessary for the healthy development and repair of bones.

Except for the pituitary, the thyroid gland is perhaps the most important in the body's complex hormone control system. When it malfunctions, the effects can be dramatic.

SEE *cretinism, hyperthyroidism, hypothyroidism, myxedema*

tibia The shinbone, one of the two bones that form the skeleton of the lower part of the leg. It is the inner and larger of these bones and extends from the ankle to the knee. COMPARE *fibula*

t.i.d. Abbreviation for the Latin phrase *ter in die* ("three times a day"), commonly used in *prescriptions*.

tinea Any *fungus* disease that occurs on various areas of the body, including tinea capitis (scalp), tinea barbae (beard), tinea cruris (upper inner surface of the thighs), tinea pedis (foot, especially between the toes, popularly athlete's foot), or on the trunk of the body (tinea corporis); such diseases are popularly called *ringworm*.

tinnitus Any condition in which a person experiences in one or both ears the sensation of noises that are not caused by external sound vibrations. It is traditionally described as a ringing sound but it can also be a hissing, roaring, buzzing, or whistling. It is a fairly common experience and may be nothing more serious than a temporary blockage of the external ear passage with too much earwax (cerumen). If the sensation is prolonged or very troublesome, however, a physician should be consulted; tinnitus may be an early symptom of some disease of the inner ear, auditory nerve, or the tiny sound-conducting bones (ossicles) of the middle ear.

It is extremely rare to suffer from prolonged bouts of tinnitus if the hearing remains unimpaired. However, since the experience is a strictly subjective one, some people may imagine they hear sounds which are merely the normal level of background noise.

Some noises are described by patients as resembling escaping steam or rushing water. This tends to suggest some disorder of the auditory nerve or part of the brain. In most cases, however, tinnitus is nothing serious and lasts only a short time. Too much aspirin or other drugs can also cause the *side effect* of tinnitus, which ordinarily disappears within an hour or so. If not—especially if tinnitus seems to be associated with a prescription drug—the physician should be consulted at once; he or she may want to modify the dosage or prescribe another drug better tolerated by the patient.

tolerance The condition of being progressively less responsive to the effects of a drug (or poison) when given in the same doses as previously.
SEE ALSO *addiction*

tomography
SEE *computerized axial tomography*

tophus A chalky deposit in the skin (often in the fleshy rim of the ear) or within a joint. It is one sign of chronic *gout*.

topical Designed for application to the surface of the body. The term is used especially in describing a medicated cream, lotion, or ointment.

Tourette's syndrome A condition that begins in childhood and is characterized by involuntary blinking and muscular twitching (tics) of the face, uncontrollable bizarre behavior, grimaces, general jerking movements of the arms and shoulders, banging of the arms, grunting sounds, barking noises, shouting, and (in about half of those afflicted) compulsive swearing. In many cases the symptoms of Tourette's syndrome become less severe during the teenage years but can flare up again in various degrees during adult life. The exact cause is unknown but is thought to be associated with some brain disorder; intellectual function, however, is rarely affected.

The disruptive symptoms of Tourette's syndrome can often be controlled by the drug haloperidol (Haldol). No specific treatment is available other than control of symptoms, since the underlying cause has not been identified.

The condition is named after the French physician Georges Gilles de la Tourette (1857–1904).

toxemia Any condition characterized by the presence in the blood of toxic (poisonous) substances.
COMPARE *septicemia*

toxicology The branch of science concerned with the study of toxic (poisonous) substances, their detection and pharmacologic properties, and methods of treating patients who have ingested or been otherwise exposed to them. A specialist in this field is known as a toxicologist.

toxic-shock syndrome A disease caused by infection with the bacteria *Staphylococcus aureus* and characterized by the sudden onset of high fever, a drop in blood pressure (hypotension), vomiting, diarrhea, and dizziness. This is typically followed by a sunburnlike rash and then peeling of the skin, especially on the hands and feet. The sudden drop in blood pressure may rarely result in fatal *shock* (circulatory collapse).

Toxic-shock syndrome (TSS) primarily affects women who use *tampons* during their menstrual periods, although it has been seen in some women who do not and (rarely) in a few men. It is thought that the bacteria gain a stronghold after entering the vagina during the insertion of a tampon. When the tampon is composed of material that is "superabsorbent," it may not be changed as often as tampons that absorb less menstrual blood; this leads to an ideal breeding ground for the bacteria.

There is still some controversy about the specific role of tampons in toxic-shock syndrome, although the statistical evidence appears overwhelming that they play a key role in the vast majority of cases. Although some people claim that no reliable evidence indicates that the disease can be prevented by changing tampons frequently, it is a wise precaution to use tampons intermittently, alternating them with sanitary napkins.

Women should seek immediate medical attention at the first sign or symptom that might be associated with toxic-shock syndrome. Treatment involves the administration of an appropriate antibiotic and the control of such potentially serious complications as a drop in blood pressure.

trachea The medical name for the windpipe, a tube about 4 inches (10 cm) long and 1 inch (2.54 cm) wide that begins at the base of the larynx and ends behind the sternum (breastbone), where it divides into the two bronchi (main air passages). The circular shape of the trachea and bronchi is maintained by sixteen to twenty bars of horseshoe-shaped cartilage.

SEE ALSO *tracheostomy, tracheotomy*

tracheostomy The surgical formation of an artificial air passage through the tissues of the neck into the *trachea*. It is usually performed as an emergency procedure when the trachea is obstructed.

SEE ALSO *tracheotomy*

tracheotomy Surgical incision into the trachea, usually as a means of forming an artificial air passage *(tracheostomy)* when the *trachea* is obstructed.

traction The act or process of pulling or drawing, specifically by means of a device. When a steady pulling force is applied to the affected parts of a dislocated joint or a fractured bone, it helps to keep them in the correct position during the healing process.

tranquilizer Any drug designed to calm the nervous system and thus relieve anxiety, depression, and general nervousness. The more powerful drugs in this group are known as the major tranquilizers and include chlorpromazine (Thorazine); they are prescribed mainly to relieve the symptoms of severe mental distress, as in *psychosis*. The so-called minor tranquilizers such as diazepam (Valium) are prescribed mainly in mild cases of nervousness or depression.

As with all drugs that can alter the mental state, tranquilizers can be misused or abused. Prolonged use of major tranquilizers can result in the development of *tolerance* and physiological dependence *(addiction)*. True addiction, may also occur with the overuse of some minor tranquilizers, and convulsions and other withdrawal symptoms may follow the abrupt termination of use.

Taken as prescribed, tranquilizers have an important place in medical treatment. Some major tranquilizers so control the symptoms of severe mental illness that institutionalization is unnecessary. Misused, tranquilizers can create more problems than they solve.

transillumination The examination of cavities or organs by permitting a light source to penetrate their walls; particularly, the examination or inspection of the nasal sinuses by placing a light in the patient's mouth. A diminution or absence of reflected light is often diagnostic evidence of pus or structural disorder.

transsexual A person who has undergone surgical modification or removal of the external sex organs with the intention of aiding psychological adjustment in assuming the identity of the opposite sex. Such surgery is rarely performed and only after extensive psychiatric or other professional counselling.

trauma Any wound or injury. The term is also used to refer to a profound and sudden emotional shock or disruptive experience, especially one that makes a lasting impression on the mind.

trichinosis A disease caused by eating undercooked pork that has been contaminated with the larvae of a roundworm, *Trichinella spiralis*. The larvae's protective walls are digested away in the human stomach and the young parasites migrate to the intestinal walls, where they eventually develop into sexually mature adults capable of reproduction.

Signs and symptoms of trichinosis during the intestinal phase include loss of appetite, abdominal discomfort, nausea, and loose or watery stools. The greatest damage of the infestation, however, is caused by the deposition of larvae in various muscles. In very severe cases this can lead to fatal complications from pneumonia, exhaustion, or heart failure.

Diagnosis of trichinosis depends largely on finding encysted larvae in a *biopsy* specimen of muscle tissue, although other diagnostic tests are available. Treatment consists of controlling the symptoms, since no drugs are effective in attacking the parasites directly. Muscular pains may persist for a long time following the onset of the disease, but most symptoms usually disappear within about three months. Prevention consists of making sure that all pork and pork products are thoroughly cooked.

trichomoniasis A disease caused by infection with the protozoa *Trichomonas vaginalis*, usually transmitted during sexual intercourse with an infected partner. It is most often found in women and may cause inflammation of the vagina (vaginitis), urethra (urethritis), and bladder (cystitis). The infection is typically accompanied by a thick, frothy, greenish-yellow discharge from the vagina, a painful or burning sensation when urinating (dysuria), and pain during sexual intercourse (dyspareunia). Male carriers of the infecting microorganisms usually have no symptoms, although some may experience a purulent (pus-filled) discharge from the tip of the penis and painful urination.

Diagnosis of trichomoniasis requires examination of vaginal or urethral secretions for the presence of the protozoa. Treatment with the antiprotozoal drug metronidazole (Flagyl) is usually effective. Any sexual partner should also be examined and treated to prevent reinfection.

tropical disease Any disease that is more common in tropical or subtropical climates, although some can occur in nearly any part of the world. Some tropical diseases are carried by organisms that only live in hotter regions, but most are a result of the low standards of living and poor sanitation typical of many tropical countries. Thus despite the name, the diseases are associated with economics rather than climate. Malnutrition also predisposes children and adults to disease by weakening the body's defenses through prolonged lack of well-balanced meals.

Diagnosis of a tropical disease contracted by a traveler is made difficult by the fact that the signs and symptoms may not appear until after the return home and may be unfamiliar to the physician who sees them.

trypanosomiasis A parasitic infectious disease also known as African trypanosomiasis and *sleeping sickness* caused by either of two distinct species of *protozoa* of the genus *Trypanosoma*. It is transmitted to humans by the bite of infected tsetse flies, which are restricted to parts of east, central, and west Africa. African trypanosomiasis is most prevalent in undeveloped rural areas where the tsetse fly thrives.

As the protozoa enter the skin following the bite of an infected tsetse fly, they typically cause an inflammation and swelling of nearby lymph glands. The microorganisms eventually invade the blood circulation and the *cerebrospinal fluid* and are carried to the brain and spinal cord, where in untreated cases they cause inflammation and occasionally death.

The incubation period is usually one to three weeks, but may be much longer. The early symptoms of the disease are not specific for sleeping sickness; they include an irregular fever, extreme weakness and lethargy, and loss of appetite. As the infection spreads, which may be over a period of months, the patient may eat so little that he or she becomes malnourished and sleepy, seemingly disinterested in survival. The potentially fatal outcome may be preceded by complications such as pneumonia, muscular tremors, convulsions, and coma.

Antibiotic drugs are often effective in treating African trypanosomiasis, especially if they are administered at an early stage.

tubal ligation A surgical procedure in which the *Fallopian tubes* are tied to prevent pregnancy. It may be performed as a means of contraception, especially when other methods involve complications or when medical or genetic conditions exist which strongly contraindicate pregnancy. In most cases the operation is considered irreversible.
COMPARE *vasectomy*

tuberculosis (TB) An infectious disease caused by the tubercle bacillus, *Mycobacterium tuberculosis*. Two main types of the bacillus may infect man: the human strain and the bovine (cattle) strain. When children become infected it is most often by the bovine strain, transmitted through the milk of infected cows. With the widespread use of pasteurized milk in developed countries and the introduction of laws requiring that cattle be tested for infection, human infection with the bovine strain is becoming increasingly rare. The human strain is spread from an infected person in sputum or in the air after a cough or sneeze.

Infection with the bacillus in someone who has not had the disease is called primary tuberculosis. As a

tuberculosis (TB)

result of the initial infection, a partial specific immunity is developed. The original area of infection may heal but can sometimes become active again, or the body may become reinfected if a subsequent infection is of sufficient strength. Reactivation or reinfection is known as postprimary tuberculosis.

The characteristic lesion (injury) caused by tuberculosis, a tubercle, is a small area of inflammation and tissue destruction that may eventually break down to form thick cheesy pus. Tubercles are said to heal if they become encased in fibrous material and hardened as the result of calcium deposits. Evidence of healed lesions is clearly seen on chest x-rays in the case of tuberculosis of the lungs (pulmonary tuberculosis).

Not all tubercles become calcified and heal. They may remain latent for months or years. When the body's resistance is lowered (as by another disease), the infection may become reactivated and spread quickly through the bloodstream to other areas of the body.

Tests exist to determine the presence of tuberculosis. Tuberculin, a protein prepared from the tubercle bacillus, is injected into the skin; if it produces a red area of inflammation it indicates that the person is or has been infected with tuberculosis.

Pulmonary tuberculosis may be mild or severe. In many cases the lungs become infected and then gradually heal without the patient's having been aware of the disease. In more severe forms the first signs and symptoms include fatigue, loss of weight and appetite, and occasionally symptoms that resemble influenza. As the infection progresses these symptoms become more severe and the patient may experience heavy sweating, especially at night. Coughing becomes progressively intense and blood-streaked mucus, phlegm, or sputum may be coughed up. This material is highly infectious, as it usually contains millions of tubercle bacilli.

Chest x-rays are essential to determine the extent and nature of the disease. The sputum must also be examined; if the bacillus is found, it is an indication that the disease is active and the patient is infectious. The physician will then have close contacts x-rayed to determine if they have contracted the disease. Often several x-rays over months or years must be taken.

Treatment of tuberculosis usually includes taking a combination of drugs, including antibiotics. The physician will also prescribe a well-balanced diet to help regain lost weight, which in severe cases may be extreme. Fresh air and comfortable surroundings aid recovery from this potentially fatal disease.

An important measure in the control of tuberculosis is vaccination with a modified strain of the tubercle bacillus called BCG (Bacille Calmette-Guérin) vaccine. Although vaccination does not guarantee protection against infection, it greatly reduces the risks of a severe form of tuberculosis.

tumor Any swelling or growth in the body caused by an abnormal multiplication of cells. It may be either benign (harmless) or malignant (life-threatening).
SEE ALSO *cancer, oncology*

tympanites Abdominal distension or bloating caused by the accumulation of gas in the intestine or peritoneal cavity.

typanitis Inflammation of the *tympanum;* also called *myringitis.*

tympanum The eardrum, a very thin and semitransparent oval layer of tissue. Foreign objects inserted into the ear can easily pierce this delicate and sensitive tissue. A ruptured or perforated eardrum can also result from a sharp blow on the ear or proximity to the shock waves from an explosion or gun blast. Even the force of heavily amplified music can injure the eardrum and result in hearing loss. In some cases an extremely loud noise will not only rupture the eardrum but also damage the tiny sound-conducting bones (ossicles) attached to its inner side.

In the absence of infection *(myringitis)*, the treatment of a ruptured eardrum consists of protecting the ear canal with a plug of absorbent cotton to keep out water and foreign particles. In most uncomplicated cases the eardrum will heal naturally.

typhoid fever A general bacterial infection caused by ingesting contaminated food, milk, or water. The bacteria responsible, *Salmonella typhosa,* are excreted in the feces and sometimes the urine of infected patients or *carriers* of the disease. Inadequate sewage disposal and general unsanitary conditions are largely responsible for the spread of the disease. Water supplies may be contaminated or the bacteria may be spread by persons who handle food. Milk and milk products are particularly fertile breeding grounds for salmonella. The incubation period varies from about ten to fourteen days.

As with most infectious diseases, the first symptoms usually include headache and fever. The temperature begins to rise daily for a few days, often reaching as high as 105°F (40.6°C). Other fairly common symptoms are chills, sweating, development of rose-colored spots on the chest and abdomen, aching in the limbs, and tiredness. Many patients experience constipation followed by severe diarrhea.

Typhoid fever (often referred to as typhoid) is potentially fatal if not treated with the appropriate antibiotic. Bed rest is important until all signs of the fever have disappeared. The physician may also prescribe a diet consisting of foods high in calories and low in roughage (dietary fiber).

Some people who recover from typhoid fever may remain carriers for years. Precaution must be taken that such people are not employed handling food.

SEE ALSO *paratyphoid fever, salmonellosis, Widal test*

typhus Any one of three related infectious diseases caused by a species of *rickettsia*. It is characterized by fever, severe headache, and a general rash. In most cases the symptoms resolve within two weeks. All infections respond well to antibiotics.

SEE *Rocky Mountain spotted fever*

u

ulcer An open sore on the body surface or on the lining of a mucous membrane, especially of the stomach or duodenum.
SEE *peptic ulcer*

ulcerative colitis Inflammation and ulceration *(ulcer* formation) of the mucous membrane that lines the large intestine (colon). The condition is characterized by acute abdominal pain and the passing of foul-smelling watery stools containing blood, mucus, and pus. The disease usually affects people between the ages of about fifteen and forty. The cause is unknown, although there is a tendency for it to occur among members of the same family.

Without prompt medical attention, an acute attack of ulcerative colitis can be fatal. In most cases, however, the condition is chronic and characterized by periods of exacerbations and remissions. Severe forms of the disease require hospitalization and the injection of *corticosteroids*, which can also be helpful in less severe cases. Massive bleeding from the intestinal tract may necessitate emergency surgery.

ulna The inner bone of the forearm, forming at its lower end a knobby projection at the wrist.
COMPARE *humerus, radius*

ultrasonics The branch of science concerned with the study and application of sound waves higher than those detectable by the human ear, above 20,000 cycles per second.
SEE *ultrasonography*

ultrasonography A technique or procedure for visualizing various organs and structures within the body by recording (or observing on an oscilloscope screen) the reflections of the echoes of a focused beam of high-frequency sound waves that is directed into the tissues. When the echoes are converted into electrical energy and amplified, structures under the skin can be identified. The procedure is used in a wide range of diagnostic applications, such as detecting possible abnormalities of a fetus within the uterus, examination of breasts, and the diagnosis of potential problems in the gallbladder, kidneys, liver, and spleen.

Ultrasonography (also known as echography or sonography) is painless and is considered a relatively safe procedure.
COMPARE *mammography, thermography*
SEE ALSO *ultrasonics*

ultraviolet radiation Electromagnetic radiation beyond the range of visible light. It is a component of sunlight. Lamps that emit this radiation can provide an artificial suntan and stimulate the skin to synthesize vitamin D. An excess of ultraviolet radiation can cause skin cancer.

umbilical cord The vascular cord connecting the fetus with its *placenta* and through which it receives nourishment. When the cord is severed after birth, the stump eventually wastes away and leaves an abdominal depression known as the umbilicus (naval).

urate A salt of *uric acid* constituting the sharp crystals that form in the joints and are deposited as a *tophus* in certain tissues in the metabolic disorder *gout*.

urea The chief nitrogen-containing waste product of protein metabolism. Formed in the liver, it is transported in the blood and lymph and is excreted from the body in the urine. An excess or prolonged retention of urea can lead to *uremia*.

uremia A toxic condition in which the *kidneys* fail to filter out various nitrogen-containing waste products in the blood, especially *urea*. It is characterized by nausea, vomiting, dizziness, impaired vision, headache, and (in severe cases) convulsions and coma.
SEE *kidney failure*

ureter The slender tube that conveys urine from the outlet of each kidney to the urinary bladder.
SEE ALSO *urethra*

urethra The passage through which urine is conveyed from the urinary bladder to the outside of the body.
SEE ALSO *ureter*

urethritis Inflammation of the *urethra*.
SEE *venereal disease*

uric acid A waste product of metabolism, usually excreted in the urine. In certain disorders, an excessive amount of uric acid accumulates in the body and can lead to gout or the formation of kidney stones.
SEE *hyperuricemia, nephrolithiasis, urate*

urinalysis Laboratory examination and analysis of a sample of *urine*. This important diagnostic procedure enables a physician to evaluate the general state of the body, specifically the urinary system.
SEE *glucose tolerance test*

urinary tract All the organs and structures concerned with the formation and excretion of urine including the *kidney*, ureter, urinary bladder, and urethra.

urine The yellowish or amber fluid secreted by the *kidneys*, composed of approximately 96 percent water and 4 percent solids. If one drinks a lot of water or urinates frequently, the urine may become diluted and be pale yellow or nearly colorless. A fresh specimen of urine, such as one taken early in the day, has a characteristic odor. (The urine of some diabetics may smell sweet due to the abnormal presence of sugar.) If a urine sample is left standing for some time it tends to become cloudy; as it cools, salts and other dissolved constituents precipitate out of solution.

Standing urine is a rich breeding ground for airborne bacteria, which cause it to decompose and give off a pungent smell of ammonia. Physicians always request a relatively fresh urine sample for *urinalysis*, since older urine is of little diagnostic value.

Normal urine is slightly acid and has a characteristic specific gravity (weight compared to distilled water); a gross change in either may be an indication of some problem in the urinary system. The color of the urine may temporarily change after taking certain drugs or eating some foods; for example, beets contain a pigment that is filtered through the kidneys and can turn the urine red. If urine continues to appear red or is abnormally discolored in any way, prompt medical attention is essential: this may be caused by blood and represent the first sign of an infection of the urethra, bladder, or kidneys.

The solids in normal urine consist largely of the waste product *urea*, salt (sodium chloride), and smaller amounts of phosphates, sulfates, potassium, calcium, and magnesium. The presence in the urine of pus cells, blood cells, protein, or glucose is an indication of some disorder of the urinary system; in the case of glucose, it may be a sign of diabetes mellitus.

The kidneys secrete an average of 50 fluid ounces of urine every twenty-four hours; approximately 38 fluid ounces of urine are secreted during the day and 12 fluid ounces during the night. The actual amount of urine voided depends on the fluid intake and other factors.

urogenital Relating to both the urinary and genital organs.
SEE ALSO *genitourinary*

urography The technique or procedure of obtaining x-rays of any part of the urinary tract following the injection into the blood vessels of an x-ray contrast *(radiopaque)* substance.
SEE *intravenous pyelogram*

urology The branch of medical science concerned with the study and treatment of diseases and disorders of the *urogenital* tract in males and the urinary tract in females. A specialist in this field is known as a urologist.

urticaria An allergic skin reaction popularly called hives or nettle rash characterized by the formation of very itchy raised red or white patches called weals. They may be restricted to a particular area or occur all over the body; as a rule the weals are temporary and are particularly likely to appear where the skin is subjected to pressure. Severe forms of this reaction are accompanied by swelling of tissues beneath the skin or of mucous membranes.

The allergic reaction that causes urticaria may be sensitivity to any of various allergens including drugs, insect stings or bites, and some foods, particularly shellfish, eggs, fruits, and nuts. Urticaria may also be caused by bacterial or viral infections, worm infestations, or an inherited enzyme deficiency.

Urticaria is fairly common in children and is usually not serious enough to require medical attention. It may come and go and then clear up spontaneously and not reappear for long periods. In persistent or especially severe cases it is wise to see a physician.

Skin tests are rarely of help in determining the cause of urticaria. However, if the condition is associated with other allergies, particularly hay fever (allergic rhinitis), the tests may reveal a common cause. Related causes and factors that tend to aggravate urticaria include emotional stress, coffee, tea, aspirin, laxatives, and tobacco.

Most symptoms of acute urticaria can be relieved with *antihistamines*. In severe reactions accompanied by potentially dangerous swelling of the tissues, a physician may prescribe other drugs as well to bring the condition under control.

uterus The organ in females designed to contain and nourish a developing embryo and fetus from the time the fertilized ovum (egg) is implanted to the time of childbirth; the womb. It is traditionally described as a pear-shaped muscular organ, with its neck *(cervix)* pointing downward into the vagina. The uterus of a woman who has not borne children is about 3 inches (7.5 cm) long, 2 inches (5 cm) wide, 1 inch (2.5 cm) thick, and most commonly lies at a right angle to the vagina. During pregnancy the uterus stretches to accommodate the growing fetus.

SEE ALSO *endometriosis, endometritis, endometrium, hysterectomy, menstruation*

uvula A projection of soft tissue hanging from the roof of the soft palate over the back of the tongue. It is composed of muscle, connective tissue, and mucous membrane.

V

vaccination Inoculation with any *vaccine* to stimulate the body to produce specific antibodies that will establish *immunity* to a specific infectious disease.

vaccine A preparation of weakened (attenuated) or dead microorganisms that is inoculated into the body to stimulate the production of specific antibodies and thus provide resistance or immunity to a future infection by that microorganism.
SEE *vaccination*

vacuum abortion
SEE *abortion*

vagina The passage that leads from a female's external genital organs (vulva) to the neck (cervix) of the uterus; popularly known as the birth canal. The flattened muscular tube of the vagina lies behind the urinary bladder and opens onto the surface of the body at the vulva. It normally secretes a very small amount of fluid; in addition, secretions from the cervix and the vulva find their way into the vagina. These natural secretions may be thin and watery or may occasionally become somewhat mucous or sticky. The amount and nature of the secretions vary among different women at various stages of their menstrual cycles. If the discharge is discolored or has an offensive odor, it may be a sign of bacterial or fungal infection. In such cases it is important to seek prompt medical attention.

In the adult woman the vagina is approximately 3 inches (7.5 cm) long at its upper surface and up to 4 inches (10 cm) long at its lower surface.
SEE ALSO *leukorrhea, trichomoniasis, vaginismus, vaginitis*

vaginismus A painful spasm of the muscles around the vagina. It may be associated with a disease or physical factor such as an injury or congenital malformation of the vagina, but the most common cause is an emotional aversion to sexual intercourse.
SEE *dyspareunia*

vaginitis Inflammation of the vagina, often accompanied by itch-

ing. It can be caused by infection with bacteria, fungus, or protozoa (as in *trichomoniasis*), irritation from chemical douches or foreign bodies, or poor hygiene of the external genitals (vulva). Treatment depends on the underlying cause.
SEE ALSO *leukorrhea, venereal disease*

vagotomy Surgical cutting or division of the vagus nerve (which in part controls the stomach's movements and acid secretions), most often performed in the treatment of severe cases of *peptic ulcer.*

valve A membranous flap or fold of tissue on the inner wall of a vessel (especially a vein) or within the *heart* or other hollow organs designed to prevent a backflow of fluid.

varicella The medical term for *chickenpox.*

varicocele An abnormal swelling or dilation of the veins of the spermatic cord, typically causing an uncomfortable feeling in the testicles. It occurs most often during the late teens and is rarely a serious problem. The symptoms may be relieved by a suspensory, a pouch to hold the testicles; in rare cases surgery may be required.

varicose veins A condition in which the veins are abnormally swollen because of damage to their one-way valves (which normally prevent a backward flow of blood) and consequent stretching of their relatively thin walls. The veins take on a characteristic twisted (varicose) appearance. The veins most often affected are those in the legs. In some cases hereditary factors are responsible; usually, however, the cause is related to standing in one position for prolonged periods, obesity, pregnancy, and certain other conditions.

Any veins that are deformed because they are abnormally distended with blood are varicose; for example, hemorrhoids are varicose veins of the rectum. When the distended veins occur in the inner walls of the esophagus, the condition is known as esophageal varices.

The first indication of varicose veins of the legs is the discolored bulging of the veins below the skin surface. A dull aching sensation and fatigue are sometimes experienced; occasionally the ankles become swollen and a skin rash appears. More rarely, open sores (ulcers) develop on the skin near the affected veins.

Although varicose veins are seldom a serious condition, it is a good idea to see a physician so that he or she can determine if any unusual problems exist. Treatment of varicose veins of the legs involves wearing supportive bandages or elastic stockings. Varicose veins can also be treated surgically or with injections of sclerosing solution. Larger varicosed veins can be tied off (ligated) and removed surgically, a minor surgical procedure

known as vein stripping. The aim of both these treatments is to cause the blood to remain in the deeper veins on its return journey to the heart and lungs as well as providing a cosmetic benefit.
SEE ALSO *phlebitis*

vas deferens The seminal duct, through which *spermatozoa* (sperm cells) are transported from the *epididymis* of the *testicles* to the urethra during ejaculation. This duct is surgically interrupted in *vasectomy*.

vasectomy Surgical removal of a section of the *vas deferens*, usually performed on the seminal ducts of both testicles as a method of sterilization. Once a vasectomy has been performed it is unlikely that it can be reversed.

Other methods of contraception must be used for three to four months after the operation or until the physician or surgeon determines that the man's *semen* (which continues to be produced following vasectomy) no longer contains sperm cells.

Vasectomy in no way impairs sexual desire or ability.
COMPARE *tubal ligation*

vasoconstrictor Any nerve, drug, or agent that acts to constrict (narrow) the inner diameter of blood vessels.
COMPARE *vasodilator*

vasodilator Any nerve, drug, or agent that acts to dilate (widen) the inner diameter of blood vessels.
COMPARE *vasoconstrictor*

vasopressin A hormone secreted by the *pituitary gland* that causes an increase in blood pressure by its *vasoconstrictor* effects on the capillaries and smallest arteries (arterioles). The main role of this hormone is to permit the reabsorption and conservation of water by the kidneys. A failure of the pituitary gland to secrete sufficient quantities of vasopressin (also known as antidiuretic hormone) can result in *diabetes insipidus.*

vasopressor Any drug or agent that stimulates the contraction of the smooth muscles in the walls of blood vessels, thus increasing the resistance to blood flow through the vessels and raising blood pressure.

VD Abbreviation for *venereal disease.*

vein Any blood vessel that carries oxygen-depleted blood (and the four *pulmonary* veins, which carry oxygen-rich blood from the lungs) toward the heart.
COMPARE *artery*
SEE *jugular veins, phlebitis*

vena cava Either of two large *veins* that empty blood into the right upper chamber (atrium) of the heart. The inferior vena cava is the principle vessel receiving venous blood from the lower part of the body; the superior vena cava is the principle vessel receiving venous blood from the upper part of the body.

venereal disease (VD) Any disease transmitted almost exclusively during sexual intercourse with an infected partner, especially *syphilis* and *gonorrhea*. Nonspecific urethritis (inflammation of the *urethra*) can also be transmitted during sexual intercourse; its exact cause is unknown. In recent years the viral infection *herpes simplex* has become a potentially serious venereal disease. Most venereal diseases (although not herpes) respond well to antibiotics.

venesection Another term for *phlebotomy*.

venipuncture The surgical puncturing of a vein for any purpose, such as to inject medication into the bloodstream or to withdraw a sample of blood for analysis.

venous Relating to veins or oxygen-depleted blood.

ventricle A cavity, especially one of the two lower chambers of the heart or one of the four cavities within the brain that contain cerebrospinal fluid.

ventricular fibrillation Abnormally rapid, irregular, and uncoordinated contractions of the *ventricles* of the heart, constituting a medical emergency.
SEE *fibrillation*

venule The smallest vessel of the venous (vein) system. Venules form a link with the *capillaries*.
COMPARE *arteriole*

verruca The medical term for *wart*.

vertebra Any of the thirty-three irregularly shaped bones that make up the spinal column. The majority of the vertebrae are in the form of a hollow ring through which the spinal cord passes.

The vertebrae are named according to the region of the body in which they occur and the number of other vertebrae in that region. There are seven vertebrae in the neck (cervical vertebrae), twelve in the chest (thoracic vertebrae), and five in the lower back (lumbar vertebrae). The remaining nine vertebrae consist of five that form the sacrum, the triangular-shaped bone just below the last lumbar vertebra, and the four that form the rudimentary tailbone, the coccyx. A typical vertebra has three rear projections to which some back muscles are attached.

The first two vertebrae in the neck, the atlas and the axis, have specific functions. The ring-shaped atlas forms the top of the neck and supports the skull; the axis, directly underneath, has a peglike projection which extends upward into the atlas. The skull and atlas rotate together on the axis, permitting the head to turn to either side. The atlas permits the head to tilt backward and forward.

Between each vertebra is an *intervertebral disk*, a flexible pad of tissue composed of cartilage. The intervertebral disks form about 25 percent of the length of the spine and act as shock absorbers when one walks or runs.

vertigo

SEE ALSO *laminectomy, scoliosis, spinal curvature*

vertigo A condition in which an individual or whatever is in the immediate environment seems to be whirling about. True vertigo (as distinguished from simple dizziness) is associated with a disturbance of the structures within the ear responsible for equilibrium. It can be caused by several factors, including a disease of the middle ear, drug *side effects*, or blood poisoning (septicemia). Treatment depends on the underlying cause.

virology The branch of science concerned with the study of viruses and viral diseases. A specialist in this field is known as a virologist.

virulent Highly infectious, poisonous, malignant, or deadly.

virus Any of a group of microorganisms (generally much smaller than bacteria) that can reproduce only within living cells, which they parasitize. In general, viruses are not affected by antibiotics or other therapeutic agents, and only the symptoms of viral diseases such as the common cold and influenza can be treated.

vocal cords
SEE *trachea*

voice box
SEE *larynx*

volvulus A twisting upon itself of a section of intestine, causing a serious obstruction. The signs and symptoms include severe and sudden abdominal pain followed by vomiting and abdominal distention. Without immediate surgical correction the condition can lead to strangulation of the twisted loop of intestine and *gangrene*, which can be fatal as the result of *peritonitis*.

Diagnosis is established by x-rays of the intestinal tract.

vomiting The forceful ejection through the mouth of stomach contents; emesis. It is distinguished from regurgitation (common in babies), in which the stomach contents return to the mouth and gently spill out. In regurgitation, the muscular valve between the esophagus and the stomach fails to retain the food in the stomach. The stomach contents may then surge upward into the mouth, usually propelled by an excess of gas in the stomach.

In true vomiting, the cause may be related to many factors, ranging in severity from a simple upset stomach to intestinal obstruction, appendicitis, or bleeding ulcers. Vomiting is a common occurrence in many childhood fevers, and during early pregnancy many women experience nausea and vomiting. Most of the common causes of vomiting are associated with a short-term disturbance of the digestive system.

Central vomiting is associated with the central nervous system rather than the digestive system. It may be caused by a disturbance in brain function caused by a tumor, inflammation of the covering membranes *(meningitis)*, a head injury, *migraine*, or a psychological disturbance. In some cases the stomach contents may be expelled through the mouth with great force, a condition of possible diagnostic importance known as projectile vomiting.

If vomiting persists it is essential to see a physician at once. If the material (vomitus) is mixed with blood or appears very dark, it may be a sign of a bleeding ulcer or another serious condition that requires prompt medical attention.

A drug or agent used to induce vomiting is an *emetic;* one used to control vomiting is an antiemetic. Vomiting that occurs as the result of motion sickness, for example, can often be prevented by taking over-the-counter antiemetics such as dimenhydrinate (Dramamine).

SEE ALSO *ipecac syrup*

vulva The external female genital organs. This collective name includes the mons pubis (mons veneris), a pad of fatty tissue overlying the bones that form the front part of the pelvis; the labia majora (large or major lips) and labia minora (small or minor lips), two pairs of elongated fleshy folds at the entrance to the *vagina* (the labia majora are the thick outer lips of the vulva, covering the slender and normally concealed labia minora); and the *clitoris*, a small structure composed of erectile tissue partly hidden beneath the upper folds of the labia minora. The urinary meatus (canal), through which urine is passed outside the body, is located just below the clitoris and above the entrance to the vagina.

Embedded within the walls of the labia minora are Bartholin's glands, whose ducts open onto the entrance to the vagina. When a woman is sexually stimulated, these glands secrete a small amount of a sticky lubricating fluid that with other vaginal secretions minimizes friction during sexual intercourse.

SEE ALSO *hymen*

vulvitis Inflammation of the *vulva*.

W

wart A small *tumor* on the skin caused by a particular group of viruses known as papillomaviruses. Warts are essentially benign (harmless) and may disappear spontaneously, especially in young adults and children; the effectiveness of over-the-counter preparations for wart removal is therefore difficult to prove. In rare cases, especially in the elderly, a wart may become malignant.

Troublesome or disfiguring warts can be removed by a minor surgical procedure under local anesthesia, destroyed by high-frequency electric sparks (fulguration), or frozen with liquid nitrogen or solid carbon dioxide.

Warts may form on the fingers, elbows, knees, face, scalp, or soles of the feet (planter warts); their location is often associated with an irritation or trauma. Despite temporarily effective treatment, warts tend to recur in the same or a new site.

Wassermann test A routine diagnostic test for *syphilis* based on a blood sample. The original procedure was described in 1906 by the German bacteriologist August Paul von Wassermann (1866–1925). It is one of several slightly different serologic (based on blood serum) tests for syphilis.

water pill
SEE *diuretic*

white blood cell
SEE *leukocyte*

whooping cough An acute infectious disease caused by bacteria of the species *Bordetella pertussis* spread in the air from the breath or cough of an infected person. It is highly *contagious* and potentially one of the most serious childhood illnesses, especially in those under one year. For that reason, all babies should be vaccinated; this ordinarily provides *immunity*, although mild forms of whooping cough may still occur.

The first signs of whooping cough, known medically as pertussis, follow about seven to fourteen days after exposure to the bacteria. At first it resembles a bad chest cold with a slight cough. During the end of the second week the coughing increases and may come in a series of spasms with cough-free intervals; the child may cough rapidly several times before being able to catch the breath. When the child inhales after such violent coughing the characteristic "whoop" is heard, consisting of a high-pitched rasping sound caused by air being sucked in over vocal cords that are in spasm and partly covered with mucus. The spitting up of mucus tends to relieve the attack for a time. The coughing may last for six weeks or more, but generally becomes milder. In many cases the intensity and frequency of the cough begin to lessen after the fourth week.

The child should be kept isolated for at least six weeks, or about four weeks after the start of intense coughing. Older children may be permitted out of bed if the symptoms are mild. It is best to offer small meals frequently rather than two or three large ones and to restrict solid foods in younger children until the violent coughing subsides.

A physician should be consulted promptly in the early stages of the illness, since complications such as inflammation of the intestines, pneumonia, and even convulsions can occur in infants.

Controversy exists among parents and some medical professionals regarding the possibility of serious *side effects* from a *DPT* vaccination against whooping cough. Most physicians feel that the risk of side effects is less dangerous than the consequences of keeping a child unprotected.

Widal test A diagnostic test for *typhoid fever* and other diseases caused by infection with bacteria of the genus *Salmonella* based on the presence of specific antibodies in the blood serum of an infected person. A positive reaction is indicated when the infectious bacteria agglutinate (clump together).

windpipe
SEE *trachea*

wisdom tooth The third molar (grinding tooth). It is the rearmost tooth on each side of both jaws and gets its name because, like wisdom, the four wisdom teeth come with age, erupting through the gums between the ages of seventeen and twenty-five. In some cases a wisdom tooth cannot erupt because of nearby teeth and must be extracted by a dentist.

withdrawal symptoms The distressing symptoms experienced for a period of time following the failure to take a substance to which one is addicted, such as a drug or alcohol. These may include violent shivering, painful contractions of the stomach, forceful vomiting, and diarrhea.
SEE *addiction, alcoholism*

womb
SEE *uterus*

X

xanthemia A condition also called carotenemia in which a yellow pigment, carotene, is present in the circulating blood. This can cause the skin to become yellow *(xanthosis)*, but it is not related to *jaundice*. Carotene is present in large amounts in such foods as carrots and squash; eating excessive quantities of these foods can result in xanthemia.

xanthine An oxidation product of metabolism and precursor of *uric acid*. An excessive amount of xanthine in the urine can, rarely, lead to the formation of stones (xanthine calculi) in the kidneys.
SEE ALSO *nephrolithiasis*

xanthosis Yellowness of the skin resulting from eating excessive quantities of foods such as carrots, squash, and egg yolks that contain a group of yellow pigments known collectively as carotenoids.
COMPARE *xanthemia*

X chromosome One of the two *chromosomes* associated with determining human gender; the other is the *Y chromosome*. All body cells except sex cells *(ova* and *spermatozoa)* contain a pair of chromosomes: two X chromosomes (XX) in females, one X and one Y chromosome (XY) in males. Each ovum contains one X chromosome and each sperm cell contains either an X chromosome or a Y chromosome. If a sperm cell with an X chromosome penetrates and fertilizes an ovum, the product of conception will be female (XX), if the sperm cell contains a Y chromosome, the embryo will develop into a male (XY).

xeropthalmia A condition in which the conjunctiva, the delicate mucous membrane that lines the eyelids and covers the front part of the eye, is abnormally dry. It is associated with chronic conjunctivitis.

x-ray contrast medium
SEE *radiopaque*

x-rays Electromagnetic radiation of a wavelength shorter than visible light or *ultraviolet* radiation able to penetrate the body and most other solids and expose photographic plates or films. X-rays are used both to diagnose various diseases and disorders (especially of the bones and lungs) and as a method of *cancer* therapy. They are also called roentgen rays after the German physicist Wilhelm Konrad Roentgen (1845–1923), who discovered x-rays in 1895.

Y

Y chromosome One of the two *chromosomes* associated with determining human gender; the other is the *X chromosome*. The Y chromosome is present only in the cells of males. In all body cells except the *spermatozoa*, it is combined with an X chromosome; the sperm cell contains either an X chromosome or a Y chromosome. Since each *ovum* contains one X chromosome, the fertilized ovum will be either male (XY) or female (XX) depending on the sperm cell's contribution.

yeast infection A popular term for any of several fungal infections, including *candidiasis*, *thrush*, and certain forms of *vaginitis*. Technically, yeasts are any of several unicellular fungi of the genus *Saccharomyces*, which reproduce asexually by budding.

Z

zinc A bluish-white metallic element that is essential to the body in minute amounts. A deficiency of zinc may lead to *anemia*, failure to achieve sexual maturity, and stunted growth. Zinc deficiency is extremely rare in developed countries since this trace element is normally present in ample amounts in the diet.

Zinc compounds have been widely used in medicine: zinc acetate as an astringent and antiseptic, zinc chloride as an antiseptic, zince oxide ointment as an astringent and to dress sores (it is also slightly antiseptic), zinc sulfate to provoke vomiting and as an astringent.

The human body contains approximately 1–2.5 grams of zinc, mainly in bones, teeth, hair, skin, and testicles. Zinc is also a constituent of red blood cells (erythrocytes), white blood cells (leukocytes), and platelets; it is thought that zinc may play a role in enabling the blood to transport and release carbon dioxide formed during metabolism. Zinc may also help the action of the hormone insulin and give strength to the outermost layer of skin, the epidermis.

Zinc is included as an ingredient in several multivitamin supplements available without prescription. It is not known how useful dietary zinc supplements may be without a diagnosed deficiency. An excessive amount of supplementary zinc can cause problems such as vomiting and diarrhea as well as interfere with the absorption of dietary iron.

Zollinger-Ellison syndrome A condition characterized by tumors of the pancreas (about 60 percent of which are *malignant*), excessive secretion of gastric juices (including hydrochloric acid) and subsequent ulceration of the lining of the stomach and small intestine.

Treatment usually involves the surgical removal of the stomach (total gastrectomy) and removal of the pancreatic tumor.

The *syndrome* is named after the American surgeons Robert M. Zollinger (born 1903) and Edwin H. Ellison (born 1918).